# Bioethics

# The Jones and Bartlett Series in Philosophy

Robert Ginsberg, General Editor

Ayer, A. J., *Metaphysics and Common Sense*, 1994 reissue with corrections and new introduction by Thomas Magnell, Drew University

Beckwith, Francis J., University of Nevada, Las Vegas, Editor, *Do the Right Thing: A Philosophical Dialogue on the Moral and Social Issues of Our Time*

Bishop, Anne H. and John R. Scudder, Jr., Lynchburg College, *Nursing Ethics: Therapeutic Caring Presence*

Caws, Peter, George Washington University, *Ethics from Experience*

DeMarco, Joseph P., Cleveland State University, *Moral Theory: A Contemporary Overview*

Gorr, Michael, Illinois State University, and Sterling Harwood, San Jose State University, Editors, *Crime and Punishment: Philosophic Explorations*

Haber, Joram Graf, Bergen Community College, Interviewer, *Ethics in the '90s*, a 26-part Video Series

Harwood, Sterling, San Jose State University, Editor, *Business as Ethical and Business as Usual: Text, Readings, and Cases*

Heil, John, Davidson College, *First-Order Logic: A Concise Introduction*

Jason, Gary, San Diego State University, *Introduction to Logic*

Minogue, Brendan, Youngstown State University, *Bioethics: A Committee Approach*

Moriarty, Marilyn, Hollins College, *Writing Science Through Critical Thinking*

Pauling, Linus, and Daisaku, Ikeda, *A Lifelong Quest for Peace, A Dialogue*, Translator and Editor, Richard L. Gage

Pojman, Louis P., The University of Mississippi, and Francis Beckwith, University of Nevada Las Vegas, Editors, *The Abortion Controversy: A Reader*

Pojman, Louis P., The University of Mississippi, Editor, *Environmental Ethics: Readings in Theory and Application*

Pojman, Louis P., The University of Mississippi, *Life and Death: Grappling with the Moral Dilemmas of Our Time*

Pojman, Louis P., The University of Mississippi, Editor, *Life and Death: A Reader in Moral Problems*

Rolston Holmes III, Colorado State University, Editor, *Biology, Ethics, and the Origins of Life*

Townsend, Dabney, The University of Texas at Arlington, Editor, *Introduction to Aesthetics: Classic Readings from the Western Tradition*

Veatch, Robert M., The Kennedy Institute of Ethics, Georgetown University, Editor, *Cross-Cultural Perspectives in Medical Ethics: Readings*

Veatch, Robert M., The Kennedy Institute of Ethics, Georgetown University, Editor, *Medical Ethics*

Verene, Donald P., Emory University, Editor, *Sexual Love and Western Morality: A Philosophical Anthology, Second Edition*

Williams, Clifford, Trinity University, Illinois, Editor, *On Love and Friendship: Philosophical Readings*

# Bioethics
## *A Committee Approach*

**Brendan Minogue**
Youngstown State University
Youngstown, Ohio

**Jones and Bartlett Publishers**
*Sudbury, Massachusetts*

Boston          London          Singapore

*Editorial, Sales, and Customer Service Offices*
Jones and Bartlett Publishers
One Exeter Plaza
Boston, MA 02116
1-800-832-0034
617-859-3900

Jones and Bartlett Publishers International
7 Melrose Terrace
London W6 7RL
England

**Library of Congress Cataloging-in-Publication Data**

Minogue, Brendan, 1945–
     Bioethics : a committee approach / Brendan Minogue.
       p.  cm. -- (Jones and Bartlett series in philosophy)
     Includes bibliographical references and index.
     ISBN 0-86720-967-4
     1. Medical ethics.   2. Ethics committees.   I . Title.   II . Series.
   R725.3.M56  1996                                  95-24320
                                                       CIP

*Acquisitions Editors:* Arthur C. Bartlett and Nancy E. Bartlett
*Production Editor:* Anne S. Noonan
*Manufacturing Buyer:* Dana L. Cerrito
*Editorial Production Service:* Book 1
*Typesetting:* Seahorse Prepress/Book 1
*Printing and Binding:* Braun-Brumfield, Inc.
*Cover Design:* Marshall Henrichs
*Cover Printing:* New England Book Components, Inc.

Printed in the United States of America
99 98 97 96 95    10 9 8 7 6 5 4 3 2 1

For Judith ,
My Friend

# Contents

# Preface

The day this book took shape in my mind was both exhilarating and challenging. It was the last day of the semester and I had just finished my bioethics class, in which I was using a well-known anthology of readings. A medical student came to me and asked what appeared to be a complimentary question. "I really enjoyed the class," she said. "The problems and ideas were really interesting, but how can I incorporate these ideas into my future practice?" This question posed an exciting challenge because many of my students were aiming at health care careers and this was a common need. This young woman admitted that she learned a good deal but she was very unclear about how she could use the information. How would she take these ethical concepts and bring them to life in her career?

## The Hospital Ethics Committee Approach

The student's question started me thinking about how to design a bioethics text that would offer a new way of incorporating ethical theory into the practice of medicine. I hit on the idea of drawing on my experiences working with hospital ethics committees. Whenever I referred to this committee work, my students seemed very attentive. The next time I taught the course I began to merge the "ethics committee" into the classroom itself. I divided the class into three different hospital ethics committees and required them to manage problems surrounding individual cases. I also required them to develop hospital policies so that they would think systematically about the problems they faced. From these assignments developed this "ethics committee approach" to bioethics, which had several distinctive and positive features.

### Student Responsibility for Cases

First, when the students accepted responsibility for a particular patient, they became more serious about the ideas in the case. The ideas came alive when they were applied to cases. The application of theory to cases not only brought them into contact with important philosophical and ethical concepts but also compelled them to think carefully about the difficulties associated with "applying theory."

### Achieving Consensus

Second, when the students had to work with others to reach consensus on a case, they became more aware of the shortcomings of "simple solutions." When their initial solutions failed to satisfy other members of the committee, they were forced to reconsider many of the most relevant problems in the case. They soon became convinced that cooperative thinking about ethics could improve the quality of their decisions.

### Cases Are Not Enough

Third, because the committees were responsible not only for individual cases but also for the hospital's policy, the students could not limit their thinking to one case. Students are often tempted to treat every problem as unique and to believe that the solution to one problem has no implications for similar difficult cases. Many students began the course thinking that all cases could be handled on a case-by-case basis! However, the committee approach enabled them to see that particular cases, while in some ways unique, are alike in many important ways. This similarity requires students to think about the implications of their solutions for other relevant cases.

### Ethics Policies Are Developed

Once the students accepted responsibility for developing "hospital policy," they were no longer permitted the luxury of thinking that each case is unique. No matter how much they resisted, they had to think systematically. The difficulties associated with policy development forced them to confront "philosophically" the major ethical aspects of modern medicine.

### The Place of Ethical Theory

But the students also need to appreciate the place of ethical theory within bioethics. This became easier to communicate within the ethics committee model. Once it was clear that the ethics committee was at the heart of contemporary bioethics practice, the place of ethical theory became apparent. Philosophical theory interprets, clarifies, criticizes. Theory attempts to make practice as coherent as possible. Ethical theory neither follows practice slavishly nor leads like a general. Ethical theory travels alongside medical practice, and each fertilizes the other. The policies presented in all the chapters contain ethical values, but these values are somewhat abstract and imprecise. Their exact meaning is open-ended, which is why competing philosophical interpretations follow the polices. The format of the book tries to correspond with ethics committee practice. In the committee, values exist before philosophizing. However, the philosopher forces us to examine and determine the meaning and implications of these values.

## Committee Dialogue and Decision Making

Practical wisdom, or what Aristotle called "phronesis," is not completely separate from theorizing, and the aim of the text is to help the students develop practical wisdom. This means that the students see the policies of Community Hospital as "first approximations" of practical wisdom. When health care providers seek advice, the ethics committee convenes and discusses the cases in the light of their "agreed upon" policy. At a certain point in time, theorizing and discussion must stop and decisions must be made. Medicine is very different from philosophy in this respect since decisions are easier to postpone in philosophy.

But intelligent decision makers often seek advice by looking to consultants. Hospital ethics committees are on the front lines of bioethical consulting, and their advice is sometimes followed. This advice is not always determined by philosophy and ethical theory alone. Past practice, past values, and the current environment profoundly influence these decisions and these factors come together in the dialogue. Clinical medicine, economics, human emotion, religion, law, politics, and cultural and professional norms are just a few of the factors that affect a committee's advice.

## Committee Decisions Are Criticized

Because of these diverse influences, committee decisions need to be reviewed. Immediately following every decision ten critical questions are raised that expose some of the limitations of the committee's decision. The text aims to be "decision oriented," but it also encourages students to revise both the policies and the case decisions of Community Hospital's ethics committee.

## Additional Cases: Opportunities for Revisions

At the end of every chapter additional cases are presented for the students to resolve. These may be addressed using Community Hospital's ethics policies. However, students may believe that the hospital's policies need revision. If so, student groups are encouraged to make the changes and to respond to the potential criticisms. Keep in mind that the philosopher will always put pressure on committee members to resolve cases in a critical and systematic fashion.

## Acknowledgments

I wish to express genuine appreciation to all who have helped in the writing of this book. Youngstown State University gave me a one-year sabbatical to write it. Without that support it would have been very difficult to complete the project. My chair, Dr. Thomas Shipka, encouraged me and supported my efforts throughout. Dr Gene Butcher, medical director of the Western Reserve Care System, gave me access to his hospital's research facilities. Professor Richard Hull of SUNY at Buffalo gave me very valuable suggestions. My colleagues Bruce Waller, Gabriel Palmer-Fernandez, Larry Udell, "Tess" Tessier , J.-C. Smith, Chris Bache, Victor Wan-Tatah, Stan Browne, and Jim Dale were always there to clear up my confusions. Also, thanks to student assistant Skip Slavik, who spent long hours in front of a computer screen proofreading and editing the text. My editor, Arthur C. Bartlett, and all the people at Jones and Bartlett "brought this baby out of the neonatal intensive care unit." Finally, my wife Judith and my children—Michael, John, and Sheila—were patient and forgiving. I appreciate all of you.

# 1

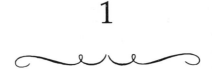

# A Committee Approach

## Introduction: What Is an Ethics Committee?

This text aims to examine the major issues of bioethics from the perspective of a hospital ethics committee. The Joint Commission on Accreditation of Health Care Organizations is the national agency that grants accreditation to hospitals and other health care institutions in the United States. Since January 1992, this agency has required that hospitals and other health care organizations establish organizational mechanisms for formulating ethics policy and addressing ethical conflicts within the health care setting. In most health care institutions this mechanism is the ethics committee. This requirement reflects in a formal way what is taking place in hospitals throughout the country. Hospital ethics committees have already become commonplace in the United States and are playing a vital role in addressing bioethical questions. These committees assist institutions and individuals to confront the major bioethical issues of the twentieth century. We will use the ethics committee as a tool for teaching bioethics.

## Bioethics and Philosophy

Bioethics is a part of philosophy. Why should we study a branch of philosophy from the viewpoint of a hospital ethics committee? The response to this question begins with a fundamental assumption: that medical decisions involve philosophical reflection and philosophical principles. For example, they involve classical questions regarding the meaning of the good life (and the good death), the nature and existence of freedom, and the extent of our obligations to others. Such decisions surely rely on philosophical foundations and philosophical arguments. Indeed, it is clear that philosophy is pervasive in contemporary medicine. Decision makers in hospitals and other health care settings are already using philosophy in their institutional

1

policies and their management of difficult cases. The critical question is not whether philosophy operates but whether decision makers will appeal to reflective philosophical assumptions and critically evaluated philosophical principles. Students need to see how pervasive philosophy is in medicine. The ethics committee approach provides this opportunity.

Indeed, the most common medical context for this philosophical reflection is the hospital or nursing home ethics committee. In the ethics committee, the challenges associated with applying the critical skills of the philosopher to medicine are recognized as central to the process of decision making. Therefore the committee approach is one of the most effective tools for demonstrating this connection.

Throughout history, philosophy and ethics have contributed to the practice of medicine. Ethical reflection helps us to refine our fundamental values, and these refinements continue to alter the face of contemporary health care. Medicine has also affected philosophy. One very influential contemporary philosopher, Stephen Toulmin, has argued that the problems associated with the emerging medical technologies have reinvigorated the study of normative ethics in the United States. The ethics committee approach effectively communicates to students the vitality of philosophy and its connection to a critical part of human existence. Furthermore, the reader can come to appreciate how the analytical skills associated with philosophy can not only clarify our moral options but also expand them. The philosophical ability to analyze ideas, criticize assumptions, and create new perspectives on issues can effectively operate within the ethics committee context. In short, both philosophy and medicine can benefit by the interaction provided by the ethics committee approach.

Throughout the text, both contemporary and historically significant ethical principles will be applied to the concrete problems that occur in the hospital setting. The ethics committee approach offers a partnership model for the relationship between medical practice and bioethics. Philosophy neither leads nor follows. Within this model, ethical principles and the critical skills of philosophy are portrayed as a full partner in case management and policy development. Cases are presented and managed not merely by using the analytical skills of the philosopher but by merging these skills with those of the other professions in order to provide the most coherent resolution to the problems that come before the ethics committee.

Cases will be presented to students in order to apply ethical theory to patients as they exist within a broad social network. Part of this wider social network is the hospital, where health care professionals encounter their patients. Therefore, understanding the hospital is crucial to understanding the ethical dilemmas that professional health care providers face. The text will apply ethical theory and philosophical analysis to realistic cases in which the hospital setting plays an important role in determining the parameters of case management. The cases that the committee works with will challenge the students to apply ethical principles, but the students will also see that applying these principles is not always as easy as it appears in the classroom.

## Description of the Committee

What then is a hospital ethics committee or, more broadly, what is an institutional ethics committee? In general terms, it is a group of professionals and lay persons who meet regularly to address ethical problems that emerge within the health care institution. These committee members come not only from professional medicine but also from other fields. Many committees include philosophers or other humanities scholars who provide the perspective of their discipline. Throughout the United States, bioethics has become not only a theoretical inquiry but a practical activity that committees practice within health care institutions. In this country, we practice bioethics within the ethics committee. This suggests that those of us who teach bioethics can use this practice within our classes. If our culture is practicing bioethics in a committee setting, then perhaps the discipline of bioethics can be taught in a committee setting.

More specifically, approaching the study of bioethics in a committee context allows us to see the product of bioethics as a multidisciplinary exercise. The discipline of philosophical ethics is central to bioethical inquiry, but by itself, philosophical ethics is not sufficient. Practical bioethical decisions require communication among individuals who have expertise in such different disciplines as clinical medicine, nursing, law, and social work, in addition to the traditional areas of philosophy, religion, and literature. Furthermore, lay persons are also represented on the committee. The voice of the lay person is vital because patients belong to this group; modern technological medicine needs to hear the opinions, values, and feelings of those it serves. The committee provides the setting for this dialogue. Finally, exploring the committee's workings also provides a realistic picture of the strengths and weaknesses of this contemporary approach to resolving bioethical dilemmas.

But why have ethics committees come into existence in the last three decades? This question is worthy of an entire book. Briefly, there are two vital reasons for this development. First, new and previously unimagined life-saving medical technologies have given health care professionals the power to extend and transform life. This new technology means new powers, and ethics committees have emerged to manage them so that they actually serve the interests and wishes of people. The technology can often prolong dying and increase suffering rather than bring genuine benefit to the patient. A second factor is that physicians, nurses, and other health professionals are practicing in settings other than the traditional private office. There are fewer and fewer individually operated health care offices. Health care professionals practice in hospitals, clinics, nursing homes, and health maintenance organizations (HMOs). The health care team is now commonplace. The health care professional has moved out of the private and largely individualized context into a very public and social one. This requires that teams develop more skills in dealing with shared ethical dilemmas.

The hospital is the most common of these public institutions. Human beings face some of life's most challenging ethical dilemmas between hospital walls. Hospitals do more than just dispense medical services. They are the settings in which we form new responses to these dilemmas.

## Practice and Bioethics

Viewed from a hospital ethics committee perspective, bioethics is a set of practical conflicts and challenges. For example, how should we approach the conflict between a patient's wish to be treated and a physician's wish to withhold treatment? If a physician knows with a high degree of certainty that a requested treatment is futile and offers no realistic benefit to the patient, should the physician be required to provide or continue that treatment? Can we dismiss the patient's desire as irrational? Can we dismiss the physician's concern to avoid futile treatment as insensitive? Neither of these simple courses of action is obviously acceptable.

Furthermore, in the hospital we address such problems in a way that is different from the way we address them in the academic setting, where leisure for reflection exists. Hospitals are "action oriented" while the university tends to be "reflection oriented." In a university classroom, one could spend hours thinking about the issues involved in the above ethical conflict between a patient and a physician. The university ethics class can concentrate on important and fundamental theoretical ideas, and the students can interpret and reinterpret ideas such as obligation, rights, goodness, and justice without the pressure of deciding how to resolve actual conflicts in a short period of time. These theoretical reflections are vital to the development of bioethics. Urgency makes the hospital significantly different from the university. Thus the requirement to act influences our thought processes. The committee context will illustrate and describe this orientation toward action.

By exploring bioethics within a committee context, we will also be illustrating how medical professionals and philosophers can work together to manage bioethical problems. We will demonstrate that often there is more than one approach to an ethical conflict and that communication about these approaches is vital to patient care. Expertise from a variety of disciplines and professions can often break a deadlock, and there is often no way of predicting how a resolution will be achieved. In effect, the guiding principle of this text is that if one wants to get a realistic vision of medical decision making, then it is necessary to appreciate not only the limits of the hospital context, but also the possibilities of developing new and innovative approaches to bioethics within the committee framework.

Traditionally hospitals, nursing homes, and other public health care institutions have dealt with bioethical problems in a variety of ways. Thirty years ago there were diverse approaches to bioethical questions, including "The medical director handles ethical problems," "Such problems are managed by the attending physician," and "Call the chaplain." Past medical practice did not offer a common model for resolving ethical conflict because our society did not recognize that hospitals should employ an institutional mechanism to address medical ethical issues. Today this is not the case. Many hospitals, nursing homes, health maintenance organizations, and the like have addressed bioethical problems institutionally using a single mechanism, namely, the institutional ethics committee. Furthermore, given the recommendations of the Joint Commission on Accreditation, it is likely that this trend will continue. To study bioethics from this perspective is, therefore, to prepare the reader to participate in the ongoing dialogue that is the practice of contemporary bioethics.

## The Functions of the Committee

Perhaps the most important thing to recognize about ethics committees is that they vary not only in composition and size but also with respect to the procedures they follow. Some, for example, do not act until they achieve complete consensus or agreement. Others will act on the basis of less than complete agreement. However, despite these variations ethics committees can be functionally defined as having all or most of the following purposes:

- First, all such committees take some responsibility for staying informed on major medical ethics issues. Committees have an informational responsibility. For example, committees will often organize educational programs aimed at both the institution's staff and the wider community.
- Second, such committees serve to develop, review, and apply the ethics policies or guidelines of the institution. In hospitals, the most common form of ethics policy is the DNR or "do not resuscitate" policy, which sets out the institution's guidelines for withholding or

withdrawing life-sustaining treatment. However, many institutions have also developed policies on "comfort measures only" orders, the treatment of severely handicapped newborns, and the rationing of scarce medical resources. We will survey examples of these policies in this text. These are the "well-traveled roads" of hospital ethics committees. In addition to examining policies that are widely discussed acr•oss the country, we will also apply the policy approach to such emerging problems as surrogacy (Chapter 5), abortion (Chapter 6), and the treatment of AIDS patients (Chapter 8). These are less-traveled roads in that many ethics committees have not yet faced these problems in a systematic fashion. In these areas, of course, there is less consensus and more uncertainty.

• Third, such committees have an educational function in the hospital. Hospitals can develop sophisticated ethics policies, but without education these policies cannot improve the quality of patient care. Furthermore, policies that are not taught are frequently not used or acted on in real-life settings, and if these policies are not acted on, they cannot be tested. Without such "clinical" testing, ethics policies can never be evaluated and rewritten.

• Fourth, such committees are responsible for case review. The kind of review varies. Frequently, the committee is directly involved in prospective case review. In prospective review, the committee becomes a consultant to assist in the ongoing management or care of specific patients. For example, John Doe, who is now on the third floor of the hospital, has a treatable disease that is terminal if left untreated. Mr. Doe is refusing treatment. The committee may be asked to offer specific recommendations concerning this case. In this context the committee is functioning as a "quasi-medical consultant." Committees may also offer retrospective case review. Retrospective cases are no longer within the institution. The goal of the retrospective review is to determine whether and how the case could have been better managed.

Each chapter will open with a brief description of a generic problem faced by an ethics committee. Imagine that you, the reader, are a member of this committee. As you consider the cases and how you would participate in the committee, keep in mind that yours is not the only voice in the decision-making process. Sitting at the table with you are physicians, nurses, hospital administrators, lay persons, attorneys, social workers, clergy, and philosophers or other humanities scholars. It is vital that members of the group represent these disciplines in order to incorporate the necessary viewpoints. We will assume that our fellow professionals, as well as the community at large, are pressing the committee not only for resolutions to these specific problems, but also for general guidelines that they can use to address future cases.

This approach may lead one to ask, "But where is the philosophical discussion? Where is the ethics discussion?" It is typical of ethics books to begin with a discussion of ethical concepts. We adopt this idea with one provision. Ethical concepts will be briefly introduced as background information, not as axioms. Bioethical problems will not be "solved" by ethical axioms. Ethical theory is part of the total background. It is not the solution to our problems. The axiomatic approach may work well within scientific contexts where there is strong agreement on what are the "best" or "right" theories. Furthermore, this approach incorrectly suggests that theories are not affected by practice.

The committee approach takes a different tack. Because there is substantive disagreement about the nature of "good" and "evil" or "right" and "wrong," hospitals have turned more to dialogue than to axioms as a means of resolving conflict. Dialogue, however, requires not only that ethical theories, principles, and concepts play a central role in decision making but also that there be a feedback mechanism between theory and practice. Just as scientific theory and scientific practice interact and thereby alter one another, so too do ethical theory and human practices such as medicine. This interaction produces theoretical and practical change. Our theories alter our practices, and our practices alter our theories.

## The Place of Theory

The committee approach to bioethics will highlight the importance of ethical theory. Throughout we will weave relevant ethical principles and concepts into the committee conversation. Differences of opinion will often be tied to different philosophical commitments. Two ethicists with opposing philosophical outlooks will serve on the committee. The first is a *consequentialist*, who holds that the effects of an action determine its moral quality and that our moral duties and rights are traceable to the desire to maximize good consequences. In effect, we grant rights and impose duties in order to secure the best possible outcomes.

The second ethicist on the committee emphasizes what philosophers call a *deontological* or *rights-based* view of ethics. Deontologists maintain that human beings have duties that should be obeyed and rights that should be respected, and that sometimes these duties and rights should be respected even if doing so does not produce the best consequences.

# Types of Consequentialism

Consequentialists argue that actions are classified on the basis of their effects or consequences. The consequences of actions, however, are usually a mixture of good and bad. In order to determine the moral worth of an act, one must weigh these consequences. Consequentialists are powerfully influenced by the work of John Stuart Mill, whose book *Utilitarianism* advances his "greatest happiness principle" as a universal decision principle in ethics. This precept states that actions are right if "they tend to promote happiness, wrong as they tend to produce the reverse of happiness."[1] This principle of utility contains Mill's answer to two fundamental questions, namely, "what things are good?" and "what actions are right?" Philosophers often distinguish between two kinds of good, extrinsic and intrinsic. Extrinsic goods are things that we desire because they produce something else. My coat is extrinsically good. I want it not for its own sake but because it keeps me warm. An intrinsic good is something that we desire for its own sake, not because it leads to other goods. Utilitarians maintain that pleasure and happiness are the only intrinsic goods. Other objects are extrinsically good or valuable because they advance happiness and pleasure, or alleviate pain and unhappiness.

Rightness is a property of actions or kinds of actions. For utilitarians, right actions are those that produce maximal happiness. Rightness is something that one calculates based on the amounts of pleasure and pain produced by an act or a rule of action. Right actions are those that produce the most happiness. Wrong actions are those that produce more pain than happiness.

## Act Utilitarianism

Mill's principle of general happiness is somewhat ambiguous because it does not explicitly state whether one should apply the greatest happiness principle to specific acts or to general rules of behavior. Act utilitarian ethical theory resolves this ambiguity by stating that the greatest happiness principle applies to specific actions. For example, if a person who is near death and competent to make decisions directs another person to kill him, then killing may be right if it maximizes benefits over harms in this particular situation. People who support voluntary active killing of terminally ill patients often argue that there are legitimate exceptions to the "do not kill" rule. The act utilitarian admits that although there is a social rule against killing and that this rule is generally legitimate, this rule should be violated in specific cases. In these limited cases, obeying the "do not kill" rule produces more harm than good. As act utilitarians we ought to apply the principle of utility directly to actions and ethically select particular actions only if they will produce more benefits than the alternatives. For the act utilitarian, social rules of conduct such as "do not kill" have exceptions, which should be identified by applying the greatest happiness rule to particular acts.

## Rule Utilitarianism

The second version of utilitarianism has a very different conception of social rules. For the rule utilitarian, what produces maximal happiness is obedience to socially useful rules. Granting people the right to selectively "pick and choose" which rules to obey in specific situations threatens the very practice of setting down rules to govern human behavior. Legislatures do not pass laws and allow citizens to decide for themselves whether to obey them. Laws apply universally. Indeed, the rule utilitarian argues that following the act utilitarian principle may produce chaos because every person would be able to decide for herself whether a rule was binding in a given situation. This freedom to disobey laws may harm society. For example, if doctors could decide for themselves to kill patients who were suffering from a terrible disease, then patients might avoid seeking medical treatment.

Another example of how act utilitarianism might be unethical involves hatred. Assume that millions of people hate Smith, who is obnoxious but innocent. This hatred may motivate Jones to kill Smith. Furthermore, Jones might do a "calculation" that establishes that killing Smith will produce more good than harm. The millions who hate Smith would be happier if Smith were dead, and no one would really be unhappy over the death of this obnoxious person. Does this justify killing Smith? The rule utilitarian says "No!"

Furthermore, according to the rule utilitarian, rules should not be broken on a case-by-case basis because this would tend to blur the distinction between what is right and what is convenient. To return to our illustration involving Jones and Smith, it may be convenient to kill Smith because it would make millions happier, but it is surely questionable whether it is morally right to kill an individual merely because doing so would produce happiness for millions.

Rule utilitarians argue that these difficulties can be avoided if we apply the greatest happiness principle to rules rather than particular acts. In addition, once a rule is judged to maximize social welfare, everyone is obliged to follow that rule. This is true even in particular cases where obedience to the rule may produce more harm than good. Rule utilitarians admit that following a rule in some circumstances can produce more harm than good. However, the rule utilitarian claims that rules bind the individual

*Explanation:*

because obedience to these rules produces more good than harm, in general. The "do not kill" rule may currently prevent us from helping a terminally ill patient who wishes to die, which, may prevent us from maximizing the good in this case. However, obedience to this rule may produce more social welfare than its alternatives.

The rule utilitarian, however, accepts the idea that rules can change. Social rules are not absolute. Our society currently has rules against the direct killing of terminally ill patients who voluntarily wish to have their lives ended. Do these rules produce more good than harm by preventing unjustified killings? The rule utilitarian would argue that it is permissible for a society to change these rules if society can demonstrate that alternative rules would advance social happiness without producing more harms. We already have three exceptions to the "do not kill" rule: self-defense, capital punishment, and just war. It may be that we can develop a rule covering a fourth exception, namely, "killing for mercy." The rule utilitarians will demand proof that the new rules will not violate the greatest happiness principle.

# Deontology

### Kant's Theory

The second approach to ethics that will be highlighted in this text is *deontology*. There are many forms of deontology, but all of them emphasize that there are traits of action other than consequences that determine whether an action is morally right. Deontologists often speak of offering a "rights-based approach to ethics" because they argue that individuals have rights that override what is best for society as a whole. For deontologists, individual rights in many cases morally override social welfare considerations.

Perhaps the most famous deontological theory is associated with the eighteenth-century philosopher Immanuel Kant.[2] Kant maintained that it is not the effects of actions that determine their moral worth but the causes. The causes of human action are motives or intentions. Morally right actions are those that flow from good intentions or motives. Wrong actions flow from bad intentions. For Kant morality is based on good intentions, not good results.

Kant noted that great harms can flow from accidental actions. But accidental actions are neither moral nor immoral. For example, a guest at your house may fall and accidentally damage your favorite chair. The act causes you harm, but is the action immoral? For Kant, this question can only be answered by examining the cause of the act. If the fall was a genuine accident, then the fall was neither moral nor immoral. It was an accident. However, if you discover that your guest intentionally slipped in order to break your favorite chair, and that your guest did this because of envy, then we have an action that may be immoral. Intentions are what make the difference between actions that are moral or immoral and actions that are neither.

What then makes a motive moral or immoral? Kant answers this question by distinguishing hypothetical from categorical imperatives. Imperatives are commands such as "break the chair!" A hypothetical imperative is one that applies only if certain other conditions are satisfied. For example, the imperative "study that philosophy book!" applies only to a person who wants to obtain a degree or become competent at philosophy. If someone does not wish to acquire knowledge of philosophy or obtain a degree or achieve other goals related to reading the book, then the imperative to "study that philosophy book" does not apply to that person. Kant claims that nearly all imperatives are hypothetical in that they are goal or condition-directed. However, for Kant, there is one imperative that is categorical in that it applies to everyone under all conditions no matter what their goals in life are. For Kant, if one obeys this imperative, then one has good intentions. If one is violating this imperative, then one has bad intentions.

Kant calls this "the categorical imperative" because he claims that it applies under all circumstances. It sounds very much like the golden rule, which states that we should treat others as we wish to be treated. Kant has several formulations of this imperative, but the most famous requires us to "act only on the basis of maxims that we could will to become universal laws." Another version commands us always to treat others as ends, never as means. For Kant, both of these formulations assert the same categorical rule, which he believes is derived not from our desire to maximize our happiness, but from reason itself.

For Kant, this single categorical rule is the source of all morality. For even if it were beneficial for society as a whole to keep slaves, it would still be wrong because keeping slaves violates the categorical imperative not to use others as means. Reason would allow us to keep slaves only if we could find a trait that distinguished slaves from persons. But for Kant, there is no such trait, and therefore reason requires that we prohibit slavery. Because we are rational, we could not will to be slaves ourselves. Therefore, we cannot rationally will that other persons be slaves even if this would produce more general happiness. The imperative to produce general happiness is hypothetical and conditional; consequently utilitarianism cannot be the basis of moral theory.

## Multi-ruled Deontology

What is critical to note about Kant's theory is that it is a single-rule deontology. All of our moral duties and rights are presented as coming from the one categorical rule. However, many deontologists have argued that we cannot account for the great variety of our duties and rights by appealing to a single rule of morality. W. D. Ross' "many-rule deontological theory"[3] pictures our moral life as resting on several rules. For Ross, utilitarianism and Kantianism both suffer from a common error: both try to derive our complex moral convictions and intuitions from a single rule. However, according to Ross, neither the greatest happiness principle nor the categorical imperative can account for the great variety of moral rules that bind us. No single moral rule is more important than the rest. We can illustrate this point by looking at two such rules: "keep your promises" and "assist the injured." These are widely accepted as duties that bind us on many occasions throughout our lives. Both these rules are vital in our moral life, but on occasion they can conflict. Suppose Jones needs to break a promise to meet you this evening because he believes that he must stop and bring aid to an injured motorist. Jones is in a state of conflict that is derived from being obligated by two different moral rules. Our moral life is complex. For Ross, we are bound by many rules, and frequently individuals and societies must choose between fundamentally opposing values. Should Jones keep his promise or assist the injured motorist? Ross asserts that rules such as "keep your promises" or "assist the injured" are "prima facie obligatory." This means that at first glance, if we have made a promise, then we are bound to keep it. However, the situation demands that we either keep our promise or aid the injured person. If we assume that we cannot do both, then we must decide what rule actually obligates us in this situation. Many-rule theories admit that there may be no precise mechanism or algorithm for doing this. Ross asserts that in given situations humans intuit which rule actually obligates them, and thus it is possible that disagreement in ethics will continue.

## Four Basic Questions

In order to more fully appreciate these different approaches to ethics, we can pose four basic ethical questions and then answer them first with a consequentialist approach in mind, then with the deontological or "rights-based" approach. It is important to note, however, that there are a wide range of consequentialist responses to these questions, and thus a variation of opinions among consequentialists and deontologists. These sample answers are not offered as the only consequentialist or deontological answers. They do represent a model of how these different perspectives determine our approach to ethical questions.

1. What makes actions right?
2. What makes things good?
3. How are conflicts between society and the individual to be reconciled?

4.  How do these answers give us procedures for addressing our bioethical problems?

## Consequentialist Answers

The rule utilitarian or social consequentialist responds to these questions by first affirming that it is kinds of action that are right or wrong rather than individual actions. Removing someone from a respirator is a kind of action. Whether it is generally right to do so is determined by examining the overall social consequences of permitting this behavior. If, in general, the consequences secure human welfare or general happiness, then the social consequentialist considers this kind of action right.

This response also contains an answer to the second question: what makes things good? The social consequentialist asserts that good is to be defined in terms of social welfare. Actions that systematically diminish this social welfare are wrong. In effect, the consequentialist defines right actions as those that, in general, lead to maximal human welfare or general happiness. For example, Martin Fisk will approach all debates about forgoing life support services in terms of whether the forgoing of treatment will maximize patient welfare in general. In so doing he asserts not only that the effects of the action are the key issue but also that it is the action's effects *on patients* that are most important.

With respect to conflicts between the individual and the state, consequentialists argue that maximal social welfare is best achieved by supporting the autonomy of the individual unless there is a "compelling" state interest to override this autonomy. Our autonomous society is thus on record as requiring a good deal of tolerance with respect to how individuals determine what is best for themselves. For example, we know that smoking decreases life expectancy, but because of our respect for autonomy we need not obligate individuals to quit smoking, though we may limit their ability to expose others to second-hand smoke. The point here is that consequentialists support autonomy as the best means for securing social welfare. One issue on which a compelling state interest currently limits autonomy is active euthanasia. Some social consequentialists have argued that there is a compelling state interest that permits us to override the wishes of patients who want euthanasia.

Finally, with respect to question 4, the consequentialist argues that procedures for resolving bioethical problems should be guided by the principle of securing the well-being of patients in general. Many consequentialists support the emergence of ethics committees because such committees bring together the parties that are involved in making decision that will maximally benefit patients. When ethical dilemmas emerge within

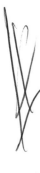

the hospital, the consequentialist frequently recommends that they be addressed by the ethics committee, not because the committee is a storehouse of ethical truth, but because the committee has the information needed to make judgments that will lead to maximal patient care.

## Rights-based Answers

The rights-based approach rejects the notion that either short-term or long-term consequences alone determine whether a particular action or kind of action is right or wrong.[4] Human beings have rights, even if the exercise of these rights conflicts with long-term social welfare. These rights are derived from a fundamental respect for the rights of individuals. Rights-based theorists argue that the presence of terrible consequences by itself is often an unreliable indicator that an unethical action has occurred; unfortunate consequences can occur without any immoral actions. For example, if one exercises one's right to quit a job, a great many people may be harmed, but the presence of harm does not necessarily indicate immorality. Furthermore, according to the rights-based approach, the production of maximally good consequences is not by itself a reliable indicator of rightness. Consider the case in which using an unwilling human subject in a medical experiment could secure a great social benefit. Imagine that this research produced a new medicine that would benefit large numbers of people. Do such potential benefits permit us to use individuals without their consent? Probably not! This illustration certainly does not logically imply that the social consequentialist view is false, but it does suggest that factors other than consequences should influence our moral evaluation of actions.

The rights-based approach also rests on the intuitive idea that it is wrong to treat persons as means to produce maximal social welfare. The social consequentialist account of our ethical life suggests that it may be permissible to coerce or use individuals, if doing so is socially beneficial. Rights-based theorists argue that using persons against their will transform persons into objects, which violates a fundamental moral intuition. Furthermore, many rights-based philosophers have used *universalizability* as the criterion for what makes actions right. What makes an action right is not that it maximizes social welfare but that it is universalizable. To say that an act is universalizable is to assert that an act could be allowed in all relevantly similar circumstances. If it is morally right for me to steal your wallet, then it must be morally right for anyone to steal anyone's wallet (including mine) in all relevantly similar situations.

To illustrate this concept we can again turn to the case of the human subject. The research director who is tempted to use or coerce a person in order to secure beneficial information must apply the universalizability rule in order to determine the rightness of the action. The universalizability rule places a condition on what it would take to make the action ethically permissible for the researcher. The condition is that if the act is right, it must be right no matter who the human subject is. If it is right to use or coerce a patient, then it is right to use or coerce anyone (including the researcher) in relevantly similar circumstances. But since the researcher would not like to be treated this way, then the action fails to pass the universalizability test and is therefore wrong.

With respect to question 2, what makes something good, there is no clear consensus among rights-based theorists. Some argue that motives are the only things that are good; some argue that happiness and social welfare are also good. The approach taken in this text is that, from the rights-based perspective, there is no clear indicator of what is good under all circumstances. The good is not universally decidable. Rather, rights-based theorists allow individuals to exercise a limited right to determine for themselves what is good. Individuals may seek God's will or they may seek pleasure, knowledge, social welfare, self-fulfillment, or power. The contemporary rights-based theorist suggests that there is no philosophical argument that will always allow us to determine decisively whether a given object is good or bad.

In resolving conflicts between individuals and society, rights-based theorists tend to be suspicious of approaches that make maximal social welfare the only criterion. Many deontologists support emerging ethics committees as tools for resolving conflict because the committees provide a forum in which the rights of the patient can be affirmed. Rights-based theorists recommend that ethics committees develop procedures for resolving conflict between individuals that either do not violate individual rights or that violate them to the least possible extent.

## Additional Ethical Perspectives

Ethical values are not, however, the exclusive domain of the philosophers on the committee. Philosophy is pervasive. In this text, the chair of the committee, a physician and the medical director of the hospital, is also very much influenced by feminist writers. She often presents a feminist perspective on the ethical challenges that the committee faces. A religious perspective is also offered. A pastor/theologian from a Christian tradition is a member of the committee. One person coming from only one religious tradition is surely inadequate to represent all varieties of religious opinion regarding medical ethics. Other theological views are also very relevant to the issues that we address in this text. You are encouraged to view the issues from these other perspectives.

You will come to appreciate these conflicting perspectives by seeing their effect on specific bioethical problems. Other committee members will frequently offer ethical opinions and values that are not tied to the consequentialist or deontological perspectives. Nurses, physicians, business professionals, hospital administrators, and attorneys will offer their ethical insights. As partners in the decision-making process the philosophers on the committee will often add clarity, precision, and critical perspective.

The major reason for approaching the study of bioethics in this manner is that this is how medical ethical problems are handled in actual hospitals and other health care institutions. Philosophy continues to make vital contributions to the management of health care dilemmas because philosophers enter into a dialogue with other professionals, and this dialogue enriches both philosophy and the other professions. The reflective attitudes fostered by philosophy can assist the physician, nurse, or hospital administrator to "think through" more carefully the pressing problems that they must face daily.

It is surely true that the urgency associated with medicine sometimes requires health care professionals to assent to positions that have significant weaknesses. But urgency need not demand that the philosopher or health care professional be silent. Criticizing weakness and imagining better ways of doing things helps improve health care. By working together to address the weaknesses, philosophers and health care professionals advance the welfare and rights of patients. Furthermore, because of the complexity of the problems they face, ethics committees are fundamentally interdisciplinary in their approach. Formal philosophy and ethics, as well as internal medicine and nursing theory, law, social work practice, and a host of other disciplines, are partners in the decision-making process. Precisely how these partners actually reach decisions is still largely unknown. But they certainly do not use a calculator or any other exact formula to reach their decisions. Statistics are involved, but their decisions are not statistical. Medicine is used, but ethics committee decisions are not purely medical; traditional ethical theory is used, but the result is not purely theoretical. Decision making on ethics committees is "messy" in the sense that there is no recipe for deciding which theory or discipline will have the most input. Although ethical theory will remain a crucial aspect of this text, it will play the role of a partner in the process. Ethical theory will thus enter into conversation with other disciplines in order to achieve the most coherent responses to the ethical challenges the committee faces.

## The Setting: Community Hospital

Our fictional hospital is called Community Hospital. It is a medium-sized hospital situated in a large American city and has about 600 beds. It is a teaching hospital, which means that much of the medical work is performed by residents who are completing postgraduate medical training. There are also highly qualified house staff physicians who are responsible for teaching as well as patient care. Like many other hospitals in the United States, Community Hospital has problems; one of the largest is financial. A new and business-like administrative staff is making every effort to keep the hospital open, but very few people are convinced that the hospital will survive in anything like its current form for very long. Many of the services the hospital provides are not profitable, and many of the patients who use the hospital are uninsured and unable to pay their bills. The nursing staff is well trained but constantly facing understaffing problems. The hospital is located in an economically depressed area of the city; the staff frequently confronts personal safety concerns faced by all residents of inner cities. Finally, because low-income residents cannot afford private health care, the emergency room is constantly being pressed to treat nonemergencies, for instance, the significant illnesses of individuals who cannot afford private medical care.

### The Members of the Committee

The nine members of the ethics committee are as follows:

*Marian Rhodes* is the head nurse in charge of nursing services in the intensive care units of the hospital. Marian has been a nurse for 20 years and in managerial positions for the last 5.

*Philip Davis* is a board-certified physician specializing in internal medicine. He is also an "intensivist," which means that he has special training in the management of the hospital's intensive care units. Dr. Davis is responsible for these care units. He has been a practicing physician for 15 years.

*Mary Collins*, the hospital's vice president in charge of medical affairs, has been a physician for over 20 years and is board-certified in family practice. She chairs the ethics committee and is widely known for her feminist convictions.

*Richard Marcus*, the pastor of a local Lutheran church, has a Ph.D. in Christian ethics, which he teaches at a local Catholic university. Pastor Marcus brings religious as well as community interests to the committee and is familiar with much that takes place in the hospital because of his experience as a hospital chaplain.

*John Quinn*, the hospital attorney, has been closely associated with the risk management department of the hospital and has served on the ethics committee since its inception. He brings to the committee an institutional concern for risk management issues in medicine. Ethics committees, he believes, must be careful to avoid developing policies that run afoul of the criminal law or civil law.

*Martin Fisk,* a professional philosopher, received his Ph.D. in applied ethics five years prior to joining the hospital staff as the ethicist. He credits the philosopher John Stuart Mill as having the largest influence on his thinking. He assists in ethics committee work by organizing the committee, manages all ethics consultation for the committee, and does ethics education with the nurses, residents, and other staff. Philosophically, he is oriented toward a consequentialist approach to ethics.

*Mary Quigley* is a lay person on the committee. Mary has been a patient at Community Hospital and offers a patient's perspective. Mary, a successful businesswoman, brings to the committee the perspective of a nonmedical professional and "ordinary citizen."

*Vivian Harris,* a social worker on staff at the hospital for the past 15 years, is often able to gather information regarding the social condition of patients. This information frequently affects committee decision making.

*Carla Thomas,* a Ph.D. in philosophy, is an associate professor of philosophy at a local university. She is also on staff at the medical school associated with the hospital. Professor Thomas is very much oriented toward a rights-based approach to ethics and often makes reference to the influence that the philosopher John Rawls has had on her thinking. She is also a feminist philosopher who brings a feminist perspective to many of the issues facing the committee.

## Further Reading

Feinberg, Joel, "The Nature and Value of Rights," *Journal of Value Inquiry* 4 (1970).

Frankena, William, *Ethics,* 2nd ed. (Englewood Cliffs, N.J.: Prentice-Hall, 1973).

Kant, Immanuel, *Groundwork for the Metaphysics of Morals,* trans. H. J. Paton (New York: Harper and Row, 1964).

McCormick, Richard A., S.J., *Ambiguity in Moral Choice* (Milwaukee: Marquette University, 1973).

Mill, John Stuart, *Utilitarianism, On Liberty, and Essay on Mill,* ed. with introduction by Mary Warnock (New York: New American Library, 1974).

Pellegrino, Edmund, and David Thomasma, *For the Patient's Good: The Restoration of Beneficence in Health Care* (New York: Oxford University Press, 1988).

President's Commission for the Study of Ethical Problems in Medicine and Biomedical and Behavioral Research, *Making Health Care Decisions* (Washington, D.C.: U.S. Government Printing Office, 1982).

Ramsey, Paul, *Ethics at the Edges of Life* (New Haven, Conn.: Yale University Press, 1978).

Ross, W.D., *The Right and the Good* (Oxford: Clarendon Press, 1930).

Singer, Marcus G., *Generalization in Ethics* (New York: Alfred A. Knopf, 1961).

Singer, Peter, *Practical Ethics* (Cambridge: Cambridge University Press, 1979).

Williams, Bernard, *The Moral Rules* (New York: Harper and Row, 1973).

## Notes

1. John Stuart Mill, *Utilitarianism, On Liberty, and Essay on Mill*, ed. with introduction by Mary Warnock (New York: New American Library, 1974).
2. Immanual Kant, *Foundations of the Metaphysics of Morals*, trans. Lewis White Beck (Indianapolis, Ind.: Bobbs Merrill, 1959)
3. W.D. Ross, *The Right and the Good* (Oxford: Clarendon Press, 1930).
4. The following authors represent this position: (1) W. D. Ross, *The Right and the Good* (Oxford: Clarendon Press, 1930); (2) John Rawls, *A Theory of Justice* (Cambridge: Harvard University Press, 1971); (3) Immanuel Kant, *Groundwork for the Metaphysics of Morals*, trans. H. J. Paton (New York: Harper and Row, 1964).

# 2

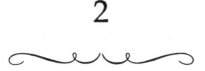

# Forgoing Treatment

## Introduction to the Problem

Hospitals are both lifeguards and lifeboats! When one's body is assaulted by disease or disaster, one goes to the hospital, just as one goes to the lifeboats when one's ship is sinking in mid ocean. The hospital often rescues the patient just as the lifeboat often rescues the passengers of a sinking ship. But before the dawn of scientific medicine, rescues were few and far between, especially with end-stage diseases. In the twentieth century this pattern has been reversed. It is not surprising, therefore, that the ethical problems associated with rescues are challenging us more now than ever before. In some sense, the problems are new because the technologies that spawned these rescues are new.

### Medical Rescues

Because the phrase "medical rescue" is ambiguous, we must identify what might be involved in common medical rescues. The idea of a medical rescue is also loaded with philosophical, ethical, and religious significance because attempting to distinguish good from bad medical rescues requires us to draw on our deepest beliefs regarding the good life, the meaning of human freedom, and death. Medical rescues also involve medical information and medical options. The interplay between medical information and ethical conviction has made the medical rescue one of the most challenging social and political issues of the twentieth century.

The most frequent rescue performed in the hospital is cardiopulmonary resuscitation (CPR). CPR is not one simple procedure. It involves a set of complex technological devices and strategies used to revive the dying patient. The list of these devices and procedures is substantial: external compression, manual ventilation by AMBU bag and mask, intubation and mechanical ventilation, electrical cardioversion, antiarrhythmic drugs, and vasopressors. Other rescues taking place in the modern hospital involve powerful antibiotics, dialysis, intravenous fluids, gastric tube feeding, hyperalimentation, blood transfusions, and a host of other technologies.

Many attempted rescues are successful, but "successful" means different things to different people. Many rescued patients survive the rescue procedure itself but die soon after . Are these rescues "successful"? Many rescued patients survive the day but not the week. Are these rescues "successful"? Others survive the week but fail to leave the hospital. Are these rescues "successful"? Some patients survive the rescue and live many years. "Successful" thus has many possible meanings, which indicates that ethical values and philosophy are present in making decisions about "the hospital rescue."[1] It is appropriate therefore that we begin with some of the major ethical questions associated with rescuing dying people within the hospital setting. The following list of questions is by no means exhaustive, but it does allow us to appreciate the complexity of the issues that we face.

1. Ought we always rescue or attempt to rescue the dying?
2. How should we define a "successful" rescue?
3. If we are not always obligated to rescue the dying, what conditions must be present to justify not attempting a rescue?
4. Since those in need of rescue are often unconscious or incompetent for one reason or other, who should make these rescue decisions if the dying person cannot?
5. What roles do the various parties in the decision-making process play? Are there clinical criteria for determining when to rescue and when not to rescue? Should the physician decide who is rescued and who is not?
6. What makes a good guardian? When the patient and/or the guardian disagree with the physician, who should decide?
7. Most rescues involve nurses. What role do they play in determining what ought to be done? Should hospital administrators who are responsible for keeping the hospital in a sound financial position play a significant role in these decisions?
8. Are there such things as futile rescues? If so, should they be performed? Who defines when a rescue is futile? What should be done when patients or their guardians want futile rescues?
9. What is the role of the state in controlling rescue policy within the hospital?
10. Is withdrawing life-sustaining treatment ethically distinct from withholding it?

Should the institutional ethics committee attempt to answer all of these questions? Surely committees by themselves cannot answer question 9. Although all of these questions are relevant to the issue of withdrawing life support in a hospital setting, institutional ethics committees usually focus on addressing a more modest question: "Under what conditions is it ethically permissible to withhold life-sustaining treatment from dying patients?"

In short, the first task of Community Hospital's ethics committee is to identify the duties and functions of the committee. The committee must select the most important questions that concern the hospital. This selection process is frequently very difficult because committee members may have different expectations. However, throughout the United States, hospital ethics committees have been able to focus on the practical concerns of the staff and patients, which continue to center on a common question: Under what conditions may the health care professional forgo treatment that is designed to rescue dying patients? Once again, it is crucial to remember that this is not the only important question. But it is the one that professionals most commonly demand that committees deal with. It will therefore be the primary concern of our committee. The committee will keep in mind that answers to this question will have implications for broader ethical concerns.

**Rescue Policy**

In addition to identifying and carrying out their tasks, institutional ethics committees must be prepared to state clearly the results of their deliberations. This requires that ethics committees formulate hospital ethics policies on forgoing life-sustaining treatments. Our first goal therefore will be to develop a hospital ethics policy on forgoing treatments that can "rescue the patient." However, the policy will be raised in the context of a specific case so that the reader will have a concrete sense of why such policies are created.

Developing such policies is a major task for any hospital ethics committee, but frequently policies yield unanticipated consequences. When policies create problems, the committee must address them. But concern about the possible unanticipated consequences of our policies need not defeat us. Rather, these may be viewed as opportunities for coming to a more comprehensive understanding of bioethical challenges. They may lead to improved hospital policies. We will therefore begin with the withholding and withdrawing policy of Community Hospital. It will be followed by a commentary on the ethical aspects of the policy. In this commentary we will clarify many of the terms and ideas used in the policy. We will then apply the policy to a case that requires us to face some of the difficult ethical issues in forgoing rescue treatment.

## Community Hospital Policy for
## Forgoing Medical Treatment

*Purpose:* The purpose of these guidelines is to offer recommendations to the staff of the hospital on questions concerning the withholding and withdrawing of life-sustaining medical care.

### For Decisions Involving Competent Patients or Patients
### Who Executed an Advance Directive
### before Becoming Incompetent

The following three guidelines are useful for managing requests from competent patients or from incompetent patients who have advance directives.

*Policy:*

1. If a competent patient rejects medically beneficial treatment, forcing such treatment upon that patient against his or her will is in most cases unethical. This guideline applies not only to withholding treatment but also to withdrawing treatment. The committee recognizes that there are profound emotional differences between withdrawing and withholding life-sustaining treatments, but we do not recognize any fundamental ethical difference between them. The goal of the institution should be to foster understanding on the part of the patient and other involved parties. Our emphasis should be on assisting these patients to appreciate the consequences of this decision. Health care professionals may help patients to explore the reasons and causes for refusal. This is often a first step toward developing more satisfying responses to this difficulty. However, the hospital staff should not unilaterally begin or continue life-sustaining treatment against the explicit wishes of the competent patient. All forms of available supportive care, however, should be continued if the patient desires.
2. Where a presently incompetent patient has expressed his or her wishes concerning withholding or withdrawing care through a living will or has appointed a representative to make decisions about refusal of treatment (for example, by means of a durable power of attorney), such advance directives should be respected by physicians and other health care workers.
3. The hospital has a traditional well-grounded obligation to respect competent patients' requests for life-prolonging treatment. However, certain qualifications are relevant:

A. The hospital does not recognize any obligation to provide medically futile treatment even if it is requested. A futile treatment is one that is not capable of "improving the patient's prognosis, comfort, well-being, or general state of health." Futile treatments do not contribute to the interests of the patient. Furthermore, the committee is very suspicious of treatments that only maintain biological existence with no hope of securing the recovery of the patient. Full and open discussion with the relevant parties should precede any declaration of futility. Guardians, of course, have the right to withdraw such patients from the hospital if they so desire.

B. Scarcity of resources may sometimes limit the ability of the hospital to meet a patient's requests for treatment.

*For Decisions Involving Presently Incompetent Patients*
*Who Were Once Competent and Who Have*
*Not Executed an Advance Directive*

These guidelines apply to patients who once were but are no longer competent, and who left no advance directive. The choices involve selection of treatment and the issue of forgoing specific treatments.

*Policy:*

1. *Medically relevant information.*
   A. A diagnosis and as accurate a prognosis as possible
   B. Information on any significant uncertainties
   C. Information on additional medical or supportive services
   D. Information on side effects of continued treatment
   E. Information on whether death will, in all likelihood, follow the discontinuation of treatment
   F. Information on possible alternative courses of action
   G. A clear statement of the patient's current social situation, and the likely future course of the disease or condition in the absence of intervention should be clearly stated. The committee wishes to emphasize that the decision makers should clearly understand that withholding or withdrawing treatment will in all probability lead to the death of the patient.
2. *The patient's values history.* The hospital maintains that the attending physician has the obligation to make reasonable efforts to determine the patient's values and preferences about forgoing treatment.
3. *Surrogate decision makers.* Surrogate decision makers are usually the patient's next of kin. This policy, however, does not exclude other competent persons who have been involved with and concerned about the patient, who are knowledgeable about the patient's values

and preferences, and who are willing to apply the patient's values to the decision at hand.

4. *"Substituted" decisions.* Guardians can authorize forgoing of treatment on the basis of either the patient's wishes or the patient's best interest. The committee holds that the *wishes of the patient* are of primary ethical importance. Therefore, guardians should be advised to make decisions that the patient would make.

5. *"Best interests" decisions.* If the patient's wishes are unknown, then the attending physician should consult with the surrogate decision makers. If the surrogate or surrogates concur that forgoing treatment achieves the best interests of the patient, then it is appropriate to formulate directives that will initiate forgoing treatment. Ordinarily, for example, persons would want to preserve identity, maintain independence and control, interact with others, have pleasurable experiences, avoid pain and suffering, and avoid being a severe burden upon others. Normally, treatment must be justified in these terms.

6. *Discord.* If there is a conflict between the attending physician and the surrogate decision makers, then decisions should be postponed. The ethics committee of the hospital is available to help the parties resolve the conflict.

7. *Socially isolated patients.* If the now-incompetent patient has no family or friends, the health care professional has an especially weighty obligation to ensure that decisions are made well. An increasing number of such individuals appear in our hospital, and getting a court-appointed guardian for all of them is impractical. It is therefore recommended that the ethics committee be consulted prior to withdrawing or withholding services from such individuals. Some cases may merit formal review by extra-institutional authorities before the decision is made.

8. *Withholding and withdrawing.* Withdrawing treatment already initiated should not be regarded as more problematic, ethically speaking, than initially withholding such treatment. Indeed, in many cases, medical diagnosis and prognosis becomes clear only after a trial of treatment. For this reason, withdrawing ineffectual or harmful treatment may often have more ethical justification than withholding the treatment at the outset.

9. *Quality review.* The decision-making process must be documented and justified in writing to facilitate regular audit by the hospital and the professional standards committees who are responsible for quality assurance.

10. *Active euthanasia.* Intervention with the sole intention of directly causing death (as distinguished from forgoing treatment) has no place in the treatment of patients. However, vigorous treatment to relieve

pain and suffering may be justified, even if these interventions lead to an earlier death. Please consult the active euthanasia policy of Community Hospital on these issues.[2]

11. *Persistent vegetative state.* The patient who is reliably diagnosed as being in the persistent vegetative state (PVS) has no self-regarding interests. It is the opinion of this committee that treatments such as ventilator support, along with nutrition and hydration, do not secure the interests of such patients. Given that the hospital's medical resources are scarce, and given that treatment is widely recognized as futile, the committee holds that continuing treatments for such patients is, therefore, generally inappropriate. This means that continuing such treatment requires extensive justification and is not viewed as the general rule or standing order of the hospital. This rule, however, will be followed in a way that meets the requirements of state and federal statute.[3]

# Commentary on the Philosophical and Ethical Aspects of the Policy

This policy incorporates many decisions made about ethical matters. We will highlight a number of ethical concepts in the policy, including autonomy, futility, competence, advance directives, guardianship, and best interests. First, the policy opens with the notion that because competent adult persons have autonomy, i.e., the right to oversee the disposition of their lives, they therefore have the right to refuse treatment, even if the treatment is medically beneficial. On the surface this emphasis on personal autonomy sounds almost prosaic in the United States. Individual autonomy is something that Americans often take for granted. However, many traditional Western and non-Western societies reject the idea that individuals possess this moral and political right, and even in the United States the extent or scope of individual autonomy continues to be a hotly contested issue. Furthermore, "autonomy" has many philosophical meanings. We must explore some of these before turning to the concrete problems involved in the forgoing of life-sustaining treatment.

### Autonomy as Noninterference

Autonomy may be viewed as *the right to self-determination or the right to make choices that do not violate the rights of others or unjustifiably harm others.* This view is most frequently associated with philosophers such as John Stuart

Mill.[4] He argued that the real meaning of freedom or autonomy is the following: To say that a person is free or autonomous requires that the person act from his own desires and that these desires not be interfered with by others. I freely go to a restaurant, if I have a desire to do so, and no one is permitted to coerce me from going to the restaurant. Black people were not free to go to certain white restaurants in the American South prior to the civil rights movement of the 1950s and 1960s. For Mill, noninterference is at the core of freedom or autonomy.[5] He viewed the free society as related to the free individual. If one lives in a society that severely inhibits one from acting on one's desires, then individual autonomy is not highly regarded in that society. A free society is critically important for the free individual. It makes respect for the individual's legitimate choices a matter of law. The free society imposes obligations to avoid interfering with many, though not all, of the autonomous choices of individuals. If a society decides that John Q. Citizen may autonomously decide to forgo life-sustaining treatment, then other people, including health care providers, are obligated to avoid interfering with John Q. Certain individuals within the society may consider John Q. a fool because they believe that all life is absolutely valuable. Others may pity John Q. for his bad ideas and encourage him to forsake them. But according to this noninterventionist view of freedom, they cannot coerce John Q. Citizen because the society considers him autonomous with respect to life-sustaining treatment.[6]

There are, of course, some criticisms of this view of autonomy as freedom from interference. Philosophers such as Immanuel Kant questioned whether one can really define freedom in terms of the absence of external or social coercion. Kant argued that freedom is grounded not on desire but on reason. Our desires often impel us to perform irrational and immoral acts. Persons often desire to eat more than is rational. They sometimes desire to murder, which is immoral. For Kant, if all of our actions are caused by our strongest desires, then we will never have the ability to follow reason or the moral law. Therefore, for Kant, free acts are not caused by desires. Free acts are "contracausal" in the sense that they are "outside" the causal order. Rather, they are acts grounded on the individual's ability to follow reason or the moral law even when desire is opposed to reason and morality. At its deepest level, freedom is understood as an act that flows from our reason.[7]

## Deliberative Autonomy

Our second sense of autonomy is related to Kant's and may be called the deliberative view.[8] Merely because an action was uncoerced does not automatically mean that it was well thought out and deliberative. According to this second account of autonomy, reason and deliberation are necessary for genuinely autonomous actions. For example, if I act without thinking carefully about the consequences involved, I may lack the requisite deliberation necessary for describing an action as autonomous. I may act impulsively or spontaneously rather than autonomously. For example, a person may start smoking cigarettes as a teenager without considering the consequences. It is common for young people to have irrational feelings about being immune to risks associated with smoking. Such a decision may not be autonomous because it was grounded on desire rather than a deliberative thought process.

However, this deliberative view of autonomy also has some weaknesses. For example, it is often difficult to distinguish an irrational decision from a decision made by someone from a different culture or religion. The health care professional often encounters patients who are psychologically, culturally, and ethically different. It is all too easy for the professional to represent these differences as irrational preferences that derive from impaired thought processes. The adult Jehovah's Witness who refuses a blood transfusion can appear irrational to the health care professional. Should we characterize such decisions as nonautonomous because they diverge from what typical university professors or doctors consider rational? There are massive difficulties with respect to defining what is a rational deliberative process.

### Existentialist Autonomy

The third version of autonomy that has had an enormous impact on philosophy during the twentieth century may be called existentialist autonomy.[9] In this view, the autonomous person is not someone who merely acts on the basis of desire or acts deliberatively. Rather, the autonomous person recognizes that her fundamental decisions cannot be proven right by any precise rational scheme. The truly autonomous person recognizes that our most basic decisions are grounded not in reason but in faith or commitment. According to this view of freedom, the will of the individual is at the root of human values, not reason, desire, or cultural conditioning. When we choose to become a doctor or a nurse, we are not making a rational decision based on a mathematically precise calculation. Instead, we are defining the person that we will become. Because there is no proof that there is a "correct type of person" that we should become, reason and deliberation cannot determine what constitutes a genuinely autonomous activity. According to the existentialists the truly autonomous person is someone who lives without rational proof that his life or preferences are best. The existentially autonomous person makes a leap of faith when she decides to be a physician, and in doing so she defines herself. Furthermore, the existentially autonomous person takes responsibility for these fundamental choices and, according to the philosopher Jean Paul Sartre, accepts the guilt or the "dirty hands" associated with becoming a doctor or a lawyer or a military officer. For example, the existentialist argues that there is no rational way to prove that the wishes of a patient are more important than her welfare. Should a doctor force treatment on an unwilling burn victim because the doctor is confident that the patient will benefit? Or should the doctor simply respect the wishes of the patient and allow the patient to die unnecessarily? Existentialists argue that there are no correct answers to such fundamental questions. Rather, these questions force us not to search for a correct answer, but to decide what kind of persons we want to become. Some people choose to become paternalistic physicians; others choose to become physicians who value patient autonomy over patient welfare. One must decide rather than deliberate.

This existentialist view of autonomy has its limits. It seems to suggest that reason and sentiment are irrelevant to fundamental decision making. But surely it is just as difficult to protect one's fundamental decisions from rational critique as it is to protect one's ordinary decisions from rational critique. Let us suppose, for example, that a young medical resident is preparing to be a burn unit physician. It is likely that he will encounter severely burned patients who wish to refuse treatment and thereby die. This young resident might make a fundamental decision to become a paternalistic physician who always chooses to disregard the burn victim's wishes. He may choose to force life-sustaining and life-preserving treatment on unwilling patients. This choice leads the young physician to become a particular kind of person: a paternalistic doctor. But surely this choice can be criticized. Its consequences can be reviewed. Random patients can be asked if they would like to be treated by a physician who systematically disregards their wishes about treatment. Or we could examine the resident's choice from the viewpoint of social policy. If legislative or judicial bodies forbid him to act paternalistically, then these would surely count as ethically relevant, though perhaps not ethically decisive. Finally, we could ask the resident whether, if he himself were severely burned, he would want his wishes to be disregarded. In short, a decision is not immune to rational criticism merely because it is a fundamental decision.

## Organic and Autonomous Societies

These three views of autonomy can all be found in current philosophical literature. In addition, there is a political or social dimension associated with the idea of autonomy. Societies may be viewed as being on a continuum with respect to individual autonomy. At one end are societies that picture individuals as existing for the good of the state. We may call this social view "the organic picture of the individual." On the other end of the continuum are societies that picture the state or government as existing for the good of the individual. This we can call the "autonomous picture of the individual."

In the organic picture, a person serves a higher purpose. In this picture, the individual's relation to the state is the relation of the part to the whole: the individual is to the state as the arm is to the body. States are superior to individuals just as whole persons are superior to arms or legs. States do not serve the cause of individual rights. The opposite is the case: individuals serve the welfare of the state. Just as the arm may be legitimately sacrificed for the good of the whole body, so too the individual may be sacrificed for the welfare of the state. For example, if an arm becomes gangrenous, then it may be removed for the good of the person as a whole.

On the other end of the continuum are "autonomous" societies. In this philosophy, individuals are viewed as independent of the social plans or goals or perceived destinies of the majority. One need not be identified with any social goal in order to be considered a legitimate member of the autonomous state. Such a state must respect the liberty of individuals and avoid direct and unjustified interference with them. This is a weak ethic in that it is silent on what defines the good life. Participation in social and religious rituals may produce a happier individual, but the individual makes the decision to identify with any set of social values.

There are virtues and vices associated with both these extremes. Members of organic societies frequently experience a sense of cohesion with other members that is often missing in autonomous societies that isolate the individual from others. This cohesion is fostered by participating in tradition and subjecting individual preferences to those of society or family. However, individuals in the organic state often lack the sense of independence that has been such a part of Western tradition, at least since the Renaissance. The point to be emphasized is that societies can be either organic or autonomous, or fall anywhere between the two on the continuum. There are advantages and disadvantages to both forms of social organization.

In many respects our society leans toward the autonomous picture of the individual. But there is a price to pay. The Western public ethic, while it aims to liberate the individual from the coercive forces of groups, can also contribute to a weak sense of community. Organic communities make demands on individuals to provide services to others, and individuals within an organic community receive services from other members of the community. This loss of community can breed the alienation and isolation that is often attributed to individuals in the West.

The autonomous state, however, does permit private communities that secure many of the values of the organic society. Private groups are free to develop within the Western state and can require, as conditions of membership, commitment to very substantial obligations. In addition, these private communities mimic organic societies in their cohesiveness; individuals are more tightly bound to one another by shared beliefs and reciprocal commitments than members of the larger society. For example, the Amish are bound to one another in ways that many Westerners find difficult to understand. But this unity comes with a price: deviation from Amish rules is often punished. In short, many of the virtues, as well as many of the vices, associated with the organic society remain within the private spheres of the contemporary Western state.[10]

### A Weak Ethic

Community Hospital's policy rejects the organic view of society and accepts only a weak public ethic. It is weak in that it is silent on major ethical issues that relate to a person's decision to forgo life-sustaining treatment. For example, it does not address the purpose of human life or the existence of God and God's plans for how we should die. It is religiously neutral. The weak ethic emphasizes that the individual is left to decide many ethical issues autonomously. It accepts that people can belong to religious groups that impose very strong requirements on their members with respect to death. Thus it allows individuals to make their own decisions regarding their deaths. Sometimes these choices are very controversial. The Jehovah's Witness, for instance, has a very distinctive view of the obligations of the good person, including the obligation that "the true witness" never accepts transfused blood. Refusing such treatment is obviously inconsistent with several contemporary values, but the hospital's policy does not forbid competent persons to refuse blood. The policy is thus committed to a broad tolerance concerning adult commitments. This tolerance is grounded in the assumption that without appeal to the wishes of patients, we cannot determine their best interest. In a very practical sense, autonomy is necessary to determine the "best interests" of dying patients.[11]

But autonomy, though it has had an important impact on our policy, is not the only relevant consideration. The policy stops short of saying that the consent of the patient is necessary in order to forgo life-sustaining treatment. The incompetency of vast numbers of end-stage patients precludes this claim and requires some method for incompetent individuals to consent by proxy. In addition, guardians are often called upon to authorize forgoing of treatment, even when they are ignorant of the patient's wishes. When a patient's wishes are unknown, we need to turn to what is in the best interest of the patient in order to make a decision.[12]

## Futility and Forgoing Treatment

But there is another reason for not taking consent as necessary in forgoing treatment. People other than the patient have interests in the issue. Forgoing life-sustaining services is both a private and a public affair. It is private in that individuals often disagree about whether it is best to have their lives extended. It is public in the sense that these life-sustaining technologies are scarce resources and hospitals are obligated to use them wisely. Thus, if consent were always considered necessary, or if the request for treatment were considered sufficient to obligate the hospital to provide the treatment, then the hospital could never say "no." Community Hospital's ethics committee rejects any obligation to provide futile treatment. In this respect, the policy is consistent with the report of the President's Commission for the Study of Ethical Problems in Medicine and Biomedical and Behavioral Research, which asserts that "a decision not to try predictably futile endeavors is ethically and legally justified."[13]

What then is futile treatment?[14] The policy does offer some definitions of the concept of medical futility that focus on the inability of a procedure to achieve its physiological objectives of contributing to the interests and recovery of the patient. A futile treatment could also be defined as a treatment whose goals cannot be achieved no matter how many times the treatment is repeated.[15]

These definitions have both strengths and weaknesses. They are patient-centered in that futility is defined in terms of a patient's best interests. This approach excludes any attempt to offer a complete catalogue of futile treatments. The policy adopts the idea that futility should be judged on a case-by-case basis. On the other hand, these definitions have the weakness of being somewhat inexact and imprecise. They leave us with some difficult clinical and ethical judgments to make about the many borderline cases. Indeed, some critics of the futility criterion have argued that because of the haziness of the concept of medical futility we must never make withdrawal and withholding judgments based on futility alone. Such critics argue that we must always supplement futility judgments with the consent of the patient or a surrogate.

Despite these problems, Community Hospital still takes a strong position on cases of treatment that secure biological existence and nothing else. Patients who are in a persistent vegetative state (PVS) meet this criterion, so the policy affirms quite clearly that the hospital does not accept any obligation to maintain merely biological existence.

This position on futility represents a major ethical decision for the hospital because our society's medical, legal, and ethical traditions lean heavily toward the view that consent is necessary in order to forgo treatment and, in the absence of patient or surrogate consent, forgoing futile treatment is unethical.

Four arguments can be offered against these traditions especially as they relate to PVS. For this class of patients, ventilation, nutrition, and hydration are nonbeneficial treatments. The concrete case that forms the backdrop for this discussion is the Wanglie case,[16] in which the husband of an 80-year-old PVS patient demanded life-sustaining treatment from health care professionals who thought that such treatment was futile.

The first argument involves counterexamples. When medical resources are scarce, forgoing treatment is permissible, even if consent is absent. If Mrs. Wanglie, for example, were in an intensive care unit and if others needed her bed, it seems clear to many that we would have the ethical right, and perhaps the duty, to withdraw life-sustaining services from her. The justification for this decision is based on the desire to save the lives of acutely ill patients who have a chance to recover. PVS patients have no reasonable hope of recovery, therefore, to favor PVS patients over patients who might recover is unjust.

A second argument appeals to the everyday practice of nurses and physicians who serve on resuscitation teams. Such teams often forgo resuscitative efforts, even when surrogates dissent and there is no scarcity of resources. Consider the patient with advanced metastatic lung cancer who wants "everything done," and consider the resuscitation team who has provided five resuscitative efforts in the last 20 hours. Are they moral monsters for giving up after five resuscitative efforts? Or is the magic number ten or twenty? To suggest that one can never give up if consent is missing contradicts common medical practice. Such multiple resuscitative efforts are often futile. Few of us would call nurses or physicians moral monsters for giving up. Quitting is justified when professionals cannot *in good conscience* continue to *batter their dying patients* with futile treatments.

The issue of professional conscience takes us to the third argument. Making guardian consent unconditionally necessary makes the health care professional a slave of the potentially irrational patient or surrogate. The provider of treatment is not obligated to give a futile treatment merely because a patient or surrogate wants it. Patients often request nonbeneficial treatments such as antibiotics for their viral infections. The mere request does not obligate the provider to obey. Patient autonomy is not patient dictatorship. In the Wanglie case, Mr. Wanglie demanded for his wife treatment that health care professionals deemed futile. They interpreted nutrition, hydration, and ventilation as useless for recovery. From their viewpoint, these treatments served merely to prolong her biological existence and thus did not secure her best interests. To coerce these professionals to provide treatment violates the professional's right to conscience. Furthermore, a requirement to provide futile treatment if requested would transform Mr. Wanglie's right to be free from interference into a right to receive from the hospital any treatment he wants. These two rights are substantially different.

The fourth argument concerns standards of care for PVS patients. It has been the standard of care to provide ventilation, nutrition, and hydration to PVS patients. Should it remain so? For some philosophers and physicians the answer is "yes" because air, food and water are ordinary necessities of life. They are not medications, and therefore we cannot withdraw them. The Society for Critical Care Medicine, in its report on forgoing life-sustaining medicine, refers to nutrition, hydration, and ventilation as "treatments that offer no benefit and serve only to prolong dying should not be employed." Food and water are provided by gastric tubes, and IVs are common. Ventilation is often secured by complex machinery that forces air into the lungs. For PVS patients, these ordinary necessities require highly technological services. This society of critical care professionals has argued that "in the light of a hopeless prognosis, the indefinite maintenance of patients diagnosed as being in a PVS state raises serious ethical concerns both for the dignity of the patient and for the diversion of limited medical resources." The report is clear that critical care physicians are under no obligation to provide futile therapy.

There is, however, an important criticism of Community Hospital's futility rule. For many critics, allowing futility judgments transforms physicians into gods who have ethical as well as medical expertise. Surely doctors are not omniscient, and therefore we should not give them this authority. This is a powerful argument, but it can be countered in three ways. First, we may admit that futility judgments are value judgments but that this does not by itself mean that the decision can only be made by the surrogate. Society may authorize physicians to refuse futile treatment if it judges that there is a compelling state interest (such as avoiding the waste of resources) to allow refusal. Second, the physician only approaches godhead status when she acts in isolation. But if futility decisions require significant consultation with other professionals, the hospital ethics committee, and the hospital administration, then the potential for unethical decisions is reduced. In short, a futility decision should be a conscious institutional decision as well as a conscious professional decision. Finally, granting the institution the right to say no does not require that surrogates stand by and do nothing. Whoever wants the futile treatment remains free to petition the court for an injunction against the hospital or the professional. They are also free to seek a transfer to another institution.

## Competence and Forgoing Treatment

Another aspect of the policy that needs to be emphasized is the concept of competence.[17] This idea plays an essential role in our policy because although it is generally unethical to force medically beneficial treatment on the competent, it is not generally considered unethical to force such treatment on the incompetent who have expressed no advance preferences on the matter. There are two reasons why competence is one of the most difficult areas of medical ethics. First, the definition of competence is subject to much debate. Second, even if competence could be precisely defined, many people are neither competent nor incompetent.

Despite this difficulty, competence can be broadly defined in terms of the following three factors:

1. The competent person has the ability to reason in a fairly coherent manner and is able to communicate in some fashion.
2. The competent person can appreciate the consequences of his/her actions or inactions.
3. The competent person can make decisions on the basis of relatively stable values. *for their culture*

For example, if a person refusing resuscitation efforts is competent, then we should be able to communicate with that person about the issues involved. Furthermore, we should be relatively confident that the individual has considered the consequences of rejecting resuscitation, i.e., death. We should also be relatively confident that the decision was reached in a manner that is not distorted by mental or physical pathology. This issue remains one of the most perplexing problems in bioethics, since there are many forms of disease and many treatments and medications that affect our ability to reason and thereby potentially diminish our competence.

Another problem associated with the issue of competence involves patients who are neither competent or incompetent. These patients have "diminished competency." Such cases need to be treated on a case-by-case basis, with special weight attached to the professional opinions of psychologists and psychiatrists who have specific training in making competency judgments. However, it was a nearly unanimous feeling of the committee that physicians should typically assume that their patients are competent, and if health care professionals decide otherwise, then they bear the burden of proof to establish incompetence. Solid evidence is required before overriding the wishes of the patient.[18]

## Advance Directives

Community Hospital's policy also employs the concept of an advance directive. The most common forms of written advance directives are the living will or the durable power of attorney. These advance directives do one of two things. In the case of the durable power of attorney, they stipulate that a given individual has the power to make health care decisions for another in the event that the other is terminally ill and becomes incompetent. In the case of the living will, the person does not name a surrogate decision maker but states specifically what he or she wishes to be done in the event that he/she becomes terminally and irreversibly ill and is also incompetent. Living will documents usually contain statements asserting that the individual does not wish any extraordinary means employed to extend life.

### Guardianship

The policy makes reference to the concept of a guardian. This idea is crucial to many problems in bioethics. Guardians speak for individuals who cannot speak for themselves. Parents are considered the guardians of their children. But parents are not the only guardians. Frequently adults who are terminally and irreversibly ill are incompetent but have not issued a living will or a durable power of attorney. In these cases hospital staff need someone to speak for the patient. In most instances the hospital looks to the next of kin, such as a spouse, an adult child, or another relative. Many of the most pressing issues of medical ethics focus around the guardian who must speak in the absence of an advance directive. It is impossible to address all the relevant issues surrounding guardianship, but it is vital to identify the functions of guardianship so that we can evaluate guardians in terms of what purpose they serve.

The function of the guardian is twofold. First, the guardian must express the wishes of the patient insofar as they are known by the guardian. Second, the guardian must decide what actions or inactions would maximize the welfare of the patient. Guardians make judgments about the wishes and the welfare of the incompetent patient. Both of these functions are very complex. For example, many individuals never express their wishes concerning "end-of-life treatments" such as resuscitation. Often even their next of kin simply do not know their wishes. Or individuals may express their wishes to people other than their next of kin. The classic problem that then emerges for the health care professional is "who should I listen to when the family does not agree?"

Another crucial problem with the concept of guardianship is the difficulty of evaluating whether the wishes of the patient are necessary to withdraw life-sustaining treatment. In cases involving infants, it is obviously unnecessary, since infants do not have wishes on these matters. But with adults there is more heated debate. Many individuals, as well as courts, have argued that guardians do not have the right to withdraw treatment based completely on the "best interests" of the patient. In the absence of explicitly expressed wishes, withdrawal is problematic. The Nancy Cruzan case illustrates this issue.

In this case a young woman was injured in an auto accident that left her in a persistent vegetative state. Her family had convinced a Missouri lower court to permit withdrawal of treatment including nutrition and hydration. However, when appealed to the state supreme court, the lower court's ruling was overturned. The Missouri Supreme Court ruled that it was not permissible to withdraw hydration and nutrition from Nancy Cruzan even though she was in a persistent vegetative state because the family had not provided "clear and convincing evidence" that it was her wish to do so. Her guardians —her parents— thought that it was not in her best interests to be kept biologically alive in the absence of any chance of regaining her cognitive life, but they were unable to convince the Missouri Supreme Court that it was Nancy's specific wish to have nutrition and hydration removed in these circumstances.

Here the question is whether guardians have the right to make welfare or best interest judgments in the absence of a proven expression of wishes. The Missouri Supreme Court was reluctant to permit withdrawal because it found "no principled legal basis" for permitting the withdrawal. It decided that there was a compelling state interest to protect individuals in a PVS from possible harms and ruled that Nancy's parents could not remove the nutrition and hydration if they had not offered "clear and convincing evidence" that this was Nancy's wish. The family could not act on what they considered Nancy's best interest because such action might, the court ruled, undermine the state's interest in preserving life.

The Cruzan case was then brought before the U.S. Supreme Court,[19] which ruled that Missouri had the constitutional right to require a very high standard of evidence (clear and convincing) to establish that it was Nancy's wish to refuse treatment. Other states may employ weaker standards, but Missouri did have the right to adopt a standard that required a high degree of evidence. However, while the Supreme Court rejected the Cruzans' request, its decision did recognize that there was a constitutional basis for the right to die. The court rested this claim on the Fourteenth Amendment's liberty interest and not on the question of the right to privacy, which was the basis of the *Roe* v. *Wade* decision regarding abortion.[20]

## Best Interests

Another crucial concept at the core of the policy concerns "the best interests of the patient," or what is often referred to as "the medical benefit criterion."[21] This criterion is often contrasted with the autonomy principle. The contrast is a vital one because many of the most significant conflicts within bioethics are related to it.

Medical practice in the United States before the 1960s was often criticized for being overly influenced by the goal of patient benefit or patient best interest (as defined by the physician) and not sufficiently concerned with patient autonomy and patient rights. Physicians were often criticized for being "paternalistic," which meant that the physician was allowed to determine what happened to the patient even if the patient's wishes conflicted with the physician's view of what was best. The criticism amounted to the charge that some physicians were forcing their own private and particular values on their patients and justifying this behavior in the name of "medical benefit." Thus, physicians occasionally withheld information from patients in the name of patient welfare, and in so doing treated their patients as if they were children who needed to be protected from the cruel realities of life. However, what makes such behavior ethically suspicious is that it may significantly restrict the patient's range of choices.[22]

Let us now turn to a case to see how we can apply our policy. Notice, however, that we are not applying any philosophical theory directly to our case. Rather, we have formulated a policy and provided opposing philosophical and ethical interpretations of the policy. We have not derived, or attempted to derive, the policy from our ethical theory simply because the members of the committee do not agree on what is the best ethical theory. Rather, we have reached partial agreement. We have compromised. We have agreed to live with what all of us consider an imperfect and, in some respects, an incomplete policy.

## The Case of William Revel

William Revel is 84 and is suffering from metastatic cancer, which has been diagnosed as terminal and irreversible by his primary care physician, Dr. Quincy. This same physician has spoken to Mr. Revel about a plan for providing comfort during the last stage of this painful disease. Mr. Revel told the physician, "Doc, I do not want to suffer but I want to hang on for as long as I can retain my awareness and my dignity."

Three weeks ago, Mr. Revel's wife brought him to the hospital when he began experiencing difficulty in breathing. The emergency room (ER) physician placed him on a ventilator. When Dr. Quincy arrived in the ER, he recommended that ventilator support be withdrawn. The emergency room physician sought the approval of Mr. Revel's wife. Mrs. Revel, however, wanted the ventilator and full support for her husband. She said that she knew that her husband would never want to commit suicide. The emergency room physician and Dr. Quincy told Mrs. Revel that the ventilator would only prolong her husband's dying and that it would probably increase his suffering. Dr. Quincy recommended that morphine be provided to Mr. Revel and that he be removed from the ventilator. Dr. Quincy claimed that Mr. Revel should be allowed to die. Mrs. Revel continued to refuse Dr. Quincy's advice.

At this time, Mr. Revel continues on a ventilator despite Dr. Quincy's objections. Dr. Quincy is visibly angry at Mrs. Revel for bringing her husband into the ER and is also angry at the emergency room physician for violating his wishes.

## Committee Discussion of the Case

| | |
|---|---|
| Dr. Mary Collins: (Chair) | This case came out of Dr. Philip Davis's internal medicine department, and I have asked him to answer any questions that you have concerning the case. I am sure the members of the committee have a number of questions for Dr. Davis. |
| Dr. Philip Davis: | I will do my best. I do not know whether I will be able to answer all your questions, but fire away! |
| Dr. Collins: | Let's get our questions on the table. Perhaps we can get maximal clarity by getting our questions clear first. And let's not forget that we do have a "do not resuscitate policy." |
| Marian Rhodes: | Did Revel's wife understand the wishes of Mr. Revel? Furthermore, what did she say when Dr. Quincy told her that her husband had expressed that he did not want his life prolonged by artificial means? |
| Dr. Collins: | Can we have more detailed information on Mr. Revel's clinical status at the time he first appeared in the emergency room? |
| Rev. Richard Marcus: | Has Mr. Revel been able to competently communicate with the health care team? And, if so, did he express any wishes concerning treatment? |
| Atty. John Quinn: | As you all know, our state has a living will law. Does the patient have a living will? And, if he does, was it referred to in the emergency room context or at later times during treatment? |
| Prof. Carla Thomas: | My question has to do with ventilator treatment. I realize that it may well extend |

his life, but would you think, Dr. Davis, that this extension of life could be viewed as a mere prolonging of the dying process? In short, could the patient genuinely benefit from this treatment? Are you or Dr. Quincy willing to certify that his condition is terminal and irreversible?

Vivian Harris: As the members of this committee know, we have talked a great deal about our hospital's obligation to provide or withhold futile treatment, and I am wondering, Dr. Quincy, whether the ventilator can be classified as futile treatment in this case? That is, should we invoke our rule about recognizing no obligation to provide futile treatment?

Dr. Davis: Well, you have certainly asked some tough questions. Let me begin by saying something about emergency care and informed consent. While I have great respect for the right of the individual patient to determine his own course of treatment, I think that the emergency room puts limits on the extent to which informed consent can operate. Informed consent is often hard to obtain in the emergency room. Answering questions like "what are the patient's real wishes?" or "what rights do next of kin have in this particular case?" requires time, and time is the one thing that is in very short supply in the emergency room. Therefore, when people come into the ER and they need ventilator support, we usually, if possible, give it to them and worry about informed consent issues at some later time. The emergency room physician does not have time to verify wishes of incompetent patients, nor does he have time to determine whether a living will is legally valid.

Prof. Martin Fisk: You mean you have no provision for dealing with Do Not Resuscitate (DNR) orders in your emergency room?

Dr. Davis:

Well, I guess if the patient came in with a DNR order strapped to his chest, that might affect our behavior, but even in this extreme case, the emergency room physician must determine the nature of the patient's illness and that requires time. But Mr. Revel had no DNR order strapped to his chest, and his wife came in with him and she wanted everything done for him. Our team of nurses and physicians are trained to provide exactly the services that Revel needed.

Regarding Mrs. Revel's understanding of her husband's wishes, I do not know. When the attending physician arrived on the scene and mentioned that Mr. Revel did not want any extraordinary means applied to extend his life, Mrs. Revel claimed that she did not know anything about this. It was the physician's decision to accept Mrs. Revel's wishes. The physician on duty simply believed her and provided the support. I assume that she thought that treatment would help him and she was very agitated by his inability to breathe.

Atty. Quinn:

Didn't Quincy ever tell Mr. Revel to fill out a living will or a durable power of attorney? Didn't Quincy ever tell Revel that he needed to inform his wife of his wishes? Talk about screwing up! Whatever possessed Quincy to ignore these considerations!

Dr. Davis:

Those are excellent questions, Mr. Quinn, and I wish that I knew the answers. But I do not. I have helped patients fill out these forms, and I encourage patients to speak to their families and share copies of the document with their next of kin.

Let me return to the question concerning Mr. Revel's clinical status upon admission to the emergency room. He was an emaciated and very elderly male who was having severe breathing problems. His

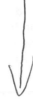

symptoms were compatible with metastatic disease. The physician on duty believed Dr. Quincy's diagnosis of metastatic disease, but our main problem was Mrs. Revel's wish that we do everything for her husband.

Regarding competency and communication, Mr. Revel was incompetent. He was at best incoherent when he did give evidence of being awake.

Regarding the living will, no such will was presented to the emergency room staff who were taking care of Mr. Revel. In effect, the issue of the living will did not emerge in this case—but allow me to say something about the living will. Even if it were presented to the emergency room physicians and it asserted that Mr. Revel did not want extraordinary means applied to his care, this in and of itself would not solve the concrete problem of the emergency room team. For if his wife did not agree with that document, we probably would have felt ourselves in a quandary. The staff would have trouble honoring such a document if Mrs. Revel insisted on treatment. I know that sounds pretty harsh, but most emergency room staff are not lawyers and we do not have any expertise to decide the legal validity of such documents, especially in the context of conflict between the document and the expressed wishes of the next of kin. Living wills can help, but I do not think that they can resolve all of our dilemmas.

Atty. Quinn:

But you would have had no problem if the family knew about the living will and if they had consented to acting on the basis of this will.

Dr. Davis:

Absolutely! If there was agreement among all the relevant parties, then I think that the physician on duty would have turned his attention to treating Mr. Revel in accordance with Dr. Quincy's orders.

Let me now turn to the issue of prolonging the dying process versus providing genuine benefit to the patient. Are we really helping Mr. Revel? I think that is a somewhat open question. In a sense, we can rescue Mr. Revel for a short time, but given the metastatic disease, I think that his quality of life is going to be minimal at best. Patients in his condition frequently request comfort treatments rather than life-prolonging treatments, and such requests are reasonable. It really was the conflict between physician and guardian that was at the bottom of this case. The emergency room team felt obligated to follow the wishes of the guardian.

Ms. Rhodes: But this has been going on for three weeks. There is no longer any question of emergency. Haven't you been able to resolve the problem during this time?

Dr. Davis: The problem still remains. Mrs. Revel wants to continue treatment. I do not know how to get past this problem.

Ms. Harris: But what about my futility question? Doesn't ventilator treatment seem futile in this case? Wouldn't you be able to withdraw treatment based on the fact that continuing such measures is futile?

Dr. Davis: I am not sure that the word "futile" is very clear. The treatment is surely futile with respect to extending Mr. Revel's life for any long period. But it is not futile with respect to prolonging his life for a short period. Given the severity of the metastatic disease, a month or two might be the most that we could expect. The question of futility, therefore, cannot be directly answered until I am given some more definite understanding of what you mean by futile.

|   | Furthermore, I hesitate to actually use the authority to withdraw patients without consent based on futility. There are real questions of legal liability. |
|---|---|
| Dr. Collins: | Thank you, Dr. Davis. Are there any other questions that the members of the committee would like to ask before we get into our discussion of the relevant ethical issues in the case? |
| Prof. Thomas: | I believe that Mr. Revel entered the emergency room about three weeks ago and that Mr. Revel is at this time still in our intensive care unit (ICU). Is that not correct, Dr. Davis? |
| Dr. Davis: | I just received a note from the nurse on duty in the intensive care unit that Mr. Revel passed away a few moments ago. He lived for three weeks in our intensive care unit. |
| Prof. Thomas: | Did Mrs. Revel persist in demanding that full treatment be provided for her husband until the very end? |
| Dr. Davis: | Yes. |
| Dr. Collins: | I think that before we begin discussing the course of this case, which is now a retrospective study, we need to review the hospital's policy on the withholding of care. I believe that all of you have a copy of that policy. |

## General Discussion of the Case

| Atty. Quinn: | Let me open the discussion by reminding everyone about what was said at the very beginning of our policy-making process. No policy can handle all cases. Repeat! No policy can handle all cases. In effect, while I think that our policy covers a lot of cases, I |
|---|---|

do not think that it covers this one. My reason for saying this is that we do not have a regulation on how to treat disagreements between the next of kin and the physician, and we certainly do not have any prescriptions on how to handle disputes between attending physicians and emergency room physicians. I myself would be very slow to criticize either the attending or the emergency room physicians for their actions. However, I think that we should contact Dr. Quincy and find out whether he had recommended that Revel speak to his wife. Other than this question, I think that both physicians acted properly from their points of view and that, ethically speaking, we did the best that could have been expected.

Rev. Marcus:  Pardon me, John, but I think that you are jumping ahead too quickly! I think we need to divide up the questions before we start to answer them, or refuse to answer them, as you seem to be suggesting. More than one question is present in this case. I think that there are at least four separate issues facing us. The separate questions are: First, how do we assess the actions of the physician in the ER? Second, how do we assess the issue of maintaining Mr. Revel for three weeks in the intensive care unit? Third, how do we assess the issue of medical futility? Finally, I think we need to speak to the issue of apparent conflict among the patient, the guardian, and the physicians.

It seems to me that what separates the emergency room from the intensive care unit is that in the emergency room there is no time to settle tough questions. But this is not the case when it comes to the intensive care unit. In effect, I might have no objections to what was done in the emergency room, but I am not so sure if I would approve of going along with the wife during the following weeks, against the wishes of the patient.

Ms. Rhodes:

I, too, am not so sure about Mr. Quinn's view that our policy is silent on this case. According to the policy, patients have the right to forgo treatment, especially when treatment does not provide a substantial benefit. I am fairly convinced, based on Dr. Quincy's report concerning Mr. Revel's wishes, that the patient did not want ventilator support during the end stages of this disease. It may be necessary to further substantiate this by interviewing Dr. Quincy, but if he is correct, and I have no reason to doubt him, I think that the hospital acted contrary to the patient's wishes. We might be excused for violating his wishes in the ER but not for the following three weeks. We kept him alive against his wishes because his wife did not approve. We harmed him unnecessarily and we violated his autonomy. Perhaps we can be excused in this case, but we should behave differently in the future.

Prof. Fisk:

If we look at this case from the view of patient welfare, I think that maybe we could have had some consultation with Mrs. Revel about her husband's wishes while he was in the ICU and perhaps we could have helped her to come to respect his wishes. Dr. Davis, was there anything done along these lines?

Dr. Davis:

As director of the ICU, I did meet with the attending physician and Mrs. Revel on the day he was admitted to my unit. We talked about what her husband had said to Dr. Quincy. She continued to demand that everything should be done to try to help her husband. I was unsatisfied at the end of this meeting but I did not feel that she had consented to withdraw her husband. I was not willing to go against her wishes.

| | |
|---|---|
| Prof. Fisk: | Why not, Phil? After all, the treatment was probably against the patient's wishes, and it was recognized as being useless for securing the patient's interests. In a sense, we may have prolonged his dying process rather than secured his best interests. As you know, I think that right and wrong actions are largely determined by the consequences of the actions, and the consequences of the actions taken at the hospital in regard to Mr. Revel did not seem to be best for him. Our treatment did not make him happier or more comfortable, nor did we secure his wishes. |
| Dr. Davis: | But Mrs. Revel is the guardian, Martin, and as much as I might disagree with the way she sees the case, I think that she has the *right* to call it as she sees it, given the incompetence of her husband. In the ICU we had the problem of acting on the basis of Dr. Quincy's evidence regarding Mr. Revel's wishes as well as on the clinical evidence that we probably could not help him. This evidence was in conflict with the explicit requests of the next of kin. We decided to go with the next of kin even though we felt that Dr. Quincy gave an honest report of the patient's wishes. To override her wishes would have involved going to court and getting involved in a very time-consuming court battle. Furthermore, I do not feel that it is my job as a physician to go to great legal lengths to secure the wishes of my incompetent patients. Finally, the medical futility question was not perfectly clear to those who were attending to Mr. Revel. I have seen patients in this or similar conditions revive for short periods of time, and I did not feel that we could initiate a withdrawal without the consent of the family. Maybe Carla Thomas can say something about these matters because I know that she and |

Fisk are constantly debating the rights versus the consequences approach to ethics.

Prof. Thomas:    Well, this is a very long story, as all of you know. If I understand Professor Fisk's analysis of the case, since the consequences of our actions were bad and since we had good reasons for thinking that the consequences would be bad, it would seem that we acted improperly in the case. Martin, is this at least an approximation of your view?

Prof. Fisk:    It is an approximation.

Prof. Thomas:    What Martin's picture of this case leaves out is that the consequences of action are frequently unknown, and, therefore, we often look to the person or persons who have the right to make a decision rather than to the question of what is the right decision. We look to procedures rather than correct outcomes in order to generate results. I think this is what is going on in this case. Since the physicians are medically uncertain in many of these cases as to what the outcome of treatment will be, they begin to look for the individual who has the decision-making authority, i.e., the one who has the right to call the hard choice. It is not uncommon for a physician to dislike the choice that the guardian makes, but the key point is that the guardian has the right to make the choice.

In this case the principle of respect for guardians seems to be operating. The physicians are not seeking a best outcome; they are aiming to respect Mrs. Revel's right to make the crucial decision. Respecting rights sometimes involves accepting bad consequences. I would agree with Martin that consequences are important in ethics, but when it comes to a conflict between rights and consequences, I am usually on the side of rights.

Furthermore, let me say that I do think that Mrs. Revel has an apparent right to make this hard choice, especially in the absence of a living will or a durable power of attorney. Also, I think that if we are going to deny her that right, we had better get a court order to act against her wishes. I agree that her action brought about less than maximally good consequences, but that doesn't mean that she was wrong or that we had a duty to resist her.

Prof. Fisk:

I sympathize with Dr. Davis's dilemma and I understand Carla's concern about rights, but I have watched enormous resources wasted in this case. The cost of his care ran at least $1,800 per day, and this situation occurs in a thousand similar cases. The social cost of respecting the so-called rights of people like Mrs. Revel is growing to what I call the gargantuan level. If this kind of case came up once or twice a year I would have no difficulty wasting small amounts of scarce resources to secure rights of guardians. But the cruel fact is that Mrs. Revel's behavior is not unique. Many guardians want "everything done" when "everything" means prolonging the dying process with technology that costs mind-boggling fortunes. Finally, I think that even if we accept the "rights" view of this case, I am not sure that guardians do have the right to override the wishes of the people they are supposed to be speaking for. In short, what exactly is the hospital's obliga-tion in cases like this? As an institution should we have some mechanism to make sure that guardians do not violate patients' wishes?

Dr. Collins:

Please, Martin, I hope that you are not suggesting another round of meetings to develop another policy on conflicts over guardianship! I don't think the committee

|  |  |
|---|---|
|  | could handle another round of policy development meetings. |
| Prof. Fisk: | I agree, Mary, that a new policy on guardianship may be an impractical expenditure of our time, but professionals, physicians, nurses, and other health care providers should do their best to secure the medical wishes of their patients regarding end-stage care, not the wishes of their patient's next of kin. |
| Dr. Collins: | Look, Martin, Quincy and Davis gave it their best shot. They met with Mrs. Revel and spoke to her. Mrs. Revel did not reach the conclusions that Davis and Quincy did. Furthermore, she did not explain her reasons for disagreeing with them. Maybe she just did not want to talk to them; maybe there were issues here that were very intimate for her and she did not wish to open up to them. I do not know why she chose to continue treatment, but I think that she is the decision maker and I do not think that it is our job to force her to go along with our wishes. Just because we are physicians, we cannot be required to secure or protect patients against their relatives. I, too, think that it was unfortunate that we provided so much end-stage care to Mr. Revel, but please do not overly obligate the hospital. We cannot protect our patients against all the evils that life hurls against them. |
|  | Furthermore, as an administrator of this hospital I have at least some responsibility to keep the place in a financially sound status. I am terribly concerned that we may have wasted resources in this case, but I am also concerned that Americans are a litigious society and that violating the wishes of Mrs. Revel may have led to a very expensive lawsuit, and I do not think the hospital could afford that. |

Prof. Fisk: Much of what you say is sound, Dr. Collins, but I will not concede your claim that Dr. Quincy "gave it his best shot." Based on the limited information that we have on this case, Quincy made some major bioethical blunders in the management of his patient. Why didn't he assist Mr. Revel to fill out a living will? Many of the problems in this case could have been avoided if such a document existed. If Revel had filled out a living will, he could have brought it to his wife and used it as a basis for expressing his wishes to her. Did Quincy really believe that his report of Revel's wishes would be "enough" for an emergency room physician to withhold services?

Ms. Quigley: Is there some way we can address some of Martin Fisk's questions to Dr. Quincy? These issues puzzle me, and I would like to know if Quincy did address these matters in his treatment of Revel.

Ms. Harris: I would like to respond to something that Dr. Collins said a moment ago regarding liability. I want to remind you that our job or function is not to do what is economically sound for the hospital. Our job is to develop ethics policies and offer advice on ethical issues confronted by the hospital. We are not here to offer advice on how to keep the hospital out of court or to give economic advice to the hospital. If we had both responsibilities, we would suffer from conflict of interest. Furthermore, I think that it is inappropriate to scare us with the assumption that a particular course of action is ethically unsound because it may lead to court action.

Dr. Collins: My remarks on the case were not intended to have the effect suggested by Ms. Harris. I merely wanted to suggest that any hospital that does not practice legally defensive

|  | medicine may have trouble staying open, and if the consequentialist view is even close to being right, then closing this hospital would be a bad consequence and, therefore, we ought to be concerned about this matter. |
|---|---|
| Prof. Thomas: | I think that we need to come to some consensus on the case and I would like to present the following recommendations: |

*Preliminary Recommendations*   The basic ethical conflict in this case involved obeying the wishes of the next of kin who wanted to continue treatment or obeying the orders of the physician who claimed to express the "real wishes" of the patient to avoid life-sustaining treatment. In the case of the emergency room, we do not believe that the physician on duty had any other course but to provide treatment. In the case of the ICU, Dr. Davis attempted to resolve the conflict between the parties but was unable to achieve agreement and acted in accord with the wishes of the primary decision maker, Mrs. Revel. The committee feels that there is significant evidence to indicate that the wishes of the patient were not consistent with his wife's, but it was not in our power to remedy this problem or to avoid the possible harm that was done without risking harm to the hospital.

   **Action:** We do not recommend any specific action except that the matter of guardianship be raised at one of the medical-ethical grand rounds and that attorneys, ethicists, and physicians be involved in the presentation.

## Discussion of the Recommendation and Action

| Ms. Quigley: | Let me put in my two cents on the question of futility. Was this treatment medically useful to Mr. Revel, or did you know from the very beginning that he was going to die? Also, is anyone going to ask Quincy about the living will issues? |
|---|---|
| Dr. Davis: | Once we had some time in the ICU to review his clinical situation, I felt that he had little or no chance of getting out of the ICU alive. I was not, however, confident that he could not revive for short periods of time. |

| | |
|---|---|
| Ms. Quigley: | Why then did you not initiate an "unconsented" withdrawal based on futility? |
| Dr. Davis: | As you know, we fought tooth and nail over that futility rule when we were formulating the policy. Although I agree in principle with the idea, I do not know how to proceed practically in a way that explicitly violates the wishes of the next of kin. Our policy is directing us to act in a way that is out of step with contemporary American medical practice. At the least I would have had to secure a court order to perform an "unconsented withdrawal," and I felt that going to court was impractical for me. Also, from my remarks about futility, Mary, I am sure you have noticed that as long as there is some chance for conscious activity, I am not willing to call a case "futile." I think that as a committee we have to think a lot more about futility, and we'd need guidance from the courts. National medical practice is not consistent with this somewhat radical idea. |
| Prof. Thomas: | Mary, do you wish to make a revision to the preliminary recommendation? |
| Ms. Quigley: | I am not going to press the futility question despite the fact that, in my opinion, futility is present in the case. Our policy is clear that physicians in our hospital are not ethically obligated to provide futile treatment. I think that at some point we need to start spelling out what this statement really means. |
| Atty. Quinn: | Mary, our ethical and legal traditions proceed as if consent were necessary in order to forgo treatment and, thus, in the absence of patient or surrogate consent, withdrawal and withholding are not ethically justifiable. I recognize that there are problems with this rule, but no rule is |

|               |                                                                                          |
| ------------- | ---------------------------------------------------------------------------------------- |
|               | going to produce only good results. We often have to live with the unhappy results associated with generally good rules. |
| Prof. Fisk:   | John, I am also very uneasy about what happened in this case. What we did to Mr. Revel does seem to have been futile, though perhaps not predictably so— and perhaps not completely futile. |
| Ms. Quigley:  | Martin and John are making important points, and I think that we need to think more about this futility principle, but I am not going to press it in this case. However, is there some way we can speak to Quincy about the living will issues? This is really important to me because he *seems* to have mismanaged the case from the viewpoint of the advance directive. |
| Ms. Rhodes:   | I agree that the ER team acted correctly, but I think that emergency room teams throughout the country are becoming more sensitive to DNR-related issues. We get lots of patients coming into the ER from nursing homes, and they frequently have expressed their wishes on end-stage care. We need to reconsider the idea that everyone who arrives in the emergency room who needs CPR gets it. This can violate wishes in some cases, and it can also look pretty futile, especially in cases where there are multiple system failures and advanced age. I know these are tough questions, but these are, after all, pretty tough times. In effect, I am recommending that in addition to doing some educational work on guardianship, I think the futility issue has to be raised in our all-too-limited educational time here at the hospital. |
| Dr. Collins:  | Mary, do you or Marian wish to make a change in our preliminary recommendation or action? |

| | |
|---|---|
| Ms. Quigley: | Yes! Marian and I would like to add to the "action" statement the following sentence: "The committee will discuss at its earliest convenience the practical implications of the futility principle that is contained within our policy, and Martin Fisk is authorized by the committee to speak with Dr. Quincy about what he did to encourage Mr. Revel to initiate a living will." |
| Dr. Collins: | Are there any objections to Mary's suggestion? |

None are raised.

| | |
|---|---|
| Dr. Collins: | It is the consensus of the committee that the following statement be entered into our minutes regarding the case of Mr. Revel. |

The basic ethical conflict in this case was the conflict over obeying the wishes of the next of kin who wanted to continue treatment or obeying the physician who expressed the wishes of the patient to avoid end-stage treatment. In the case of the emergency room, we do not believe that the physician on duty had any other course but to provide treatment. In the case of the ICU, Dr. Davis attempted to resolve the conflict between the parties but was unable to achieve agreement and acted in accord with the wishes of the primary decision maker, Mrs. Revel. The committee feels that there is significant evidence to indicate that the wishes of the patient were not consistent with his wife's, but that it was not in our power to remedy this problem or to avoid the possible harm that was done.

*Committee Recommendations*    **Action:** We do not recommend any specific action except that the matter of guardianship be raised at one of the medical-ethical grand rounds and that attorneys, ethicists, and physicians be involved in the presentation. The committee will discuss at its earliest convenience the practical implications of the futility principle that is contained within our policy, and Martin Fisk is authorized by the committee to speak with Dr. Quincy about what he did to encourage Mr. Revel to initiate a living will.

## Further Questions Regarding the Ethics of the Case

1. Did ethics or law govern the committee's decision? Do you think that Mrs. Revel really does have the right to make this decision?

2. Can you describe what might be required of the physicians if they tried to withdraw Mr. Revel from further ventilator support without the consent of the next of kin?
3. Should the committee have taken upon itself to interview Mrs. Revel, Dr. Quincy, or any of the other participants in the conflict? Give reasons for your answer.
4. Should members have gathered more information before they made their decision?
5. The committee meets once a week, and it is sometimes difficult to get everyone to spend even this much time on the issues that come before it. How might these limitations on time affect the handling of this case? Do you think that, given these restraints, they can still do an adequate job of handling cases that are as difficult as Mr. Revel's?
6. If we were to assume that the bad consequences of treating Mr. Revel in the intensive care unit outweigh the good consequences, would this indicate that his wife should not have the right to mandate such treatment?
7. What responses might Dr. Quincy offer to the questions Martin Fisk is going to ask him?
8. What might have happened in this case if everything remained the same except that Dr. Quincy brought with him to the ER a living will expressing Mr. Revel's wishes to avoid life-sustaining treatment?
9. What is the legal status of living wills in your state?
10. Was the desire to avoid liability overly influential in the management of this case? Why or why not?

## More Cases for Examination

### The Smith Case

Mary Smith was an 82-year-old resident of a nursing home when she was taken to Community Hospital for emergency treatment of dyspnea. She had expressed in writing to her family and doctor that she wanted everything done to prolong her life. She was intubated in the emergency room and placed on a respirator. After six months in the hospital she was still on the respirator, efforts at weaning having been unsuccessful. She was discharged to a chronic care institution. A week later, she suffered a cardiac arrest, was resuscitated, and was brought to another hospital for intensive care. At that hospital a doctor suggested to the family —her husband was the principal spokesperson— that withdrawal of life support be considered.

Mary's family transferred her back to Community Hospital. There, physicians concluded that she was in persistent vegetative state (PVS). She was maintained on a respirator with repeated courses of antibiotic therapy, tube feedings, and other intensive care. She never regained consciousness, and when physicians suggested discontinuing treatment, the family rejected the recommendation and showed them her written requests to be kept alive. Months passed. A new attending physician told the family that he was no longer willing to prescribe the respirator because it could not serve her medical interests. The doctor also argued that her PVS precluded the possibility of her appreciating life. The family did reluctantly accept a do not resuscitate (DNR) order in the patient's chart but argued that the doctors should not play God and kill Mary.

### Possible Senility and the Duty to Resuscitate

Warren Carlson is a 76-year-old resident of Good Faith Nursing Home. He has a history of chronic obstructive pulmonary disease and diabetes. During the past few months he has been complaining about his environment. He complains about the food, the living quarters, his fellow nursing home residents, and the care that he is receiving. According to the nurses he is becoming withdrawn and uncooperative, especially with regard to his medication for diabetes. Sometimes he speaks coherently but sometimes he lapses into incoherent conversation with his wife, who died six years ago. Two days ago while he was coherently conversing with the nurses, he indicated that he did not want any attempt to revive him if he began to have trouble breathing. He asked the nurses if he could fill out one of those living wills so that he could prevent them from keeping him alive in what he called a "living hell." His adult children are unsure as to whether he should be allowed to fill out a living will since his thinking is occasionally incoherent. What should the nurses do if tonight his breathing becomes difficult? If they do resuscitate him and he survives, what should they say to him?

### Withdrawal without Autonomous Consent

Martin Fliecher is suffering from ALS or Lou Gehrig's Disease. He is currently on a ventilator at Community Hospital but he cannot communicate. According to his physician, Martin is dying, but with aggressive ventilator support, he can be maintained for an extended period. He has not filled out a durable power of attorney or a living will, but his brother is his next of kin. His brother has expressed the wish that Martin be allowed to die, but he does not want him merely to be removed from the ventilator. He wants Martin's attending physician give Martin a sufficient amount of morphine to make him unconscious and then he wants Martin removed from the ventilator. When asked whether this was his or Martin's wish, the brother responds that Martin always avoided these discussions and never expressed a clear wish regarding any desire to die. However, Martin's brother asserts that it is clearly not in his brother's best interest to continue on the ventilator and he wants him removed from support.

## Family Wishes and Harm to the Patient

Katherine is a 72-year-old woman who had a severe stroke with multiple complications. She was weaned from the ventilator and ready to go home, but arrested for unknown reasons. Katherine was resuscitated and had an outcome of comatose state, with ventilation, tube feed dependency, and ongoing seizure activity. The patient was returned to a long term care facility with her family's wish for full treatment. She was weaned again from the ventilator but remained comatose. She arrested again with successful resuscitation. She was still comatose, weaned partially from ventilation and stabilized for one month. She developed recurrent infectious complications leading to slow multisystem failure.

Ongoing discussions with her family disclosed a difference of opinions; some wanted termination of life support, and others wanted all available treatment. Ethics committee consultation clarified this, but no solution was obtained. The patient continued with a slow dying process. Over time, the family as a whole reached agreement on cessation of invasive treatment such as surgery, ICU transfer, or acute hospital transfer. They continued to desire resuscitation and medical treatment of problems as well as continued feeding. The patient eventually developed paralysis of the gut and feeding ceased. She was given nutrients intravenously. The family eventually decided to resume feeding despite the problems associated with ileus. The patient developed feculent emesis and massive aspiration. The family was contacted and desired no further effort at prolonging life except mechanical ventilation. The patient died four hours later. Did the physician act rightly in following the family's wishes?

## Further Reading

Bedell, S. E., T. L. Delbanco, E. F. Cook, and F. H. Epstein, "Survival after Cardiopulmonary Resuscitation in the Hospital,"*New England Journal of Medicine* 309 (1983): 469–76.

Berlin, Isaiah, "Two Concepts of Liberty," in *Four Essays on Liberty* (Oxford: Oxford University Press, 1969), pp. 118–72.

Blackhall, J. L., "Must We Always Use CPR?" *New England Journal of Medicine* 317 (1987): 1281–5.

Capron, M. A., "In re Helga Wanglie," *Hastings Center Report* 21 (5) (1991).

Childress, James F., Who Should Decide? Paternalism in Health Care (New York: Oxford University Press, 1983).

Childress, Joanne Lynn and James F., "Must Patients Always Be Given Food and Water?" *Hastings Center Report* 13.

Council on Ethical and Judicial Affairs, American Medical Association, "Guidelines for the Appropriate Use of Do-Not-Resuscitate Orders," *Journal of the American Medical Association* 265 (1991): 1868–71.

Dworkin, Gerald, "Autonomy and Behavior Control," *Hastings Center Report* 6 (February 1976): 23.

Feinberg, Joel, *Harm to Self*, Vol. III in *The Moral Limits of Criminal Law* (New York: Oxford University Press, 1986).

The Hastings Center, *Guidelines on the Termination of Life-Sustaining Treatment and the Care of the Dying* (Bloomington: Indiana University Press, 1987), p. 32.

Miles, S. H., "Informed Demand for "'Nonbeneficial'" medical treatment," *New England Journal of Medicine* 325 (1991): 512–5.

President's Commission for the Study of Ethical Problems in Medicine and Biomedical and Behavioral Research, *Deciding to Forego Life-Sustaining Treatment* (Washington, D.C.: U.S. Government Printing Office, 1983).

Schneiderman, L. J., N. S. Jecker, and A. R. Jonsen, "Medical Futility: Its Meaning and Ethical Implications," *Annals of Internal Medicine* 112 (1990) 949–54.

Schwartz, David, ed., *Withholding and Withdrawing Care: Practical Strategies for Clinical Decision Making* (Atlanta: American Health Consultants, Inc., 1986).

"Standards for Cardiopulmonary Resuscitation (CPR) and Emergency Cardiac Care (ECC), V., Medicolegal Considerations and Recommendations, *Journal of the American Medical Association* 227 (1974 Suppl.): 864–6.

## Notes

1. For a good discussion of the effectiveness of cardiopulmonary resuscitation, see Leslie Blackhall, "Must We Always Use CPR?" Sounding Board, *New England Journal of Medicine* 317 (20) (Nov. 12, 1987).

2. This policy is presented in Chapter 3 of this text.

3. This policy is influenced by "The Appleton Consensus: Suggested International Guidelines for Decisions to Forego Medical Treatment," *Journal of Medical Ethics* 15 (1989): 129–136.

4. A good discussion of this topic is found in John Stuart Mill, *An Examination of Sir William Hamilton's Philosophy*, Chapter 26, London (1867).

5. For a criticism of this view and an argument for indeterminism, see William James, *The Will to Believe and Other Essays in Popular Philosophy*, (New York: Longman, 1897).

6. For a good discussion of this noninterventionist view of freedom, see John Stuart Mill's *On Liberty*, ed. Mary Warnock (New York: New American Library, 1974).

7. For a good discussion of Kant's views, see Immanuel Kant, *Groundwork for the Metaphysics of Morals*, trans. H. J. Paton (New York: Harper and Row, 1964).

8. For a good discussion of this sense of autonomy, see Gerald Dworkin, *The Theory and Practice of Autonomy* (Cambridge: Cambridge University Press, 1988) and Harry G. Frankfurt, "Alternative Possibilities and Moral Responsibility," *The Journal of Philosophy* 66: 829–839.

9. For a good discussion of existential freedom, see Albert Camus, *The Myth of Sisyphus*, trans. J. O'Brien, (New York: Knopf, 1955). Also Jean Paul Sartre, "Existentialism," in *Existentialism and Human Emotions* (New York: Philosophical Library, 1948).

10. For an interesting discussion of the relationship between private and public communities as they affect medicine, see H. Tristram Engelhardt, *The Foundations of Bioethics* (New York: Oxford University Press, 1986), esp. Chapter 2.

11. The issue of children raises special problems for the hospital. Chapter 10 is exclusively related to this topic. For a very solid discussion of the legal aspects of terminating life-sustaining treatments, see Alan Meisel, "Legal Myths about Terminating Life Support," *Archives of Internal Medicine* (August 1991).

12. Chapter 10 will focus exclusively on the problem of infants and children, where the concept of best interests dominates decision making.

13. President's Commission for the Study of Ethical Problems in Medicine and Biomedical and Behavioral Research, *Deciding to Forego Life-Sustaining Treatment* (Washington, D.C.: U.S. Government Printing Office, 1982), p. 219.

14. The following articles provide a good discussion of relevant information on this topic.

American Medical Association, Council on Ethical and Judicial Affairs, "Guidelines for the Appropriate Use of Do-Not-Resuscitate Orders," *Journal of the American Medical Association* 265 (14) 1868–71.

A.S. Brett and L.B. McCullough, "When Patients Request Specific Interventions: Defining the Limits of the Physician's Obligation, *New England Journal of Medicine* 315 (21) (1986): 1347–51

D. Callahan, "Medical Futility, Medical Necessity: The Problem-without-a-Name," *Hastings Center Report* 21 (4) (1991): 30–35.

A.M. Capron, "In re Helga Wanglie." *Hastings Center Report* 21 (5) (1991): 26-8.14.

In re *Conservatorship of Helga M. Wanglie*, Fourth Judicial District (Dist. Ct., Probate Ct. Div.) PX-91-283. Minnesota, Hennepin County.

R. E. Cranford, "Helga Wanglie's Ventilator," *Hastings Center Report* 21 (4) (1991): 23–24.

J. A. Gold, D. F. Jablonski, P. J. Christensen, R. S. Shapiro, and D. L. Schiedermayer, "Is There a Right to Futile Treatment? The Case of a Dying Patient with AIDS," *Journal of Clinical Ethics* 1 (1) (1990): 19–23.

J. C. Hackler, and F. C. Hiller, "Family Consent to Orders Not to Resuscitate: Reconsidering Hospital Policy," *Journal of the American Medical Association* 264 (10) (1990): 1281–83.

N. S. Jecker and L. J. Schneiderman, "Futility and Rationing," *American Journal of Medicine* 92 (2) (1992): 189–96.

N. S. Jecker and R. A. Pearlman, "Medical Futility, Who Decides?" *Archives of Internal Medicine* 152 (June 1992): 1140–44.

E. Haavi Morreim, "Profoundly Diminished Life: The Casualties of Coercion," *Hastings Center Report* 24 (1) (1994): 33.

15. The case is discussed in the *Hastings Center Report* 21 (4) (1991).

16. For a good discussion of the issues in medical competence and decision-making capacity, see Jonsen, Siegler, and Winslade, *Clinical Ethics* (New York: Macmillan, 1982), esp. Chapter 2.

17. More information on incompetence will be offered in Chapter 4, which covers informed consent.

18. See the U.S. Supreme Court decision *Cruzan v. Director, Missouri Dept. of Health* 580 U.S. SLW 4916 (June 25, 1990).

19. For a criticism of the court's ruling, see the dissenting opinions of Judges Brennan and Stevens, which follow the majority opinion in the case.

20. For a good defense of the primacy of the principle of medical benefit, see Edmund Pellegrino and David Thomasma, *For the Patient's Good: The Restoration of Beneficence in Health Care* (New York: Oxford University Press, 1988).

21. For a thorough discussion of the issues involved in withdrawing treatment, see the President's Commission Report, *Deciding to Forego Life-Sustaining Treatment*, Chapter 2.

# 3

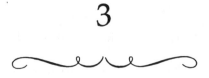

# Euthanasia

## Introduction to the Problem

In the previous chapter we were concerned with a policy covering passive euthanasia. Passive euthanasia may be defined as omitting medical actions that extend the life of a dying patient. Passive euthanasia involves allowing an individual to die. In the most obvious cases of passive euthanasia, one is not committing an action. One is doing nothing to extend the dying process. No one, for example, is injecting strychnine into anyone's veins. No one is infusing a patient with an overdose of morphine. No one is providing information about suicide. Rather, the physician or nurse is forgoing services that serve only to extend the dying process of a patient who has in some way refused these services. Our policy on forgoing treatment was based on the assumption that there were many instances in which saving a life violates two of our most cherished moral values. When we save someone's life contrary to the wishes of that person, we are risk violating that person's autonomy. Furthermore, when we save a life and succeed only in prolonging the dying process, we risk harming the person. However, contemporary law as well as contemporary medical practice has extended this concept of passive euthanasia to include treatments that have already been initiated. Therefore the problem of withdrawing treatment, which appears to be an action, emerges. For example, if a terminally ill patient has been placed on a ventilator in an emergency room and the medical team later finds out that this patient has filled out a living will or other advance directive refusing this treatment, then removing or withdrawing this ventilator is considered passive euthanasia, even though the health care professional is acting when he withdraws the ventilator. This extension of the concept of passive euthanasia from withholding (an omission) to withdrawing (an action) suggests that the concept of passive euthanasia is not precise, and that there are borderline cases of allowing to die that look like active euthanasia.

## A Definition

*Active euthanasia* may be defined as directly and intentionally acting to bring about the death of a patient for reasons of compassion. Active euthanasia involves commission, not omission. Many philosophers, jurists, and medical ethicists maintain that while passive euthanasia is under some conditions morally right, active euthanasia is morally wrong. Until recently, the Western tradition had not spelled out any conditions under which active euthanasia was permissible.

Passive euthanasia is widely practiced in the United States. Whenever a "DNR" (do not resuscitate) is written on a patient's chart, the parties involved are practicing passive euthanasia. Whenever families and physicians agree that giving a dying patient dialysis would only increase her suffering, they are practicing passive euthanasia. Whenever physicians withhold antibiotics at the request of the dying AIDS patient, they are practicing passive euthanasia. However, acting to bring about the desired death in these circumstances is currently forbidden by law and by our fictional hospital's policy. For example, to give a willing terminal cancer patient an injection of strychnine is an action that directly and intentionally kills him. It is forbidden by Community Hospital's policy as well as by current law.

## Active Euthanasia and Murder

But many readers may ask why the question of active euthanasia is a problem. Why not treat active euthanasia as murder, and those who commit it as murderers? One response is that our society simply does not treat individuals who commit active euthanasia as murderers. No physician or nurse in the United States has been convicted of first degree murder in any case involving active euthanasia. Even when individuals are convicted of active euthanasia, they are not convicted of first degree murder, nor are they punished as severely as murderers.

There seem to be three reasons why our society distinguishes active euthanasia from murder. First, those who commit active euthanasia are not motivated by greed, jealousy, lust for power, or any of the other classical motives for murder. In legal terminology, they do not have evil intent. Rather, they are motivated by one of the highest of motives—namely, mercy. Indeed, a popular synonym for "active euthanasia" is "mercy killing."

The second reason is that murder victims do not consent to being murdered. They do not ask to be killed. Murder is always a violation of the victim's autonomy. However, active euthanasia is initiated by the person who is killed. When one is committing active euthanasia, one has been given permission by the dying person to mercifully end that person's life.

Finally, active euthanasia, unlike murder, has at least some good consequences for the person who is killed. Murder victims lose something that they want, i.e., their lives. But those in the terminal stage of an irreversible disease do not always consider their lives valuable. Some victims of painful and terminal disease hold that death is far preferable to life. In the words of the poet Baudelaire, life "weighs them down and breaks their shoulders." Supporters of active euthanasia claim that this practice respects the autonomy of the patient and leads to less harm for the patient than the alternative of a long and painful death.

However, while granting that active euthanasia is not murder, a society may agree to oppose active euthanasia. Principle 10 of the hospital's policy on forgoing treatment expresses this opposition to active euthanasia, but it is incomplete in some respects. For example, our chapter on forgoing treatment does not address any of the arguments for or against active euthanasia. Principle 10 does not say anything about the use of narcotics and other comfort measures in the treatment of the terminally ill. Nor does it address the question of assisted suicide and whether or not it is ethically the same as active euthanasia. In short, Community Hospital's policy on forgoing treatment leaves a lot unsaid. This chapter is aimed at clarifying and limiting this rule against active euthanasia.

---

### Community Hospital's Policy on Active Euthanasia

*Purpose:*   The purpose of this policy is to clarify the position of the hospital on active euthanasia.

*Definition:*   Active euthanasia is the commission of any act that directly leads to the death of a patient. The intention of the act is to mercifully cause the death of the patient.

*Principles:*

1. Intervention with the solitary intent of causing death (as distinguished from forgoing treatment) has no place in the treatment of terminally and irreversibly ill patients at Community Hospital.
2. Principle 1 should not be viewed as forbidding the provision of pain medications that are reasonable and adequate for reducing pain in the terminally ill. It is ethically permissible with the informed consent of the patient or his guardian to provide pain medications sufficient to secure the comfort of the dying patient. The concern that adequate and

reasonable amounts of pain control medication may hasten the death of a consenting patient is not a satisfactory basis for withholding adequate medication. The committee recommends that any physician unwilling to act on the basis of this principle should consider referring his or her patient to the hospital's pain control unit. Furthermore, with the terminally ill, there ought to be no resistance to the use of adequate and reasonable doses of pain-controlling medications, even if these doses are addictive. Such a principle does not, of course, apply to the nonterminally ill individual.

3. Principle 1 should not be viewed as implying anything about the withdrawal of patients from end-stage life support. It remains the position of the committee that withdrawing patients from life support in the face of terminal and irreversible disease is permissible within the guidelines set by the hospital's policy on forgoing treatment.

4. Nothing in this policy should be interpreted as implying any reduction in the rights of competent patients to refuse treatment. Refusing treatment is fundamentally different from asking a physician to commit medical murder. Reduced levels of treatment for the terminally ill remain permissible within the guidelines set forth in the hospital's policy on the forgoing of treatment.

5. The fact that active euthanasia is based on the merciful intention to relieve the suffering of a patient is not considered by this committee a justifiable basis for committing this act.

6. The fact that a patient has autonomously asked to be actively euthanized is not considered a justifiable basis for committing this act.

7. Patients who seek active euthanasia are frequently those whose pain is being undertreated and undermedicated. Often this is related to health care providers' concerns about the potential of pain-controlling medications to hasten death. These concerns can be addressed by principle 8.

8. Any employee of the hospital who is aware of or believes that active euthanasia is being practiced at this hospital should immediately contact and inform his superior of this fact.

9. The committee sees important ethical differences between active euthanasia and physician-assisted suicide. In the latter case the physician provides information. He does not act directly to bring about death. The committee is very reluctant to forbid any forms of patient-physician communication. Furthermore, the committee believes that in many cases patient welfare and patient autonomy could significantly be enhanced without producing the harms associated with active euthanasia. The committee continues to research and develop policies on physician-assisted suicide.

# Commentary on the Philosophical and Ethical Aspects of the Policy

There are five basic questions that dominate the ethical and philosophical background to the active euthanasia debate. First, is the distinction itself between active and passive euthanasia a clear and precise one? The philosopher James Rachels[1] has argued that the boundaries that separate active from passive euthanasia are vague and therefore some instances of active euthanasia may be seen as wrongful killing and some as justifiable killing.[2] Second, how does the autonomy principle—especially the restriction on the principle involving "compelling state interests"—determine the ethical status of active euthanasia? Third, how do "slippery slope" considerations, i.e., the possibility of terrible harm resulting from the legalization of active euthanasia, determine the ethical status of mercy killing? Fourth, how does the health care professional's commitment to provide help to patients and avoid harming them determine the ethical status of active euthanasia? More specifically, is the reluctance of the medical profession to become "medical killers" relevant to the debate? Finally, the question of the relationship between active euthanasia and physician-assisted suicide needs to be addressed.

## The Distinction between Active and Passive Euthanasia

Let us begin, therefore, with the assumption that the distinction between active and passive euthanasia is clear and precise, even though there are reasons for thinking that it is not. The President's Commission for the Study of Ethical Problems in Medicine and Biomedical and Behavioral Research tackled this issue and concluded that the distinction between active and passive euthanasia is vague. The following passage captures the sentiments of the commission:

> The distinction between acting and omitting to act provides a useful rule-of-thumb by separating cases that probably deserve more scrutiny from those that are likely not to need it. Although not all decisions to omit treatment and allow death to occur are acceptable, such a choice, when made by a patient or surrogate, is usually morally acceptable and in compliance with the law on homicide. Conversely, active steps to end life, such as by administering a poison, are likely to be serious moral and legal wrongs. Nonetheless, the mere difference between acts and omissions—which is often hard to draw in any case—never by itself determines what is morally acceptable. Rather, the acceptability of particular actions or omissions turns on other morally significant considerations such as the balance of harms and benefits likely to be achieved, the duties owed by others to a dying person, the risks imposed on others in acting or refraining, and the certainty of outcome.[3]

The reason for doubting the distinction is that acts of omission can be morally wrong just as acts of commission can be morally right. The physician who doesn't provide antibiotics to an otherwise healthy 20-year-old who later dies is surely guilty of wrongful death just as the physician who withdraws a consenting, terminally and irreversibly ill patient from a respirator is morally innocent. According to the President's Commission, being passive is in itself no indicator of moral innocence nor is being active a reliable indicator of moral guilt. Both forms of behavior can lead to ethically justified or ethically unjustified death.

The commission, however, did not totally reject the traditional distinction between active and passive euthanasia. Rather, its view seems to be that, although the distinction is not one of kind, it is one of degree. The commission viewed the distinction as a "useful rule-of-thumb" in that "the commonly accepted prohibition against active killing helps to produce the correct decision in the great majority of cases."[4]

There are, however, some difficulties with this view. First, good rules of thumb are provable. For example, checking the blood pressure of an unconscious person who is brought to the emergency room improves medical outcome. This is a good rule of thumb, and it is provable. But, how does one prove that most deaths brought about by action are wrongful deaths and that most deaths brought about by omission are rightful deaths? This claim is not an empirical claim because the concept of wrongful or rightful death is a moral, not scientific, one. Whether something is or is not a rightful death can not settled by observation alone. Therefore, it is simply not something that can be determined to be a good or a bad rule of thumb.

Second, if avoiding active euthanasia were a good rule of thumb, and if rightful death were an empirical concept, then this would automatically imply that the commission's rule of thumb could be tested. In short, it should be possible to run a clinical trial comparing active with passive euthanasia to determine which would lead to "better clinical results." But in the United States this is absurd because active euthanasia is presently illegal. To run such a test would be illegal, and, to my knowledge, no such controlled studies have been performed. The point here is that the commission has no evidence or clinical trials to justify empirically its claim that avoiding active euthanasia is a useful rule of thumb.

But if the commission's preference for passive euthanasia over active euthanasia is not based on empirical evidence such as clinical trials, then what is the basis for this preference? Supporters as well as critics of active euthanasia interpret this preference as a **moral or ethical commitment**. However, the reasons for accepting this preference rest on considerations that are independent of the distinction itself. For example, there is a conviction that terrible consequences will occur if we allow active euthanasia.

How then should we summarize our findings on the moral status of the distinction between active and passive euthanasia? As the President's Commission noted, the distinction cannot be viewed as one of kind. There are simply too many counterexamples. But can it be viewed as one of degree? Are most passive euthanasia behaviors right and most active euthanasia behaviors wrong? The President's Commission said yes, but we have indicated there are significant problems associated with this view. Therefore we need to turn to other considerations that ground opposition to active euthanasia.

### Autonomy and Active Euthanasia

Perhaps the strongest arguments in favor of active euthanasia are based on the principle that individuals have the right to determine the course of their own lives and this right should be extended to authorizing others to kill them. Autonomy justifies active euthanasia. This principle maintains that because it is difficult to determine what is best, the individual should be empowered to decide for herself. If a patient authorizes a doctor to kill her because she is terminally ill, then this falls under her individual authority. The argument proceeds by showing that if we disregard an individual's autonomy in this area, then we transform that person into an object. Disregarding autonomy requires us to force or coerce the person to live against her will. Disregarding autonomy in this area involves disrespect for persons.

For many consequentialist philosophers, the notion of autonomy is justified, by appeal not to the distinction between persons and objects, but to the notion that society can achieve maximal happiness only if the individuals within it are maximally autonomous. The consequentialist view of freedom or autonomy is an instrumentalist view in that individual freedom is represented as the best means for securing social well-being. Most of us will be happier if we have free choice. Applied to active euthanasia, the position suggests that society will be better off if the individual's right to active euthanasia is respected.

However, it is vital to note that although consequentialists and rights-based theorists disagree over fundamental issues in the philosophy of freedom, neither would require that only autonomous choices that produce personal welfare are to be respected. Even if a competent person's choices lead to his own unhappiness, they still need to be respected. An illustration can help. What career should you pursue, and who has the right to make that decision? The traditional Western answer is that "the individual has the right to answer this question." For Kant, the reason is because you, the individual, are not a tool of our society. Furthermore, you are the one who will be most affected by the decision. You may be able to make a great contribution to our society by becoming an architect, but we cannot force you to follow that career path. To force you to become an architect would be to treat you as an instrument for social welfare. Kant maintains that persons are subjects and not instruments, and therefore they cannot be treated as a means to social welfare. For Kantians, women and men do not exist for society. They exist for themselves. Therefore, the individual person must be given the right to make her own choices, not because they will lead to what is best for the individual (individuals often do not exercise their rights wisely), but because denying individuals the right to make these choices reduces them to nonpersons.

John Stuart Mill and other nineteenth-century consequentialists agree with Kant that all choices need not be prudent and wise, but they have a different reason for asserting why we must respect the individual's choices. According to Mill, we must respect choices that may prove harmful to the very individuals who make them because this policy will have the best social results. For example, my friends may think it a mistake for me to invest all my savings in a pharmaceutical stock that has just been issued. They may speak against this investment. They may give me all manner of reasons that this investment will lead to my ruin. However, even if they have the best of intentions, provided that I am competent, they may not ethically coerce me or limit my choices in this context. The consequentialist argues that thousands of benefits to society have been secured in precisely these circumstances. Free choices that seem harmful to the individual occasionally wind up being not only good for the individual but also for society as a whole.

Is mercy killing best for a particular person and society at large? Some consequentialist philosophers have argued that granting individuals the liberty to be euthanized is substantially different from allowing them to make risky investments. According to these philosophers, social harm will result if we permit active euthanasia. Unlike thinkers influenced by religious traditions who believe that mercy killing is alien to God's will because it robs God of the power to end life, these consequentialist thinkers maintain that social harm or, perhaps, social chaos will result from permitting active euthanasia.

Susan Wolf, who was an associate for law at the Hastings Center, has argued that a terrible judicial result would occur if legislatures or voters permitted active euthanasia.[5] Courts would immediately begin reexamining their willingness to allow passive euthanasia. According to Wolf, courts have generally given physicians and families wide latitude in allowing patients to die without court interference. However, if legislatures began experimenting with active euthanasia, courts would quickly rescind their former consent and begin interfering with passive euthanasia cases on the ground that passive euthanasia may conflict with a compelling state interest.

Another critic of active euthanasia, Leon Kass, has also argued that the right to be assisted in suicide or the right to be actively euthanized is a myth.[6] One of his main arguments involves potential consequences. One might be tempted to allow competent persons to authorize others to kill them or to assist in their suicide, but because there are such difficulties associated with distinguishing competent from incompetent persons, especially at the end of life, this temptation ought to be resisted. Active euthanasia and assisted-suicide policies could quickly become the tools of ill-intentioned, cost-conscious families or hospital administrators to dispatch unconsenting patients from this life.

But the philosopher H. Tristram Englehardt criticizes such consequentialist approaches to active euthanasia.[7] He employs a set of neo-Kantian ideas to counter the suggestion that we justify using state authority to either coerce or forbid individuals to secure assistance in suicide or active euthanasia. Englehardt emphasizes that many of the ethical principles established in the eighteenth and nineteenth centuries have fallen into disrepute. Among these are the consequentialist concepts that it is better to allow people to suffer than to permit active euthanasia. Englehardt argues that prior to the eighteenth-century movement called the Enlightenment, states employed religious conviction as a basis for social prohibitions. Active euthanasia was forbidden by the state because it was abhorred by God. With the coming of the Enlightenment and the idea that reason could rule human affairs, it was argued that active euthanasia was forbidden because it would produce harmful social results. One could coerce people to prevent them from euthanizing themselves because one could presumably prove that, although euthanasia might benefit the individual, the general practice of euthanasia would be socially harmful.

But Englehardt argues that this consequentialist strategy assumes that one can secure agreement on the idea that allowing an individual to suffer is better than euthanizing him. This is what he calls a "thick vision of the good." A thick vision of the good leads to priorities among goods and evils. For Englehardt, agreement on these priorities was possible in the nineteenth century, but in our profoundly pluralistic culture such agreement is no longer possible.

Despite the difficulties, Englehardt argues that a thin moral project is still possible. He calls this a quasi-Kantian program, in which individuals agree to resolve conflicts without resorting to violence in order to create a public life. All that is required is mutual respect and a commitment to avoid "using others without their consent."[8] He argues that in the absence of a shared thick vision of the good, one cannot coercively prevent others from establishing suicide or euthanasia agreements. To do so would involve using the public power of the state to endorse a particular private, thick vision of the good. This may have been politically possible prior to the Enlightenment as a result of religion's influence over the state, but in the twentieth century this shared, thick vision of the good is absent. For Engelhardt, we must accept active euthanasia "by default" as a consequence of our general commitment to avoid using persons.

Engelhardt expresses in philosophical terminology a sentiment shared by many people that the laws against active euthanasia unethically coerce:

1. individuals who do not think great social harm will follow from legalization of euthanasia.
2. individuals who are not religious.
3 individuals who believe in a God who does not punish.
4. individuals who believe in a God who has not necessarily outlawed mercy killing.

According to many supporters of active euthanasia, the current laws against active euthanasia coerce the individual to adopt an ethical view that he has not freely chosen for himself. In doing so, current law transforms the individual into an object that cannot act freely according to the dictates of his own conscience. In effect, the law imposes on everyone the ethical views of religious traditions within the society without proving that these laws are necessary for public welfare. To require the patient to suffer against her wishes involves determining what the course of her life should be. According to proponents of active euthanasia, this is a violation of the principle of autonomy.

It is clear that the major reason for opposition is that there is a compelling state interest to limit the individual's right of autonomy to be actively euthanized. Our policy on forgoing life-sustaining services was largely based on the principle of autonomy. In that context there did not seem to be a compelling state interest in preventing people from refusing care. Autonomy seemed to place in the hands of the individual a great deal of authority to refuse treatment, even if it was life-prolonging. But refusing treatment does not involve direct killing. This distinction makes all the difference.

Let us turn to an obvious case of restricting freedom in order to get a clearer picture of what is involved in the appeal to the notion of a compelling state interest as a basis for limiting individual rights. In 1950, if one owned property on the shore of Lake Erie and wished to use that property as a dump site for toxic chemicals, one would have had the right to do so with minimal restrictions. In short, one had a largely unrestricted liberty. At the time, few perceived that there was a compelling state interest to limit this right. Today, of course, there are very serious restrictions on the right to dump toxic wastes in Lake Erie, but that is because evidence was offered that dumping toxic wastes was inconsistent with a compelling state interest.

It is instructive to note that the right to dispose of toxic wastes was restricted *after* evidence was presented to indicate that social harm resulted from unregulated disposal. Evidence of harm was necessary in order to undermine the right to use one's property as a dump site. The fear that the dumping might lead to harm was not enough to restrict the right to dump. This policy of requiring evidence of social harm before an individual right is limited is based on the Western suspicion of the power of the state. Large and powerful states have often used social fears to undermine the rights of the individual. States are likely to use that power unless we place on the state the burden of establishing that restricting a right is necessary in order to achieve a compelling state interest. The rule then is that when restricting an individual's right or liberty, one must offer evidence that the exercise of the liberty would in fact undermine public welfare. It is not enough to establish that granting a right *may* undermine public welfare. Supporters of active euthanasia argue that this rule of evidence is being violated in the issue of active euthanasia. The state fears that permitting active euthanasia *may* undermine the safety of weak, vulnerable, poor, or socially disliked citizens. If this resulted from legitimizing active euthanasia, then surely it would be unethical to do so. However, the fear that something bad will happen if we allow active euthanasia is different from evidence that something bad has happened.

Opponents of active euthanasia disagree with this interpretation. They argue that the burden of proof is not necessarily borne by those who wish to limit liberties. Rather, the burden of proof is on those who wish to change the law. Environmentalists had to prove that indiscriminate dumping was harmful to the society. They were demanding a change, so they had to prove that the change was necessary. Replacing the current law that opposes active euthanasia with one that permits it is a change in the law; thus, the burden of proof rests on those who desire change. Proponents must prove that active euthanasia will not undermine the safety of those who lack power in society.

This issue of who bears the burden of proof is an important one because evidence about the social consequences of active euthanasia is hard to come by. How much suffering would actually be avoided by those who would exercise the right if they had it? How many individuals would be unjustly killed if we permitted active euthanasia? These questions are difficult to answer because active euthanasia is currently illegal. Therefore, it is impossible to perform clinical experiments, and without some basis for comparison, it is hard to justify one's beliefs.

## The Slippery Slope and Active Euthanasia

Considerations concerning compelling state interests take us to our third question surrounding the active euthanasia debate. Philosophers call this "the slippery slope argument." This argument suggests that once we take our first step out onto a slippery slope, a terrible result will shortly follow. If we start killing terminally ill people, we will inevitably start killing healthy but burdensome people. Critics of active euthanasia argue that once we permit patient-requested medical killing for mercy, we will not be able to prevent a range of other killings such as medical killing of the incompetent. This is the compelling state interest that Western cultures have employed to reject mercy killing.

The aim in this section is to point out that there is not just one slippery slope argument. Philosophers and logicians have argued that there are at least three. More importantly, failure to distinguish among these closely related arguments can produce confusion among all participants in the debate. The first two analyses of the argument suggest that the argument is rationally accessible in the sense that it is possible to offer "reasons" for and against a particular slippery slope argument. The third version suggests that so-called slippery slope arguments are arguments in name only and that they are best viewed as rhetorical devices that can persuade people with certain attitudes to support one side of an issue rather than another.

The first interpretation of the slippery slope argument may be called the empirical analysis. It maintains that slippery slope arguments are empirical in nature. This empirical analysis is illustrated when opponents of active euthanasia use the Nazi case to illustrate that small beginnings with active euthanasia may generate a holocaust. The argument proceeds analogically by mentioning similarities between German society in 1933 and Western culture today. It aims to prove that the legalization of euthanasia in Germany led to terrible results by desensitizing the German people to the horrors that followed, i.e., the holocaust. Defenders of this reasoning conclude that the legalization of active euthanasia in our culture will similarly desensitize our people and lead to horrendous consequences.

In effect, the argument proceeds by providing some evidence that two societies or cultures (Germany of 1933 and the contemporary West) are empirically similar. Additional evidence is provided to show that legalization led to horrendous consequences in the first case (Germany) and, by virtue of the similarities between the two cultures, is likely to lead to similar horrendous consequences in the second (contemporary Western societies). Proponents maintain that we need not assume that a specifically Jewish holocaust will result, but that active euthanasia will lead to an assault on one or more vulnerable subgroups within society. We may discriminate against the elderly who consume so much of our limited health care budget. Or perhaps we will not assault the elderly but we will target racial minorities that white Westerners have negative attitudes toward. The empirical version of the slippery slope argument claims that we are not that different from the Germans of 1933 and that allowing active euthanasia puts everyone at increased risk because tomorrow any one of us may belong to a socially despised group.

If we view slippery slope arguments as empirical and analogical, then we must be ready to submit them to empirical verification. This means that we must be able to deliver a solid inductive or scientifically sound argument that the terrible result will actually follow. Are the similarities between the two cultures *sufficient* to establish the probability that horrendous consequences will follow from legalization? Although there is little doubt that some significant similarities exist between Germany of 1933 and contemporary Western culture, there are significant dissimilarities as well. If the similarities increase the probability of the dire conclusion, then the dissimilarities decrease it. To determine the probability, we must assign weights to similarities and dissimilarities and then, by comparison, base the probability on the relative weights. But meeting this requirement is very difficult. How does one assign a numerical weight to the cultural and political similarities between Germany of 1933 and America of 1996? Or to the dissimilarities? This seems to be a case of attempting to quantify what is not a quantity. Because of these difficulties historians seldom make predictions.

But perhaps the empirical interpretation of the slippery slope argument is misguided. There is another interpretation of the argument, called the *logical interpretation*, which disregards the empirical and quantitative considerations and turns to matters of definition. A definition of unjust killing is presented, then it is shown that killing even consenting patients for reasons of compassion violates this definition. For example, if we suppose that unjust killing always involves intentionally and directly killing the innocent, and if intentionally and directly killing terminally and irreversibly ill people who are suffering is killing the innocent, then we have crossed the line into unjust killing. Actively killing a willing patient crosses a semantic or definitional barrier. Once this semantic barrier is crossed, the moral argument for active euthanasia is undermined.

This type of slippery slope argument does not concern itself with predictions, probabilities, analogies, facts, causes, or comparing cases with contrasting similarities and dissimilarities. No empirical claim is made. The question is reduced to whether or not the rule "Do not directly and intentionally kill the innocent" is a social rule that is being violated by active euthanasia. Supporters of the conceptual version of the slippery slope argument claim that once we accept that the above rule is violated, the unethical character of active euthanasia follows. No other information is needed. Direct and intentional killing of the innocent is wrong; therefore, active euthanasia is wrong.

The difficulty with this version is, while it is fairly obvious that most instances of direct and intentional killing of the innocent are wrong, it is not so clear that *all* instances of killing the innocent are wrong. Surely the German or Japanese children who were killed by Allied bombing during World War II were innocent. Furthermore, it looks as if these children were directly killed by the bombs dropped in Allied air raids. Furthermore, these killings seem to have been intentional. Since it is difficult to hold that two-year-old children were responsible for the war, it seems that they were indeed innocent. But if they were innocent and if they were intentionally killed, and if we accept the premise that killing the innocent is always wrong, then it was surely wrong to bomb those cities, since bombing involves the direct and intentional killing of the innocent.

This conclusion, however, is not universally obvious. It was surely horribly unfortunate that these innocent children were killed and maimed, but do we want to hold the fliers of the bombers responsible for murder? Some people may want to go this far, but it is not obvious to everyone that these fliers were murderers. What we must draw from this case is that one can doubt that all instances of intentional killing of the innocent are wrong. Innocence is surely an important aspect of unjust killing. It may even be a necessary condition of unjust killing. But innocence by itself is not considered sufficient to make a killing unjust. The argument may therefore be criticized for mistaking a necessary for a sufficient condition for unjust killing.

The empirical and logical interpretations of the argument both suffer from significant weaknesses, which suggests that there is a hidden source behind the attractiveness of the slippery slope argument. This is the third interpretation of the argument. In this third view, slippery slope arguments are pictured as having rhetorical force behind them rather than having the force of reason. Slippery slope considerations often reinforce belief without justifying it. In effect, this view treats slippery slope arguments as apparent, rather than real, arguments.

The distinction between causing and justifying a belief is a complex one. It is a distinction that is vital but difficult to generalize. For example, it is clear that parents and peers have enormous power to cause children to believe things. But merely because they have power to cause belief does not mean they have power to justify the belief. Many of us remember discovering that Santa Claus did not exist. This simple example illustrates that we were caused to believe something that we later discovered was not true.

Another example can be drawn from the world of advertising. It is clear that an advertiser can cause me to believe that buying a flashy red sports car is in my interest by showing pictures of beautiful starlets standing next to the car. These advertisements can work. But are they *reasons* for believing that buying the car is in my interest? Probably not! Not all advertisements function in this way, of course. Many advertisements inform and justify belief, but a good many do little but cause, or at least influence, belief and behavior. In short, advertisements, especially those that are artistically powerful, can cause belief without justifying belief.

This third interpretation suggests that some slippery slope arguments are rhetorical devices that, when crafted with subtlety and depth, can reinforce or perhaps even change a person's attitudes. Supporters of active euthanasia, for example, are horrified when pictures of the holocaust are presented. Associating the holocaust with active euthanasia can be an enormously effective strategy for controlling belief. These events in the history of Western culture are so real and so heinous that once we associate active euthanasia with the holocaust in the minds of men and women, there is little doubt that they will resist the legalization of active euthanasia. But such associations are rhetorical rather than rational. These associations cannot be considered rational until solid causal or inductive evidence is presented that legalization will actually lead to the terrible consequence.

This third interpretation of the argument is neutral in that proponents and opponents of any issue can use slippery slope considerations to cause, reinforce, or change belief. Slippery slope considerations can function by attempting to associate a belief with something either positive or negative in the minds of the listener. The reader is cautioned not to reject all slippery slope arguments out of hand but rather to become aware that they can and do influence one's moral and ethical attitudes. In effect, this view recommends that we interpret the arguments as having significant causal influence on beliefs, attitudes, and behaviors without necessarily having rational significance. These slippery slope considerations gain rational value only when they can be replaced by plausible causal or inductive arguments.

## Holland and Active Euthanasia

Let us now turn to the issue of whether there is any evidence that active euthanasia will not produce terrible consequences. Proponents of active euthanasia can appeal to a test case that is currently taking place in the Netherlands. There, at this time, active euthanasia is legal. Furthermore, it is a widely practiced activity that is protected by legal precedents and public opinion that favors it. It is estimated that 2,000 people per year are actively euthanized. The Dutch Medical Association and a government-appointed commission developed stringent guidelines for the initiation of euthanasia; the aim of these guidelines was to prevent the slippery slope. These guidelines are "steps" that prevent the Dutch from sliding down the slope.

The first of these restrictions or guidelines is that no patient who is incompetent may be actively euthanized. Since vast numbers of dying people are comatose or otherwise rendered unconscious, this is a very strong requirement because it clearly rules out the possibility of writing an advance directive that would authorize a guardian or surrogate to initiate active euthanasia on an incompetent patient. For example, end-stage victims of Alzheimer's disease or persons in persistent vegetative states cannot be euthanized because they are incompetent. The reason for this is that the Dutch wish to establish a barrier against guardians' attempts to free themselves of the responsibilities and burdens of caring for incompetent patients. For the Dutch, this is the step that will prevent them from sliding down the slippery slope. This very restrictive stipulation obviously separates active from passive euthanasia. However, the Dutch believe that this restriction is necessary if assaults against the weak are to be prevented and respect for individuality preserved.

The second condition is that the patient must freely request numerous times to be actively euthanized. The request must be voluntary and consistently made. This prevents impulsive or ill-considered requests from being taken as an adequate basis for action.

These first two conditions effectively prohibit guardians from playing any role in initiating active euthanasia. They also seem to indicate that advance directives can play no role in the process. These are limitations of the Dutch system that many American supporters of active euthanasia have opposed, but the Dutch Medical Association maintains that they are required in order to protect the rights of the ill. One does not need to have a negative attitude toward human nature to accept the idea that guardians might be tempted to abandon their responsibilities to the old and the infirm by employing active euthanasia. To legalize active euthanasia might motivate and encourage guardians to act in their own interest and not in the best interests of the patient. The Dutch system is explicitly designed to avoid this possibility. It does so by taking the radical step of excluding guardians and advance directives from any role in the process.

The third requirement is that the patient be suffering from an incurable disease and intolerable pain for which there is no possible remedy or relief. It is very important to notice, however, that the guidelines do not require that the patient be suffering from a terminal and irreversible disease that will imminently lead to death. No time limit is specified. The certifying physician doesn't have to affirm that the patient will die within three or six months. This prevents the Dutch physician from actively euthanizing anyone who has a treatable disease, but allows the physician to actively euthanize individuals who have untreatable diseases that are profoundly painful but not terminal.

The fourth guideline is that euthanasia be performed only after the case has been reviewed by a second physician who has confirmed that the first three guidelines have been satisfied. The method used involves the use of a barbiturate to put the patient to sleep. When the patient is fully unconscious, a lethal dose of curare is injected.

These restrictions do not, of course, guarantee that harms will not result from the legalization of active euthanasia. The only protection against abuse is constant vigilance. However, supporters say that arguments against the early use of passive euthanasia took the same form as the current arguments against active euthanasia. Fears that harm would result from the use of passive euthanasia were realistic since we did not have much experience with technologies that could extend the life of the dying person. Many argued that if we did not do everything to extend the life of the dying patient, then blatant discrimination against socially disliked individuals would be inevitable. At this point there are no indications that permitting passive euthanasia has brought about any widespread, terrible consequences. Proponents argue, in effect, that just as we have responsibly used passive euthanasia without violating any human rights, so too we can responsibly employ active euthanasia without violating human rights in the future.

The Dutch government has recently completed an extensive study of active euthanasia within the Netherlands.[9] This investigation was by no means an exhaustive or complete study of Dutch euthanasia, so the results obviously cannot be accepted without qualification. However, the study does provide some evidence that Dutch provisions and restrictions regarding active euthanasia are not leading to widespread abuse. We can summarize the results in the following way. Of the deaths taking place in one year, 35 percent involved a nontreatment decision. Passive euthanasia, or letting a patient die, is still the most practiced form of euthanasia. Some of these deaths involved the use of pain-relieving narcotics that may have hastened the dying process. Only 1.8 percent of the deaths that occurred in Holland during a one-year period were associated with active euthanasia, and only 0.3 percent were physician-assisted suicide. Approximately 1,900 deaths were associated with active euthanasia or physician-assisted suicide. These cases of active euthanasia and physician-assisted suicide were carefully studied, and in only 0.8 percent of the cases was one of the above restrictions violated. Thus, in 152 deaths some violation occurred.

What were these violations? More than half involved incompetent patients who had professed to their physicians that they wanted to be actively euthanized but who lapsed into incompetence before the procedure could be initiated. The remaining cases were associated with unbearable pain and the double effect of narcotic use among the terminally ill. However, this last group of cases that violated the rules is still ethically troublesome. For this reason, it is wise to withhold any final assessment of the Dutch experiment with active euthanasia until more detailed and comprehensive data become available. However, one can say that this study does indicate with some reliability that the Dutch restrictions are being followed in the vast majority of instances and that these restrictions form solid steps that prevent the Dutch from sliding down the slippery slope.[10]

## Euthanasia and the Patient-Doctor Relationship

Let us now turn to the fourth question that provides important background to the euthanasia debate. The patient-doctor relationship is one that is traditionally marked by trust and caring. Opponents of active euthanasia argue that this trusting relationship is threatened by legalization because the weak and vulnerable patient with a possibly terminal illness will not seek medical help if the medical helper is legally entitled to kill him. Who would go for help to someone who was legally permitted to kill those who seek help? The legalization proposal thus undermines the trust that is assumed to exist between the patient and the health care professional.

This argument is deliberately phrased in a way that disregards the absolute necessity for the patient to initiate and autonomously consent to euthanasia. Proponents of active euthanasia may consider it an unfair question, but it seems eminently possible that despite every effort to inform patients that physicians cannot medically kill without the patient's authorization and without the presence of a terminally ill and irreversibly painful illness, many patients will not get that message. For these patients, legalization will provide another barrier for them in seeking help. The context of this concern is what may be called the self-image of the medical profession as well as the self-image of individual physicians and other health care providers. What does it mean for physicians or health care professionals (such as nurses or physical therapists) if they became known as "medical killers"? Notice that this has nothing to do with whether great evils will result or whether the autonomy of individuals is being respected or violated. It has to do with public relations. By saying this I do not mean to cast aspersions on the profession. A profession unconcerned with its self-image or the public's image of it is hardly worth the title "profession." One's image is the set of expectations that a client brings into the office. These expectations can profoundly affect the quality of care provided. But if the patient's expectations are at least partially influenced by a fear that the physician may kill them, then legalization may be more harmful than beneficial.

These concerns suggest that if active euthanasia were legalized, it should be administered by a social mechanism that is completely separate from health care providers. For example, just as funeral directors are distinct from physicians, it may be best to establish a new institution for euthanasia that is as separate from medicine as funeral homes are. There is good reason for keeping the two institutions separate, just as there is good reason for keeping the physician separate from the mortician. Those who perform euthanasia need not be physicians or health care providers. They should function on sites separate from medical sites that are constructed so as to provide no incentive to commit active euthanasia. Medical verification for the terminal and irreversible nature of a patient's disease should be provided by third-party physicians, but in no way should the physicians or any other health care provider be actively involved in the process of active euthanasia.

### Physician-Assisted Suicide

Finally, no discussion of active euthanasia would be complete without a more thorough discussion of doctor-assisted suicide. And no discussion of this topic would be complete without some reference to the activities of Dr. Jack Kevorkian, whose license to practice medicine in Michigan was revoked because he assisted over 30 people to commit suicide.

On February 15, 1993, Michigan passed a law prohibiting anyone with knowledge that another person is going to commit suicide from "intentionally providing the means" or intentionally participating in the physical act by which the patient commits suicide. Assisted suicide occurs when a physician facilitates a patient's death by providing the necessary means and/or information to enable the patient to end his or her life. For example, the physician provides sleeping pills and information about the lethal dose while aware of the patient's intent.[11] In these cases, doctors do not withhold or withdraw life-sustaining treatment (passive euthanasia) nor do they directly inject lethal poisons into patients who voluntarily request that they be euthanized (active euthanasia). Instead the doctor provides assistance (usually information and prescriptions or other means) to a competent and physically capacitated individual. This difference has suggested to some that assisted suicide may be an effective compromise between supporters and critics of active euthanasia. Physician-assisted suicide is aid in dying, but it appears to some physicians and philosophers that it is less than direct killing by doctors.

Another physician who has engaged in assisted suicide is Dr. Timothy Quill. In a well-known article in *The New England Journal of Medicine,* Dr. Quill openly informed the public that he had prescribed barbiturates as well as provided suicide information to at least one terminally ill, competent patient who requested this assistance. Upon reading this article, the prosecutor of Rochester, New York, brought Dr. Quill before the grand jury, which reviewed the case for possible indictment. The grand jury did not indict Dr. Quill. This decision is not atypical. Indeed H. L. Glantz argues that there are no instances when a physician has been convicted of prescribing medications that could assist a patient to commit suicide.[12] However, the fact that such laws against assisted suicide remain on the books in many states constitutes a genuine deterrent to physicians who are ethically sympathetic to assisted suicide.

Derek Humphry's *Final Exit* was a national best-seller that amounts to a "how to" book on how to commit suicide. Finally, *The New England Journal of Medicine* recently published an article entitled "Care of the Hopelessly Ill: Potential Clinical Criteria for Physician Assisted Suicide" by doctors Christine Cassel, Diane Meier, and Timothy Quill.[13] In this essay they lay out the following seven criteria, which they consider to be sound ethical guidelines for regulating physician-assisted suicide. We may summarize these criteria as follows:

1. The decision must be a voluntary one that the patient repeatedly initiates.
2. The patient must be competent and capacitated.
3. The patient must be suffering from an incurable disease.
4. The physician must know that the patient is not suffering from inadequate comfort care.
5. There must be a meaningful relationship between the doctor and the patient.
6. Second opinions are necessary prior to assistance in suicide.
7. Clear documentation that the above criteria have been satisfied is both prudent and ethically mandatory.

We cannot at this point comment on the multiple ethical issues raised by Quill, Cassel, and Meier's suggestions. However, it is vital to note that these approaches to the care of the terminally ill are not, in their opinion, straightforward active euthanasia. Assisting in suicide is ethically problematic, but it does not draw the physician into direct and intentional killing in the way that active euthanasia does.

## The Case of Debbie II[14]

A 20-year-old woman whom we will call Debbie II is dying in Room 402 of Community Hospital from ovarian cancer. She is in a great deal of pain. She is emaciated and weighs about 90 pounds. An IV line has been inserted. She is receiving nasal oxygen but is still suffering from air hunger. She has not eaten or slept in two days. She makes a request of the resident who has been caring for her for the past week. She asks, "Can we get this over with?" The resident then asks her to be more explicit. She says that she wants to die and that she would like the resident "to give her a lot of morphine" because she knows that will bring a permanent end to her suffering. Her parents are in the room with her, and both of them tell the resident that they want her request to be honored. The resident says that he understands her request but such an action is not permitted by medical practice. He does, however, tell her that he would be willing to call an emergency meeting of the hospital's ethics committee so that it can discuss this matter at length. She agrees and closes their conversation with, "If you could feel the pain that I feel, if you knew the depth of my depression, the sense of utter hopelessness that I feel, you would honor my request no matter what the committee says."

## Committee Discussion of the Case

| | |
|---|---|
| Dr. Mary Collins: (Chair) | A resident, Dr. Thomas Henderson, called me this morning and reported that a patient had requested that he actively euthanize her. I have given you a report of the case that was prepared by Dr. Henderson, and I would like to initiate discussion of the case. Why don't we begin as we usually do by getting our questions on the table? I asked Dr. Eric Warren, our staff oncologist, to do a medical review of the case and assist Dr. Henderson in answering your questions. |
| Atty. John Quinn: | Given the position stated within our policy, these questions are really unnecessary. The euthanasia policy of the hospital, to say nothing of the present law in our state, makes granting this request impossible. It is an open-and-shut case. I do not see why you called this meeting, Dr. Collins. |
| Dr. Collins: | I am perfectly aware of the hospital policy and the law. Perhaps the conclusion is one that is forgone, but this woman is dying and her situation is something that we have to face in order to appreciate the impact and significance of both the law and the policy. |
| Rev. Richard Marcus: | I agree with Dr. Collins. I think that it is very easy to pass policies and laws and to view the problem from a great distance, but I think we need to get "up close" and see the impact of a policy decision in order to understand it. It is one thing to pass a policy and something very different to examine how it affects patient care. Allow me to make an analogy. Pilots who drop bombs on cities never feel, see, or hear the effects. They never see the children or the ordinary people suffer because they are so distant from the effects of their actions. I think as health care providers and policy |

makers we had better acquire "hands-on" knowledge of the consequences of our policy actions.

Vivian Harris:

I have four questions. Just how sick is this woman? Is she terminal and irreversible? And what is her level of discomfort? Finally, as her physician, have you discussed assisted suicide with her?

Dr. Collins:

I can see that Dr. Warren is anxious to answer Vivian's question, but our protocol, Dr. Warren, is to put all the relevant questions on the table prior to responding to them. Prof. Thomas wanted to raise some concerns.

Prof. Carla Thomas:

Yes. I think we need to know something about this woman's competence at the time of her request, since, if the request was based on incompetent judgment, it would not qualify as even possibly legitimate. Also, what about the family? In the case report it is said that they want her request to be honored. Do they fully understand what they are asking?

Dr. Philip Davis:

I have not heard from Dr. Warren yet, but I would bet that he has altered her medication to reduce the pain and depression. What impact will this have in terms of reducing her expected life span? Also, what is the treatment plan if she should develop any other life-threatening diseases, for example, pneumonia?

Mary Quigley:

Has this woman been fully informed concerning the nature of her disease, its prognosis, and the treatment plan that has been adopted? Does she understand that she can be deeply medicated to prevent this discomfort? In short, does she understand that there are alternatives open to her? Finally, our policy admits a distinction between active euthanasia and assisted suicide. Does that recognition come into play here?

Atty. Quinn:

Allow me to step in here. Our policy does recognize an ethical distinction between these activities. But I interpret that principle as a theoretical idea without practical import. The law considers active euthanasia illegal, and physician-assisted suicide is also very close to being illegal. I have no problem discussing the differences from a theoretical or philosophical viewpoint, but I want to caution everyone that endorsing the active killing of this woman would place the institution at significant legal risk. Furthermore, the whole issue of assisting her suicide is a legal nightmare. I know we make some statements in principle 9 of the policy, but I would caution us that entering the domain of physician-assisted suicide is legally and ethically treacherous.

Dr. Collins:

Atty. Quinn has done his job by informing us of the law. We thank you, John. If there are no other questions, I will ask Dr. Warren to provide us with some responses to the relevant questions.

Dr. Warren:

The patient was informed of the nature and prognosis of the disease by her attending physician over four months ago. I reviewed her disease and there is no doubt that she has ovarian cancer and that her disease is fatal. It is a terminal and irreversible cancer. Her death is also relatively imminent, and I would guess that a month would be the limit of her life expectancy. In my conversations with her I found that she was very well informed about her disease and that she understands her medical situation quite well. With respect to her competence: although I am not a psychiatrist, I had no indication of irrationality or mental illness. She is depressed and I have treated that depression, but this kind of depression is very often associated with this disease process. In fact, I would call it realistic depression. I have treated her for this depression, and I have managed to alleviate some of it. The depression medication that I have given her might, in a court of law, count as mind-altering, and therefore, this might compromise my belief that she is fully competent, but despite this legal consideration, I have no doubt that she is fully competent.

Regarding the comfort treatment: I have placed her on a morphine regimen that has been quite effective in managing the severe pain. The regimen will increase over time and it may well slightly hasten her death, but I cannot prove that it will. I have recommended to her that she return to her home and that she be cared for by the local hospice nursing team. They can visit her on a regular basis and educate the family on caring for her.

She is a very persistent person regarding active euthanasia. She admits that her pain is decreased, but she is still very uncomfortable and believes that it is needless and pointless pain. She has asked me on two occasions to give her a lethal dose of morphine and I have refused. She has also asked me to assist her in committing suicide, and I am very troubled by the request. I see her point, but this would be very difficult for me. I simply do not know what to do about this request. I have spoken to her about the possibility that these requests are derived from the depression that she feels, but she insists that it is based on strong feelings that she has had all her life. Her parents have verified that she has always held that a person had the right to be actively euthanized if she were terminally and irreversibly ill. One of her main complaints is that she is being forced to stay alive and suffer by a society that is very influenced by a Judeo-Christian ethic that prohibits euthanasia. She insists that she sees nothing immoral or unethical about it and that she is being coerced to suffer because the religious prohibitions against euthanasia have been written into the law. She said that it is wrong to transform religious preferences into legal obligations. I am not well versed in ethics and so I had a difficult time responding. I spent most of the time listening.

Prof. Martin Fisk:    I think that, given the present policy of the hospital and the present law, we are offering her the only solution that lies within our power. To actively euthanize this woman would force us into the position of committing civil disobedience, and although as individuals we may support changes in the law, few of us want to endorse the idea that the hospital as an institution should violate the law. Given these circumstances, hospice and an aggressive plan of palliation is her best option and the only thing that we can offer her. The value of this case, as far as I am concerned, is that it does illustrate how the law and the policy of our hospital may be in conflict with the patient's autonomy, her moral intuitions, and her medical welfare. I might add that the law is at odds with my moral intuitions as well. I have absolutely no doubt that if this woman were receiving treatment in the Netherlands, then her request would be honored. The Dutch respect the woman's right to be euthanized, and it is a scandal, in my opinion, that we will sit by and let this woman needlessly suffer against her will. However, the law is clear and the policy of the hospital is clear, and I do not think it is appropriate for us to violate these rules.

Atty. Quinn:

Martin's view of this case is certainly not mine. I think that what is happening to this woman is very unfortunate. But I do not see that physicians, therefore, have the obligation to medically kill her merely because she requests it. Nor do physicians, in my opinion, have the right to perform medical murder. Finally, in the light of this, I think that her competence and her understanding are irrelevant because, even if they were present, we still could not honor her request.

But there is a much more important issue that is present in cases involving active euthanasia. Currently, courts across the nation have been more than liberal in extending to patients, hospitals, and physicians extraordinary control within the area of passive euthanasia. They have granted to physicians the right to withdraw and withhold services from consenting patients who are terminal and irreversible. In some cases they have granted to guardians the right to withdraw life-sustaining treatment even from patients who are not terminal and irreversible. Nancy Cruzan was not terminally ill even though she was in a persistent vegetative state. There is, in short, wide discretion granted to patients and their guardians in the domain of passive euthanasia. But if hospitals or physicians were to cross the barrier that divides active from passive euthanasia, then I believe that courts would be far less willing to trust families and physicians to engage in passive euthanasia.

Prof. Fisk:

Dr. Warren, let me change the topic slightly. Suppose Debbie develops a treatable pneumonia. Are you going to treat it?

Dr. Warren:

I might make some changes in her palliative treatment to accommodate the infection. Air hunger is a very painful experience. But

I will not try to cure the infection unless curing it is directly related to her palliative plan. I believe that this is her wish. It's an overused expression, but there is a good deal of truth to the old saying that pneumonia can be a person's best friend.

Prof. Fisk: In other words, you would be very happy to see the infection develop and grow and kill her quickly.

Dr. Warren: "Happy" is the wrong word to describe my feelings. This is a tragic situation that could never make anyone happy, but I would be relieved and thankful that she developed the infection and I would do nothing to fight the infection, unless she changed her mind.

Prof. Fisk: You might even increase her morphine, which might further reduce her respiration reflex and thus lead to an increase in her carbon dioxide levels, and that might directly lead to her death.

Dr. Warren: I would have no problem increasing those morphine levels, even if they led to this consequence. My job is to comfort this woman. I have given up hope of curing or saving her.

Prof. Fisk: Wouldn't you say, Dr. Warren, that this action of increasing these morphine levels would directly lead to her death, and thereby violate the injunction against actions that directly lead to death?

Dr. Warren: I see your point. Society allows physicians to perform this kind of medical killing but it forbids other kinds of medical killing. This seems inconsistent.

Atty. Quinn: Slow down a minute. You are giving Fisk more than you have to.

Dr. Warren: Atty. Quinn, I am not trying to win a debate. I am trying my best to be honest.

| | |
|---|---|
| Atty. Quinn: | I understand, Dr. Warren, that your actions may seem inconsistent, but they are not. There is a double effect associated with pneumonia. The morphine reduces pain, but it can also decrease respiration. The intent in using the morphine is to reduce pain, not to decrease the respiration. As long as the intent is clear, then we do not have murder. |
| Prof. Fisk: | What is your intent, Dr. Warren, in using the morphine in this case? |
| Dr. Warren: | I have done this on many occasions, and I have been trained to say that my intent is to reduce the pain and not to inhibit the respiration reflex. But I am very relieved to be able to use the morphine and to free a person from so much suffering. What I have got is a defense for what I am doing— but I know what I am doing. The two intentions are distinct, but they are also so closely connected that it is hard for me to separate them. To separate them seems so abstract. |
| Prof. Thomas: | I think that Dr. Warren is legitimately skeptical of the principle of the double effect, and, when you see the elements of the principle, I think that you will understand his skepticism. Basically, the principle asserts that it is sometimes ethically permissible to perform an action that has both a good result and a bad result. The good result is treated as both intended and foreseen, but the bad result is treated as something that is foreseen but not intended. Supporters of the principle, such as Attorney Quinn, argue that such double effect actions are permitted under the following four conditions:<br><br>**First:** The action that is performed is not bad in itself. In our case, the administration of morphine is not in itself evil. |

**Second:** The agent only intends the good result. In our case the sedation is intended and the hastened death is unintended.

**Third:** The evil effect is not the means by which the good effect is achieved. In our case the death is not the means to relieve the pain.

**Fourth:** The good result outweighs the bad result. Palliation is worth the price of shortening the life.

Attorney Quinn, is this a fair representation of the principle?

Atty. Quinn:  It is a bit brief, but it does capture the idea.

Prof. Thomas:  There are a number of problems with this distinction. For example, what counts as an action that is bad in itself? Is giving someone an amount of morphine sufficient to hasten their death bad in itself? It seems to me that there is no clear way to determine what is bad in itself. In other words, there is no clear definition of this idea and so it is best to drop the very idea of "wrong in itself." If we had a list of the actions that are bad in themselves, condition one might be useful, but without a clear list, the rule seems useless. Secondly, what is an intended action? Is it an action that is desired or wanted? If that is the definition of being intended, then perhaps we need to ask Dr. Warren if he wants his patient to die. I know what my answer is, but perhaps we can ask Dr. Warren.

Dr. Warren:  Death is the only thing that is going to put an end to this suffering at this time, and so I think I do want this woman to die. Especially given the fact that she obviously wants to die.

Prof. Thomas:  But if he wants it, then maybe he intends it. And if this is so, then maybe he is violating the second condition. Furthermore, we often remove terminally and irreversibly ill persons from ventilators, and this directly leads to their death. Their death seems to be the intended effect. But this does not make the removal of patients from ventilators immoral under all circumstances. This is certainly hard to believe. My point here is that distinguishing between intended and unintended actions is difficult at best and this principle of the double effect assumes that it is a simple distinction to negotiate. But this last assumption is clearly false. Finally, the last criticism that I would offer is that Dr. Warren has emphasized that death is this woman's only way out of her torment. The death seems to be the means by which the pain is brought to an end and, thus, principle 3 is being violated.

Ms. Quigley:     It seems to me that if we accept what Carla is saying we have a choice to make. We either have to condemn Dr. Warren for his palliative treatment, which seems really dumb to me, or we have to excuse Dr. Warren and drop the principle of the double effect.

Prof. Thomas:     That is correct. It seems to me far more reasonable to give up the principle of the double effect since Dr. Warren is obviously acting in an ethically correct way when he administers reasonable and adequate amounts of morphine.

Atty. Quinn:     Well, what are you going to replace the double effect rule with?

Rev. Marcus:     I agree with the criticisms of the double effect principle, and I think that we need to emphasize that the principle is tightly connected historically to religious notions of right and wrong. Traditional theologians have often tried to give us a clear picture of right or wrong by claiming that they know what God's will is. What God wills is what is wrong in itself! Many modern theologians, including myself, reject this notion and argue that God's will is harder to determine than the tradition has assumed. There is a personal or individual element that cannot be overlooked, and finding God's will cannot be reduced to a "cookbook" or catechism concerning the will of God. Things are more complicated than this.

Dr. Collins:

I would like to turn our attention to another aspect of this case. I am not sure that Rev. Marcus is right when he suggests that the law has a religious foundation. I believe that slippery slope considerations are at the foundation of the laws against active euthanasia. The potential consequences of permitting active euthanasia are what concerns most health care professionals and most citizens. What happened in Hitler's Third Reich terrifies me and I worry that if we were to permit this kind of active killing for medical reasons, then we would be opening the door to all sorts of frightening consequences. If we can kill the consenting terminally ill, then we might act against the unconsenting nonterminally ill patients who are burdensome for us.

Prof. Fisk:

This is an important matter because the central question is whether a society like ours could responsibly exercise the power to actively euthanize. I share these concerns and I believe that we need to consider very carefully what kinds of restrictions should be imposed on active euthanasia. For example, while I support a change in the law, I am not all that happy with the Dutch model. Two weaknesses that I see are that the Dutch allow physicians to do the active killing and they permit it for nonterminally ill patients who have chronic and profound pain. I have serious doubts about these cases. However, I think they are quite wise to exclude patients' guardians from exercising any role in the initiation of active euthanasia.

Atty. Quinn:

Martin, I do not understand how you can support this medical killing idea, given your consequentialist version of what makes an act right. The consequences of allowing this seem to me to be very profound and very dangerous. I simply do not trust other people to have the right to kill me.

Prof. Fisk:

Twenty years ago, John, I would have been with you, but since then we have taken some steps out onto the slippery slope by permitting many types of withholding and withdrawing of life-sustaining treatment. These kinds of behaviors were opposed by many who claimed that forgoing treatment would lead to terrible results. These fears were unfounded. Permitting withholding and withdrawal of life-sustaining services has not led to any of the widespread terrible consequences that we worried about 10 or 20 years ago. Furthermore, John, I have given up the notion that there is a significant moral difference between acting and omitting. I know that the law still accepts that there is a significant difference, but there is no philosophical basis for this conviction. The law, I think, is lagging behind the philosophy.

Atty. Quinn:

What led you to this change of mind, Martin?

Prof. Fisk:

Experience and philosophy! The experience here at the hospital with the way our forgoing policy is operating gives me every confidence that we could also manage a policy involving active euthanasia. There would certainly be problems, but I do not think that they would be any more difficult than the problems that we face in the context of withholding and withdrawing life-sustaining care.

The philosophical argument hails from a philosopher named James Rachels. He argued that there are cases of murdering someone by omission and that there is no moral difference between these murders by omission and acts in which we murder someone by commission. The example that he uses is gruesome, but it effectively makes the point. Suppose that two different people have every intention of murdering their young cousin in order to receive an inheritance. The first plans to drown the cousin while the child is taking his bath. As the vicious relative enters the bathroom with every intention of drowning his cousin, the boy slips and falls into the water. He receives a severe blow to the head that renders him unconscious. He dies as a result while the vicious cousin just looks on.

Rachels asks us to evaluate the vicious cousin's refusal to help. Is it an omission? Yes! Is his omission murder? Most of us would say, "Yes!" He had evil intent. The consequences of his omission were awful. And he could have easily prevented the boy from dying. Furthermore, Rachels asks whether this case of murder by omission is morally different from a case in which the cousin grabbed the child and forcibly drowned him. Rachels convinced me that there was no moral difference between the two cases and therefore that there was nothing fundamental about the omission/commission distinction.

But he argues that there would have to be a difference in the two cases if committing an action were to be morally more significant than omitting an action. Rachels convinced me that, since we cannot make the distinction in this case, we cannot make it in any case. I gradually came to the opinion that there was no intrinsic and ethically significant difference between committing and omitting and that, if we couldn't make good on this abstract difference, we could not justify our cultural assumption that committing was morally more significant than omitting. Without this cultural assumption I was unable to justify my simultaneous approval of passive euthanasia and disapproval of active euthanasia.

My inability to find a general difference that separated active from passive euthanasia really influenced my practical opinions on the matter.

This argument helped convince me, John, that if it is permissible to *passively* euthanize people under certain conditions, then it may be permissible to *actively* euthanize people under certain conditions. What do you think of this argument?

Atty. Quinn:

It's interesting, but I am not convinced. Merely because a philosopher can come up with a case in which there is no difference between acting and omitting, that does not mean that the practice of active euthanasia is permissible. The general practice of killing people on demand scares me, and it threatens the social fabric. If this is a limitation on individual freedom, then I am willing to live with this limitation. To believe in individual freedom is not the same as believing in unlimited individual freedom.

Dr. Davis:

May I turn to the Hitler analogy for a moment? I am a bit of a history buff. It is important to note that Hitler's regime perverted most of the principles of constitutional government. For example, most of us would admit that, for reasons of national

security, the president of the United States
does not always have to reveal military
secrets to the press. Democracies sometimes
allow military secrets to be kept from the
public. Hitler took this sensible rule and
perverted it by using it to justify all sorts of
immoral actions. I could give you many
examples like this drawn from the history
of the Third Reich. Merely because a rule
can be perverted by a powerful and vicious
government does not mean that the rule is
not a good one. Who among us would say
that generals must publish their war plans
in *The New York Times* before they can
execute them? And yet this limited rule
could be used by a monster like Hitler to
profoundly harm society.

Dr. Collins:    What is your point, Philip?

Dr. Davis:    My point is that, while I share your concerns, I do not think that we can continue to
base opposition to active euthanasia solely
on the Hitler analogy. I agree that he
perverted the idea of active euthanasia, but
he and his gangsters also polluted every
decent rule of democracy and if we objected
to these rules because they might be
polluted by a monster like Hitler, then we
would have to give up a lot of what we call
reasonable government. I want to emphasize that currently I am opposed to active
euthanasia, but I think we need more solid
evidence than mere possibility that an
active euthanasia law would lead to the
destruction of the burdensome.

Ms. Quigley:    I agree with Dr. Davis, and I recommend
that the committee oppose this woman's
request, but I think that we need to keep
our eyes and our minds open to what is
happening in Holland, where active
euthanasia has been legalized. We need to
see whether legalization leads to terrible

consequences. If it does, we need to continue and perhaps even increase our opposition. But if these terrible consequences do not follow, then perhaps we need to reconsider the issue. I think that this is the least that we can do for this woman.

Atty. Quinn:    But look, there is another matter that you have not yet discussed. Do physicians and other health care professionals really want to become known as killers? Would it benefit the medical profession's image to get involved in this practice? I think not. I think patients would become even more skeptical if health care professionals became involved in active euthanasia.

Ms. Quigley:    Is the image of the physician declining in Holland as a result of their involvement in active euthanasia?

Dr. Davis:    I do not know this, and I do not think any studies have been done on this matter.

Dr. Collins:    Are there any other matters that need to be discussed regarding this case? Our meeting has already gone over our scheduled time period, and I am anxious to entertain a motion regarding this request. Would someone consider presenting a motion?

Atty. Quinn:    Yes! I move that Dr. Warren inform the patient that the law of our country, the ethics of his profession, and the policy of the hospital forbid him to honor this request.

Ms. Harris:    I think that we should say a bit more than this to her. First, we need to assure her that we will not abandon her in her last weeks and that we will do everything we can to ease the pain and discomfort. I think we need to inform her about the hospice service and the possibility of going home to die. Frequently, getting out of this hospital and returning to the home environment can really help a patient. Finally, I think that we can tell her that we are going to continue to monitor the active euthanasia experiment that is taking place in the Netherlands to see whether it is possible to honor these requests without endangering society.

Atty. Quinn: These changes in my motion are completely acceptable to me. Dr. Warren, can you live with this motion or is there anything that you would like to add?

Dr. Warren: I suspect that I am going to have an extended conversation with Debbie, and so I might not raise the Netherlands issue if I think it would make her feel worse.

Atty. Quinn: Our recommendations, Dr. Warren, are always to be understood as advisory to you. The final say about the conversation that you have with Debbie is up to you and Debbie. We do not wish to interfere or manage or control the patient-doctor relationship.

Dr. Collins: Carla, do you wish to make a final comment on this resolution?

Prof. Thomas: As you know, I have no doubt that Debbie's request falls under the category of being an autonomous act that should not be restrained unless we can demonstrate that respecting it would unjustifiably harm other human beings. We have not met that standard, in my opinion, but obviously I have not succeeded in convincing you or society of that opinion. Women like Debbie, as well as thousands of other human beings, will continue to suffer needlessly until we change the law. So I will vote against this resolution and continue to press this committee and society as a whole to reconsider this matter.

Dr. Collins: Are there any other comments? If not, I will read the motion as I understand it:

*Committee Recommendations:*    Dr. Warren should inform the patient that the current law and ethics of the medical profession and the policy of the hospital forbid him to honor this request. Furthermore, he should assure her that he and the hospital will not abandon her in her last weeks. We will do everything that we can to ease her pain and discomfort. He will inform her about the hospice service and the possibility of going home to die. Finally, he should tell her that we are going to continue to monitor the active euthanasia experiment that is taking place in the Netherlands to see whether it is possible to honor these requests in the future without endangering society.

**The vote is eight in favor and one opposed.**

### Further Questions Concerning the Case and the Policy

1. What is the difference between refusing to give a lethal dose of morphine and giving a dose of morphine that will relieve Debbie's pain but inhibit her respiration sufficiently to kill her?
2. Did the committee adequately address the possibility of assisting Debbie to commit suicide? If you were Debbie's health care provider, how would you respond if she asked you to assist her in committing suicide?
3. Granting to doctors the right to kill their patients for mercy gives a great deal of authority to physicians. How might this authority be misused? How might a supporter of active euthanasia respond to this issue?
4. There have been a few instances when physicians claimed that they assisted a patient in committing suicide. Is assisting suicide ethically distinct from active euthanasia?
5. If active euthanasia were permitted, what role should guardians have in the initiation of the procedure?
6. Nonterminally ill people frequently have chronic and profound pain and discomfort. Should these people have the right to be actively euthanized?
7. Select either a rights-based version or a consequentialist version of moral rights and explore its implications for whether it is right to permit active euthanasia.
8. Patients without adequate finances place a real financial burden on health care institutions. Is it reasonable to believe that these people would be placed in jeopardy if we legalized active euthanasia? How might supporters of active euthanasia respond to this concern?
9. One critic of active euthanasia has claimed that granting such a right would increase the burden on the dying patient by pressuring the dying patient "to get out of the way" and relieve his loved ones of the

responsibility for caring for him. Support for active euthanasia is a way for young people to avoid their responsibility to the aged who are weak and infirm. Is there any substance to this critique?
10. Assume that you support active euthanasia. What restrictions should be placed on this option to protect society from possible harm?

# More Cases Involving the Policy

### Assisted Suicide

Jennifer Kent has been suffering from severe depression for 11 years. Her physician is psychiatrist Dr. Harvey Spicer. According to Dr. Spicer, Jennifer's depression has not responded well to pharmaceutical or conversational treatment and Jennifer has refused further treatment. She has told him that she wants to die because "nothing seems to be working."

Dr. Spicer has told her that she does not have any underlying disease that will cause her death and refusing treatment will not bring about her death. Dr. Spicer has a long-term relationship with her, and he believes that she has tried everything to overcome this disease but that nothing seems to be effective. She asks Dr. Spicer about how she could kill herself. At first, Dr. Spicer merely ignores the request and begins to discus another medication that might be of some help. She says that she has tried enough medications and that she has no hope that this constant suffering can be decreased. Dr. Spicer and Jennifer have talked about Derek Humphry's book *Final Exit,* which contains many "suicide prescriptions."

Dr. Spicer is concerned that Jennifer will kill herself. He is wondering whether he should initiate a court procedure that will force her into the hospital. His concern is that while she is depressed, she does not seem incompetent. Indeed, he feels that if he were in Jennifer's medical position he too might want to die. In short, her desire to die, given her condition, seems somewhat reasonable to him. However, he is also concerned that Jennifer's desire to die might be a manifestation of the disease. What course of action should Dr. Spicer take?

### A Decision to Assist Suicide

Let us assume that in the above case Dr. Spicer has judged that there is nothing more that he can do for Jennifer and that her decision to die is reasonable. He decides to give her information about how she can effectively end her life. He gives her a prescription for barbiturates and writes into her chart that he has prescribed them because of her difficulties with sleeping (which she actually has). He then gives her the page numbers in Humphry's book that describe how to end her life using the barbiturate.

### Dr. Spicer's Nurse

Let us assume that you are Dr. Spicer's office nurse and that you have discovered that he is assisting Jennifer Kent in her suicide. You strongly disapprove of his actions and you are trying to determine your next course of action. How should you respond to this situation? Among your options are the following:

- Report him to county medical society or state licensure department.
- Report him to the police.
- Speak to him about your feelings.
- Do nothing.

### Further Reading

Battin, M. Pabst, *Ethical Issues in Suicide* (Englewood Cliffs, N.J.: Prentice-Hall, 1982).

Barnard, Christiaan. *Good Life/Good Death: A Doctor's Case for Euthanasia and Suicide* (Englewood Cliffs, N.J.: Prentice-Hall, 1980).

Cassell, E., and M. Siegler, *Changing Values in Medicine*. (Frederick, Md.: University Publications of America, 1985).

Engelhardt, Tristram, Jr., H. *The Foundations of Bioethics* (New York: Oxford University Press, 1986).

Fletcher, J. *Humanhood: Essays in Biomedical Ethics* (Buffalo, N.Y.: Prometheus Books, 1979).

Flew, Antony, "The Principle of Euthanasia," in *Euthanasia and the Right to Death: The Case of Voluntary Euthanasia*, ed. A. B. Downing (London: Peter Owen, 1959).

Humphry, Derek, *Final Exit*, (Secaucus, N.J.: Carol Publishing, 1991).

"It's Over, Debbie," *Journal of the American Medical Association* 259 (1988): 272.

Lifton, Robert Jay, *The Nazi Doctors: Medical Killing and the Psychology of Genocide* (New York: Basic Books, 1986).

Kevorkian, Jack, *Prescription Medicine: The Goodness of Planned Death* (Buffalo, N.Y.: Prometheus Books, 1991).

McCarthy, D., and A. Moraczewski, eds., *Moral Responsibility in Prolonging Life*. (St. Louis: Pope John XIII Center, 1981).

Meilaender, Gilbert, "The Distinction between Killing and Allowing to Die," *Theological Studies* 37 (1976): 467–70.

President's Commission for the Study of Ethical Problems in Medicine and Biomedical and Behavioral Research, *Deciding to Forego Life-Sustaining Treatment* (Washington, D.C.: U.S. Government Printing Office, 1983).

Quill, Timothy, *Death and Dignity*. (New York: W. W. Norton & Co., 1993).

Rachels, James, *The End of Life: Euthanasia and Morality* (Oxford: Oxford University Press, 1986).

Rachels, James, "Active and Passive Euthanasia," *New England Journal of Medicine* 292 (1975): 78–80.

Steinbock, Bonnie, *Killing and Letting Die* (Englewood Cliffs, N.J.: Prentice-Hall, 1980).

Trammell, Richard L., "Saving Life and Taking Life," *Journal of Philosophy* 72 (1975): 131–37.

Winslade, W., And J. Ross, *Choosing Life or Death* (New York: The Free Press, 1986).

## Notes

1. James Rachels, *The End of Life: Euthanasia and Morality* (Oxford: Oxford University Press, 1986).
2. This argument will come up in the committee deliberations.
3. President's Commission for the Study of Ethical Problems in Medicine and Biomedical and Behavioral Research, *Deciding to Forego Life Sustaining Treatments* (Washington, D.C.: U.S. Government Printing Office, 1982), p. 62.
4. Ibid., p. 72.
5. Susan Wolf, "Mercy Murder and Morality, Perspectives on Euthanasia," Special Supplement, *Hastings Center Report* 19 (1) (January 1989): 1–32.
6. Leon Kass, "Is There a Right to Die," *Hastings Center Report* (January 1993): 34.
7. H. T. Engelhardt, "Fashioning an Ethic for Life and Death in a Postmodern Society," *Hastings Center Report* (January-February 1989): 7–9.
8. Ibid., p. 8.
9. P. J. van der Maass, et al., "Euthanasia and Other Medical Decisions Concerning the End of Life," *Lancet* 338 (1991): 669–74.
10. For a follow-up review of the Remmelink Study see Johannes van Delden, Loes Pijinenborg, and Paul van der Maas, "The Remmelink Study: Two Years Later," *Hastings Center Report* 23 (6): 24.
11. This definition appears in the *Journal of the American Medical Association*, April 22, 1992.
12. H. L. Glanz, "Withholding and Withdrawing Treatment: The Role of the Criminal Law," *Law Medicine Health Care* 15 (1987-88): 231–41.
13. Timothy Quill, C. K. Cassel, and D. E. Meier, "Care of the Hopelessly Ill: Potential Clinical Criteria for Physician Assisted Suicide," *New England Journal of Medicine* 327 (19) (November 5, 1992): 1380–84.
14. This is a variation on a famous case entitled "It's Over, Debbie," *Journal of the American Medical Association* 259 (1988): 272.

# 4

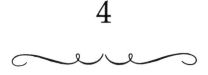

# Informed Consent

## Introduction to the Problem Area

What should the health care professional tell the patient? As our earlier chapters have already illustrated, hard choices abound in contemporary medicine, but health care professionals do not face these problems on a daily basis. We now turn to a problem that every health care professional who has patient contact does confront every day: the challenge of informed consent. What makes the issue of informed consent even more significant is that it is actually a cluster of problems that are somewhat artificially united under one banner. What unites them is the felt obligation to provide information in a way that will enhance both patient liberty and patient welfare. These goals can sometimes lead us in conflicting directions. We will begin, therefore, by identifying some specific problems that fall under the banner of informed consent.

### Explain Everything!

Medical information is unintelligible without a great deal of preparation and study. Medicine is an applied science and an applied art that requires knowledge of at least a dozen other scientific and humanistic systems. The difficulty of the material is simply staggering. Given these difficulties, can we require the physician or the nurse to reveal and explain "everything" to the patient? "Everything" may mean different things to different people. More importantly, requiring the health care professional to reveal and explain everything may involve requiring the physician or the nurse to do the impossible— and we ought not require the impossible.

## Explain Nothing!

The difficulties associated with revealing "everything" may tempt us to move to the opposite extreme, in which the physician only diagnoses and treats and never informs. In this scenario, the health care provider is a mechanic who "fixes" what is broken and never engages the patient as a partner in the healing process.

The challenge of informed consent is to find a reasonable middle ground between the extremes of explaining everything and explaining nothing. This middle ground is often referred to as *adequate disclosure*. There is little doubt that the term *adequate* is ambiguous. Courts have attempted to define it in a variety of ways.

## Selecting Terminology

To use words or ideas that the patient does not understand is to utter nearly meaningless sounds that do not contribute to informed consent, but to boil down the information to lay language frequently requires the professional to eliminate relevant facts. The professional is truly "between a rock and a hard place." The art of medicine may involve the struggle to find the middle ground between them.

Furthermore, no matter how clearly the physician presents information, the patients may still fail to understand what is disclosed. There are many possible causes for this. Understanding can be inhibited by anxiety, language difficulties, or the patient's disease. The list of causes is nearly limitless, yet the health care professional is still obligated to secure the patient's understanding. Cognitive difficulties frequently block this goal.

## Harming the Patient

Although information can benefit patients and increase their autonomy, it can also harm them. The values of enhancing patient control, enhancing welfare, and avoiding unnecessary harm often conflict when managing a patient. For example, a diagnosis may reveal a terminal and irreversible illness. If this information is revealed, the patient and the physician may use it to plan a beneficial palliative care plan. The patient may also freely use this information to reorder the remainder of his life in a way that is very rewarding to him. But this same information may also send the patient into a depression from which he may suffer significantly. The health care professional must face the choice of revealing information that may have both beneficial and harmful consequences. Is the professional always obligated to weigh these possible results and do whatever produces the best results? Or is the professional obligated to respect the patient's "right to know" regardless of the consequences?

## Competence and Informed Consent

Difficulties surrounding patient harm are matched by the challenges surrounding patient competence. A 15-year-old probably cannot give informed consent to an operation because he is not legally competent to do so. He may have been given adequate information, and indeed he may have understood the information at least as well as, or perhaps better than, his parents. He may be the kind of young man who manages most of his own affairs. Yet he is not legally competent to give consent. In short, there are legislative and judicial limitations on informed consent that can make the task of respecting the patient's right to know more difficult.

## Manipulation

Another problem with informed consent derives from the psychological authority that health care providers have in relation to patients. This authority can be used to comfort and support patients, but it can also be used to undermine patient autonomy by transferring the locus of control from the patient to the provider. When physician authority is used to undermine patient autonomy, we may see "manipulation"; when it is used to enhance welfare and autonomy, we may call it "cooperative."

If the manipulative uses of authority were as obvious as illegal coercion, threats, or blackmail, then manipulation would not be the pervasive and challenging problem that it is. However, the subtle and illusive nature of manipulation makes it difficult to manage within a legal framework. The following comment gleaned from a conversation with a physician friend captures the reality of the physician's control over patients: "I can control most patients, period! I can get them to do what I want them to do! I do it all the time and I am good at it. The problem is that I do not always feel good about manipulating them so much!" Physicians and nurses have a great deal of authority in relation to their patients, and it is easy for the experienced physician or nurse to exercise that authority at the expense of the patient's autonomy and welfare.

## Informed Consent Documents

Finally, there is a very practical reason for our concerns with informed consent. Hospitals and other health care institutions must get patients to sign "informed consent" documents prior to surgery or participation in a medical experiment that is going on at the hospital. Both problems are riddled with informed consent concerns frequently because nurses, who are often required to get these documents signed, have no guarantee that the patient has been fully informed.

---

### Informed Consent Policy of Community Hospital

*Purpose:*    The purpose of this policy is to express Community Hospital's informed consent guidelines for medical treatments.

*Definition:*    Informed consent is the voluntary, competent, and comprehended authorization of medical treatment.

*Principles:*

1. Informed consent for significant, nonemergency medical procedures such as surgery should be secured using written documents. Informed consent may be bypassed if it is impossible to secure in an emergency context.
2. Documents that merely assert that a physician has disclosed relevant information are viewed by the committee as ethically perilous.
3. Informed consent documents should address the following issues:
   A. A description of the treatment with an emphasis on its purpose.
   B. A description of any actual harms that will result from the procedure.
   C. A description of any significant risks associated with the procedure.
   D. A significant harm or risk is one that a reasonable person would want to know.
   E. A description of significant benefits that can reasonably be expected from the treatment.
   F. A physician's recommendation that the benefits outweigh the risks.
   G. A description of any alternatives to the proposed treatment, including nontreatment.
   H. The document should encourage the patient to ask any questions that he or she may have regarding the procedure. The document should also inform the patient that he or she may withdraw from the treatment where this is possible.
   I. The document should affirm that if the patient refuses the recommended treatment or withdraws from the treatment once initiated, no one at the hospital will abandon him/her.

  J. The document should affirm that the information contained in it will be kept in confidence.

4. The committee encourages physicians to develop informed consent documents that are intelligible to the medical lay person.

5. Physicians are encouraged to delay, if possible, any significant medical procedure if there is reason for thinking that the patient does not adequately comprehend the issues that confront him or her.

6. Guardians may sign informed consent documents for incompetent persons. Such guardians are encouraged to express the wishes and determine the best interests of the incompetent patient.

7. We recommend that patients or their guardians sign informed consent documents in the presence of a witness and that the witness sign the document.

8. In cases where there is doubt regarding the patient's competence, or cases when the patient is episodically incompetent, every effort should be made to respect the decision-making capacity of the patient subject to the following condition: Restrictions on decision-making capacity should be as minimal as possible and should be governed by the rule that those who make high-risk or directly harmful decisions must satisfy a high standard of capacity.

9. The committee recognizes that there are significant problems associated with adolescents. Although they are legally incompetent to *consent* to medical procedures, they often possess the cognitive skills of competent adults. Many courts advocate that adolescents, where possible, should participate in critical medical decisions. We endorse the principle that physicians secure the assent of adolescents for treatment as well as the consent of their guardians.

---

## Commentary on the Philosophical and Ethical Aspects of the Policy

This Informed Consent Policy poses a number of important practical problems for medicine, all of which have philosophical dimensions. But before we can turn to a thorough discussion of the concept of informed consent, some attempt must be made to define the idea.

  An initial affirmation of the right to informed consent was offered in a landmark 1914 case by Judge Cardozo.[1] Cardozo wrote that "Every human being of adult years and sound mind has a right to determine what shall be done with his own body; and a surgeon who performs an operation without his patient's consent commits an assault for which he is liable for damages." But this decision, important as it was, did not create the modern concern with informed consent. Another legal definition that is more specific regarding the actual duties of the physician, called *Nishi* v. *Hartwell*, gave the following definition of the legal duty to secure informed consent: "The Doctrine of informed consent imposes on a physician a duty to disclose to his patient all relevant information concerning a proposed treatment including the collateral hazards attendant thereto, so that the patient's consent to the treatment would be an intelligent one based on complete information."[2]

## Therapeutic Privilege

However, Nishi v. Hartwell imposed a limitation that provides a profound ambiguity to the doctrine of informed consent. The judge admits that since the physician's primary duty is to do what is best for the patient, the physician is permitted to "withhold disclosure of information regarding any untoward consequences where full disclosure would be detrimental to the patient's total care and best interest." This is called *therapeutic privilege.*

These initial definitions of informed consent and therapeutic privilege leave many issues unresolved. For example, what justifies the use of therapeutic privilege? Also, who has the privilege? Can the physician withhold information in order to avoid harming the patient? Can the physician also withhold information in order to benefit the patient? The latter situation occurs when placebos are used in treatment. A *placebo* is a chemical substance that is known to be biologically ineffective for the treatment of a given disease. By *biologically ineffective* we mean that there is no known biological mechanism that explains why a sugar pill, for example, should reduce headache pain. Yet some studies that indicate placebos do reduce headache pain under specific conditions.[3] Assume for the sake of discussion that a patient is given a sugar pill and told by a physician in authority that it is "clinically indicated" for pain reduction. The physician may justify this decision by saying that there is clinical data that the placebo is effective for this kind of pain.

The two main objections to the use of placebos are consequential and rights-based. First, although some patients may benefit from their use, the use of placebos threatens to undermine the trust that exists between health care providers and patients. This consequence threatens the general welfare of patients. In the rights-based argument against placebos, the patient has a right to be treated respectfully, even when the consequences of respectful treatment are harmful. One tells the truth to a terminally ill patient not because this will not harm the patient, but because withholding the truth involves deception. One can make a strong case that placebos involve implicit deception.

## The Critics of Informed Consent

Our introduction to informed consent has emphasized the legal definition of informed consent. Is this legal concept appropriate in medicine? Many authors have argued that the legal requirements surrounding informed consent and the threat of malpractice suits have done more harm than good to patients. Eugene Laforet, in an essay suggestively entitled "The Fiction of Informed Consent,"[4] has argued that the *Nishi* v. *Hartwell* definition is profoundly "ambivalent." In one sentence the physician is duty bound to reveal all relevant information. In the next sentence the physician is given the right to withhold information if doing so is in the interest of the patient. The duty "to reveal" and the right "to withhold" information impose an impossible task on the physician because it would take the wisdom of Solomon to know whether information is going to be beneficial or harmful in all cases.

Laforet would probably reject Community Hospital's requirement that informed consent documents are necessary for invasive treatments. Such documents would have to contain detailed information regarding the scientific basis for medical decisions and also not only all the alternatives to a treatment, but also an evaluation of the validity of the studies that support these alternatives. The creation and required use of such documents would transform the physician's office into a courtroom, which would result in the harm of patients. For Laforet there can be "no rigid prescription" regarding the information that the physician should reveal to the patient. Rather, the "patient should be told enough to permit him and his physician to reach a consensus."

Jay Katz, another critic of both the legal doctrine of informed consent and the medical practice of informed consent, criticizes both medicine and the legal profession by suggesting that they have failed to create a climate in which patients and physicians can "share the burden of making joint decisions."[5] The tradition of medicine, according to Katz, is one that has expressed very little interest in the value of genuine communication between patient and professional. He illustrates this point by referring to the following advice to physicians by Hippocrates: "Perform (your duties) calmly and adroitly, concealing most things from the patient while you are attending to him."[6] Furthermore, the Hippocratic oath itself says nothing about the duty to communicate with patients and obtain their informed consent before initiating treatment. Indeed, Katz maintains that recent concessions on the part of the medical profession to improve consent procedures are aimed at avoiding malpractice suits. They are not aimed at redirecting the profession toward informed communication.

## The Roots of Informed Consent

But with so many assaults against the doctrine of informed consent, why has the significance of this principle skyrocketed in the last 40 years? One reason is that informed consent has been connected with the idea of individual autonomy and the assumption that the individual has the right to authorize medical intervention. If we are to respect individuals as self-governing persons, then medical professionals ought not prescribe therapies without the patient's informed consent.[7] But how exactly are these ideas linked?

One response to this question comes from the philosopher Tom Beauchamp, who claims that the bridge that links autonomy and informed consent is the notion that human beings do not forsake their "personal self-governance" because they enter into a doctor-patient relationship.[8] For Beauchamp, respecting the patient's autonomy involves accepting that a patient's personal values, perspectives, and beliefs rightfully influence medical decisions. For Beauchamp, informed consent requires respecting the patient's right to actually authorize a treatment. Patients do not merely submit to a physician's orders, they must actually authorize the treatment. The patient is not obligated to consent to the wishes of the physician. Philosophers like Beauchamp argue that the only reasonable way for a patient to retain the right of authorization is to obligate physicians to respect informed consent. Autonomy is nearly useless without information.

But informed consent is also rooted in the desire to avoid harming the patient. As we have seen in the context of withdrawing and withholding care, the question of what is in an individual's best interest varies with that person's values and circumstances. The patient must determine what is best.

## Informed Consent as a Right

However, the phrase that is most frequently used in connection with the concept of informed consent is the *patient's right to know*. Many argue that the primary reason for the proliferation of concern regarding informed consent is the popular assumption that the patient has a right to informed consent. This is a powerful claim. For if it is accepted that the patient has a right to informed consent, then an institution, such as a hospital, or individual, such as a physician or nurse, has the duty to provide this information. Rights are usually viewed as meaningless unless there is an authority that imposes obligations on others to respect and perhaps secure those rights.

Furthermore, some traditions in medicine have not recognized the right of informed consent. The Hippocratic tradition that flourished in early Greece and Rome and has had a powerful influence on contemporary medicine does not recognize this right. The notion that individuals have rights and that government exists in order to secure these rights is a political philosophy that would have been alien to the Romans and the Greeks. It is not surprising, therefore, that the medical tradition that flourished in these cultures did not recognize informed consent. Rather, the Hippocratic tradition emphasizes that the purpose of the physician is to secure the welfare of the patient and to avoid doing what makes the patient's condition worse. The language of rights, information, and voluntary consent is foreign both to this tradition and to the culture in which it is embedded.

Proponents of the right of informed consent argue that the Hippocratic tradition errs in granting an excessive authority to the health care provider and places the professional in a position of significant advantage over the patient.[9] By withholding information, the professional can hinder the patient from securing what the patient considers to be valuable. Furthermore, withholding or misrepresenting information can undermine another important right of the patient, namely, his right to avoid what he considers harmful. For example, if physicians or other professionals have the right to determine that it is not good for patients to know the specific dangers associated with surgeries, then the patient is not able to refuse the surgery based on his own preferences to avoid these risks. One can express preferences only if one has relevant information.

The use of anesthetics in surgery represents a case where there is heated debate concerning what the patient needs to know. Certain anesthetics have a very low probability of causing death, and many physicians are reluctant to share this information with the patient because the dangers are so minuscule. Proponents of informed consent, however, respond that while the possibility may be very low, the final decision to risk death should rest with the patient. If the decision to inform the patient of this very low probability of harm resides with the professional, then the patient loses the opportunity to say "no" to the treatment. When a competent person says "no" to surgery based on these concerns, it may seem irrational to health care professionals. But according to proponents of the right to informed consent, the authority to decide still resides with the individual.

But what exactly is a right and how do rights function in the health care setting? Philosophically, rights may be viewed as legitimate claims against some other person or institution. If a person P has a right, then P has a legitimate claim against some other person or institution. One needs to be very careful when granting rights to people because doing so entails that someone or some institution has the obligation or duty to satisfy or respect these rights. In the context of informed consent the patient is said to have a right to informed consent and the health care provider has the obligation to secure or respect that right. There is vast debate within philosophy as to whether rights are basic and obligations are to be defined with reference to rights, or whether the duties of individuals and professionals should be determined first and rights selected in the light of these obligations. Our tack throughout this text is to assume that there is a dialectical relationship between rights and obligations and that, although one might want maximal rights, one does not want the maximal obligations that accompany them. Citizens frequently want maximal health care rights but are reluctant to accept the associated financial obligations. One must dialectically adjust the assignment of rights to the willingness and resources of others to accept the corresponding obligations.

Rights may also be classified as positive or negative. *Positive rights* are claims against other parties to provide services of a specific kind. For example, the citizen of the United States has a right to primary and secondary education; this right is a claim against the government to provide that service. The government has the obligation to provide that service to the individual. In many cases, positive rights are limited by resources. Thus, citizens do not have a right to a college education at Harvard University simply because the government could not afford the of cost. The right to go to college is a limited right, one that is primarily limited by social resources.

*Negative rights,* on the other hand, do not require that any positive services be provided to the individual citizen. Rather, what they require is that others refrain from interfering with behavior. For example, the right to religious freedom is a negative right in that, if an individual has this right, then others are obligated to avoid interfering with his religious activity. The government is not required to provide the individual with a church, a synagogue, or a mosque, but merely to prevent anyone from interfering with his religious choices. This involves a commitment on the part of government to avoid making laws that establish one religion over the others or taking action that favors one religion over others. However, the primary function of the negative right is to obligate government to use its considerable power and authority to guarantee that other members of the state avoid interfering with the exercise of this right to freedom of religion.

The right to informed consent involves both a positive and a negative right. To say that a patient has a right to know means that the physician has the duty to provide an information service. Violating this duty involves a breach of the relationship that binds the patient and the physician. But informed consent also involves a negative right in the sense that the physician must avoid interfering unjustifiably with the patient's decisions.

## Informed Consent and the Physician-Patient Relationship

The practice of informed consent is thus closely connected to the larger question of the nature of the relationship between the physician and the quite appropriate to allow the physician to control the flow of information based on the parent's authority and assumed affection for the child. Thus, it is necessary to turn to a more comprehensive discussion of this relationship.

Three distinct models of the patient-physician relationship are present within medicine: the traditional paternalism model, the contractual model, and the fiduciary model.

*The Paternalism Model*    In the paternalistic model, the patient comes to the physician or other health care professional seeking help, as a child comes to its parent. As the child is weak and vulnerable and easily controlled, so too is the patient. As the child is ignorant, so too is the patient. As the child is in need, so too is the patient. As the child assumes the good will of the parent, so too the patient assumes the good will of the physician. As the child should accept the parent's authority, so should the patient accept the physician's. As the parent has the right to determine what is good for the child, so too the physician should have the right to determine what is good for the patient. As the parent has the right to override the child's wishes for the child's own good, so the doctor has the right to override the wishes of the patient for the patient's own good. The image of the physician embodied in the paternalistic model is of one who knows the real interests of another person and is devoted to securing that person's interests rather than his own or those of some third party. The doctor is a "pater"—a father.[10]

There are three chief difficulties with this model. First, the paternalistic model fails to recognize that although adult patients are vulnerable and often medically ignorant, society still recognizes that they are autonomous. One does not need to be invulnerable or completely independent or well informed in order to be accorded the right to control one's life. What is wrong with the paternalistic model is not only its assumption that "doctor knows best" but also its failure to recognize that weak, vulnerable, and dependent people retain their autonomy. Ignorance, vulnerability, and need are not sufficient for incompetence.

The second difficulty associated with the paternalistic model concerns the parent-child analogy. Although there are similarities between many patients and children, there are also vast dissimilarities. The patient may be ignorant of the specific cardiac mechanisms that explain her chest pain but this ignorance is, for the most part, irrelevant to the exercise of her right to authorize the cardiologist's recommendations. The cardiologist may have a well-grounded, professional opinion regarding the care of a patient, and the patient may refuse to accept that opinion based on values that are not shared by the physician. Technical knowledge about how and why hearts fail does not automatically produce in the physician the knowledge of when it is permissible to refuse life-sustaining treatment. In short, ignorance of the scientific and technical aspects of medicine is vastly different from the kind of generalized ignorance that little children have.

*A Contractual Model*    The second philosophical picture of the relationship between doctors and patients is in many respects the opposite of the paternalistic model. Rather than viewing doctors as mothers or fathers and patients as children, we can view patients and health care providers as free and autonomous individuals who enter into a contract with each other in order to secure their mutual benefit. This contract places new obligations on both parties. For example, the physician has the duty to provide competent medical services; the patient has the duty to pay his bill. Patients are equal in all relevant respects to the health care professionals who treat them. As equals, the parties enter into a cooperative contract that can benefit both of them. But there also remains a good deal of competition and conflict between the parties because they often have conflicting interests. The physician-patient contract is similar to a business contract in which free and equal parties become duty bound to one another in order to secure mutually beneficial ends. This model rejects the central idea of the paternalistic model, that patients are children. Patients are free but in need of services. According to this model, one enters a physician's office with the same assumptions that one takes into a car dealership. The patient is not asking for help from a parent. Rather he is contracting with another free and equal person to enter into a cooperative relationship. The patient freely gives money to the professional, and, in return, the professional freely provides services.

But just as the "buyer should beware" in the car dealer's showroom, the contractual model suggests that the patient should beware in the doctor's office. As the car dealer is not one's mother, neither is, the doctor or the nurse. Within medicine there is cooperation, but there is also the constant specter of conflict, not only because both parties are trying to get the most for the least but also because there are third parties that mediate the relationship between the doctor and the patient. For example, the physician has an interest in minimizing the amount of time he spends with each patient so that he can maximize the number of patients he sees. Patients, on the other hand, often wish to communicate with physicians in ways that require significant amounts of time.

The contractual model of the relationship pictures the patient as attempting to maximize required medical services while minimizing payments while the professional tries to maximize payments and minimize services. However, neither the interests of the provider nor the interests of the patients can be fully realized; thus, contracts are developed as a way of mediating this conflict. Supporters of this model argue that just as good car dealers attempt to provide beneficial services to their customers and attempt to do what is reasonable to keep their customers happy and satisfied, so too good doctors provide very important services to their customers and do everything within reason to please them.

However, just as car dealers can refuse to enter into a business relationship for a wide variety of reasons, so too can a doctor or a nurse. The car dealer may refuse to sell a car to a customer who cannot pay for it. The doctor can refuse to provide services without payment. Just as a car is transferred to a customer on the basis of a contract that spells out the obligations imposed on both parties, so too health care services should be transferred on the basis of such a contract. Without contracts neither   party can understand what is expected of it in the relationship. Contracts can facilitate the transfer of services by making the *expectations* and *rights* of both parties explicit.

Like the paternalistic model, the contractual model has much to recommend it. Primary among its virtues is that it highlights the autonomy of both the patient and the physician. A prospective customer is free to refuse to purchase a car; a patient is free to refuse the recommendations of the health care provider. The contractual or business model offers another attractive feature. Business contracts often produce efficient provision of services because both parties are trying to minimize their own costs. Thus the patient who pays for services is motivated to purchase only those services that she needs. Minimizing costs often requires reducing needs. In like fashion, the physician is motivated to provide only services that are paid for so as to maximize his profits. One might prefer that doctors provide their services without charge, but fees often have the unexpected but beneficial result of reducing the number of needless services.

But the virtues of the contractual model are matched by significant vices. Critics argue that the model is woefully inadequate as a description of what actually takes place between real doctors and real patients. The real patient and the real doctor never, in fact, develop or sign these contracts.[11] The doctor's commitments to the patient go beyond what can be explicitly expressed in a formal contract.

There are other deeper problems with this model. The doctor, like the car dealer, has no trusting relationship with the patient. If the car dealer and the physician are comparable, then it would be as inappropriate for the patient to trust the physician as for the customer to trust the car dealer. But many commentators argue that entering professional relationships is fundamentally different from entering business relationships.[12]

The contractual model surely requires us to compare the patient with the customer, but this comparison is troublesome. The customer should beware, rather than trust, the car dealer because the customer is a mere instrument by which the dealer secures his interest, i.e., profits. But, for many commentators, trust is at the heart of the physician-patient relationship. For example, the car dealer is not obligated to inform the customer about all of a car's shortcomings. More specifically, car dealers may withhold information regarding crash tests if they think that these results will decrease sales. We may not like it, but one is wise to realize that salesmen often withhold relevant information. But while such withholding of information is frequently permitted within ordinary contractual relations, it is widely disapproved of in medicine. The health care provider is widely viewed as having obligations that transcend contractual relations. Physicians have a strong obligation to their patients to reveal the harmful effects associated with treatment.

*The Fiduciary Model*   Many authors have attempted to develop a compromise position that incorporates the values associated with the contractual and the paternalistic models of the patient–health care professional relationship. The paternalistic model emphasizes the health care professional's duty to secure the welfare of and avoid harming the patient. The contractual model emphasizes the autonomy of the patient. A third view, the fiduciary model, represents the health care professional as aiming to secure both the welfare and the autonomy of the patient. In this model the physician is viewed as superior to the patient only in terms of specialized, scientific knowledge. No ethical or moral superiority is assumed. The professional is not represented as being in a better position to make value judgments concerning the patient. Within the fiduciary model, whenever the physician is confronted with a significant moral decision that will affect the patient, he must turn to the patient or his surrogate for input and, frequently, resolution. In addition, the health care professional is pictured as trustworthy. Indeed, a fiduciary is someone whom society identifies as having the right to practice. In being granted this right, a person implicitly accepts obligations that are associated with being trustworthy. But what are these obligations?

The first implication of being a trustworthy health care professional is the professional's implicit promise to be loyal to the patient. Loyalty involves a number of traits but primarily means that the physician or other health care professional will not abandon patients when they become inconvenient or difficult to manage. Another duty of the fiduciary is to be both competent and diligent in carrying out fiduciary responsibilities. If the physician presents himself as trustworthy, then he is recommending himself as knowledgeable in a specific area of medicine. The duty to present information honestly to the patient without misrepresenting it is also vital. One could not systematically misrepresent information and still be trustworthy. The right to informed consent is thus derived from the fiduciary relationship between the professional and the patient.

Contemporary Western culture views the physician not as a father or as a car dealer but as a fiduciary. The doctor is recognized by society as having the responsibility to secure not just the autonomy of a patient, but also the patient's medical welfare. Like the father, the fiduciary is not free to do whatever maximizes his self-interest. Accepting a person as a patient involves a limited commitment to resist actions based on self-interest. For example, the temptation to perform unnecessary tests or procedures is real in medicine because these tests often produce income for the professional. But the fiduciary nature of the relationship would outlaw such self-interested decisions since they are not those of a trustworthy professional. Once the professional accepts a patient, the patient's medical welfare and medical autonomy must be regarded as primary. Sacrificing the patient's welfare for his own interest borders on conflict of interest and a violation of the physician's promise to be a faithful fiduciary for the patient. While the fiduciary lacks the freedom of a car dealer to keep her own self-interest primary, she is very different from the parent. The fiduciary lacks the power to comprehensively determine what is good for her patient.

This compromise view incorporates many of the virtues of the paternalistic and contractual models and attempts to do so without including their vices. As we return to the problems of informed consent, it is important to remember that these models of the patient-physician relationship will come into play. Indeed, many of the most important controversies surrounding informed consent derive their power from different and opposing images of the relationship between health care professional and patient.

With this background in mind, let us now turn to a detailed review of the actual elements of informed consent. We may speak of the general idea of informed consent as containing four separate elements: (a) adequate disclosure, (b) competence, (c) patient understanding, and (d) voluntary consent. Each condition is necessary for achieving informed consent. If all of them are satisfied, we may say that a health care provider has obeyed the rule of informed consent.

## Adequate Disclosure

It is tempting to suggest that adequate disclosure can be easily defined, but, as we will see, the concept is riddled with debate and conflict. For a patient to give informed consent to a procedure, most theorists believe that the professional must adequately disclose the relevant information associated with the procedure. Many of the most difficult issues about informed consent concern how one defines *adequacy*. The traditional definition held that "adequate information" was the information that professional health care providers normally reveal. This "professional standard" meant that if most health care providers did not reveal that drug X has the occasional side effect of causing sleeplessness, then health care providers were not obligated to do so. According to this definition, the typical behavior of health care providers was defined as adequate. This is somewhat ambiguous because among health care providers three exists a range of opinion about what information ought to be revealed. Furthermore, courts have recently become skeptical of this definition because it tends to emphasize the authority of the professional within the patient-provider relationship. If a local group of professionals tended to agree that withholding certain information was permitted, then patient convictions on the matter were irrelevant. The professional criterion of disclosure thus tended to place the professional in a position of advantage over the patient, as in the paternalism view of the patient-professional relationship.

A new and equally challenging definition of adequate disclosure has been introduced in many states, though the professional standard remains an important consideration when deciding whether a given disclosure was adequate. This definition is called the *reasonable person standard*. Its aim is to redress the imbalance of power that the professional definition permitted. It requires that if a hypothetical reasonable person would want to have a piece of information related to a treatment, then the provider is obligated to provide this information. Principle 3D of the hospital's informed consent guidelines, which defines "a significant harm or risk" as "one that a reasonable person would want to know," explicitly assumes this standard.

The main argument for this standard is that it enhances the autonomy of the patient. A physician may be reluctant to inform a patient that a procedure has a very low probability of causing death, lest revealing this information prevent the patient from securing the benefits of the procedure. What should the physician do? The reasonable person standard requires that the physician prove to himself and perhaps to a court that a reasonable person would not want this information. This requirement creates a high standard of justification for nondisclosure. The reasonable person standard is thus weighted toward disclosure, and disclosure preferences are usually justified by autonomy considerations.

This standard is ambiguous because it assumes that all reasonable persons would want the same information. This is unlikely because as actual—as opposed to hypothetical—reasonable persons frequently disagree over what information they actually require. Health care providers tend to view this new standard as one that makes them very vulnerable to litigation because it is not precise. It also opens the door to the notion that "reasonable" has no definition other than what a jury says is reasonable. Hypothetical persons are, at best, imprecise objects of study.

Finally, a third definition, *the subjective standard* of adequate disclosure, emphasizes that real patients (as opposed to hypothetical reasonable persons) have distinctive informational needs. The subjective standard does not impose a general definition of what every patient needs to know. Because the life circumstances of individual patients differ, so do their informational needs. This standard requires the physician to tailor, to the extent possible, her presentation of information so that it meets the specific and occasionally idiosyncratic informational needs of her patient.

There is much that recommends the subjective standard of adequacy, especially the widely held sentiment that each patient is unique. For example, if a patient is a horse-racing jockey and his physician is prescribing a medication that is associated with weight gain, he may have a distinctive need to know this because jockeys are very concerned about their weight. The subjective standard thus encourages the physician or nurse to come to know the patient as a distinctive individual and to give the person information accordingly.

What is troubling about the subjective standard is the assumption that health care professionals have solid information about the particular informational needs of their patients. In the past, many physicians had long-term relationships with patients and their families, which afforded deeper understanding of the patients. However, the doctor-patient relationship tends to be more episodic and short-term. As a result, the health care professional often does not know the patient well enough to make unique assessments of the patient's idiosyncratic informational needs. If the professional is ignorant of the patient's unique character and circumstances, it is therefore difficult to obligate the professional to provide distinctive information to the patient.

### Diminished Capacity

Throughout our discussion of informed consent we have often qualified the principle by saying that only the *competent* patient needs to consent. Although the concept of competence was partially defined in Chapter 2, the problem of diminished capacity or reduced competence was treated as one that needed to be handled on a case-by-case basis. No rules were suggested for managing the cases of patients who are legally competent but whose competence is diminished. In Chapter 2, individuals were depicted as either competent or incompetent. Competence can be treated as a minimum set of cognitive and psychological capacities. Persons who have this minimum set ought to be treated as competent. According to this minimum threshold view, the only facts that are relevant to a patient's competency are facts about the person herself. The complexity or seriousness of the decision itself is not relevant.

This qualitative view of competence accords well with the widely held assumption that patients are to be treated as competent and that physicians and other health care providers should not be continuously trying to assess degrees of competence. Furthermore, the health care professional bears the burden of proving that a patient falls below the fixed minimum standard for competence. The qualitative character of competence is grounded in our society's desire to minimize the ability of professionals, such as physicians and nurses, and institutions, such as hospitals and nursing homes, to treat individuals without adequate respect for their autonomy. It is feared that if we were to move toward a quantitative view of competence and view it as a matter of degree rather than as a quality that one either has or does not have, this would increase the control that institutions have over individuals. It is easy to prove diminished competence and thereby restrict the wishes of patients, but it is far more difficult to establish complete incompetence. Therefore, this more demanding standard represents a constitutionally justified preference for individual liberty.

However, as many health care professionals know, competence is, in many respects, a nonqualitative concept that admits of degrees. *Competence has quantitative aspects.* To treat competence as a quantitative, nonqualitative concept involves viewing it as a continuum. Some examples can help to illustrate this quantitative understanding of competence.

An 85-year-old man who is having episodic memory loss may be incompetent to run a complex business. However, this man's incompetence to run a business does not necessarily imply that he is incompetent to make his own end-of-life decisions. Age is not the only factor that affects capacity for decision making. Psychiatric disorders can also alter this ability. Often it is difficult to determine whether the psychiatric patient has the capacity to make critical decisions for himself.

Another class of patients affected by the issue of diminished capacity is the adolescent. Although adolescents are legally incompetent to make health care decisions, it seems clear that they are often able to reason effectively about the consequences of treatment. They are able to appreciate alternative treatments. They can make decisions on the basis of reasonable values and yet, legally, they are incompetent.

Ethical considerations enter into such situations because the health care professional faces a human dilemma. Should the professional recognize or refuse to recognize the capacity of patients to make decisions? Often the health care professional who is primarily concerned with protecting the safety of psychiatric patients or providing beneficial medical intervention for patients with diminished capacity chooses to override the patient's wishes. Thus the professional experiences conflict between her actions and her commitment to the principle of patient autonomy.

The philosophers Dan Brock and Allan Buchanan have developed a "decision relative" theory of competence that attempts to address these problems.[13] To say that competence is "decision relative" means that the decision to treat a patient as competent depends on factors that include not only the cognitive ability of the patient, but the nature of the decision itself. Many would assume that the advanced Alzheimer's victim whose capacity for understanding is very low is still competent to choose what television programs to watch. Relative to television choices, he is competent. His competence thus extends to areas that do not have a profound impact on his overall best interest. However, if a decision involves understanding a large amount of complex information and if the decision will have a significant impact on the patient's life, then, according to Brock and Buchanan, we are permitted to require the patient to satisfy a higher standard of cognitive capacity. Deciding whether to have a surgical procedure is such a decision. In this situation we may not regard the Alzheimer's victim as competent to decide.

Another factor that affects our choice to treat the patient as sufficiently capacitated to make the decision is the risk associated with the procedure. If the procedure involves little risk, then we frequently permit those with diminished capacity to exercise authority.

This decision relative approach to competency has a number of important virtues, but it has some drawbacks as well. Chief among the former is that it permits us to say that a person is incompetent in some areas of decisionmaking without implying she is incompetent in all areas. This relativistic view of competence can thus enhance the limited autonomy of psychiatric patients or patients whose capacity is compromised by asserting that surrogates and professionals must specify particular restrictions on the patient's decision-making capacity. Having limitations placed on one's autonomy is not equivalent to losing it completely.

However, this decision relative concept of competency is not without its problems. Primary among its defects is its potential for being unwittingly employed to justify paternalistic restrictions on the rights of patients. Brock and Buchanan admit that it works well with cases where paternalism is strongest, but it is easy to imagine that it could also permit paternalistic decisions where the arguments for paternalism are very weak. Patients who make decisions that are inconsistent with their physician's wishes are often suspected of being incompetent precisely because the patients are placing themselves at great risk of harm. If decisions that involve significant risk of harm require a high standard of capacity, then the physician may exercise his power and rule that the patient lacks sufficient capacity to make a decision. Instead of making violations of autonomy less frequent, the relativistic interpretation of competence may increase them, since it is the physician who judges the patient's capacity.

Finally, this view of decision making seems to assume that there are decent objective tests for grading capacity and that one can compare the grades scored on these tests against the risks and benefits associated with a variety of specific medical procedures. Even if this were possible, it seems to imply that patients must score very high on their competence test before they can consent to medically risky procedures. This, however, seems inconsistent with the practice of assuming that individuals are competent until proven otherwise. Few things are more risky than driving race cars, and yet we do not require that race car drivers score high marks on a rigorous competence test. If we do not require race car drivers to score high on capacity tests, why should we require this of patients?

## Patient Understanding

For health care professionals, one of the most frustrating aspects of the informed consent doctrine is that a physician can often do a first-rate job of disclosing relevant information to competent patients but still fail to secure the informed consent of the patient. For if the competent patient fails to understand the information that is disclosed, then he has not given informed consent. To understand information is to possess an accurate appreciation of its meaning and implications. In medicine, understanding is associated especially with appreciating the consequences of action. The professional has a duty not only to disclose information but also to do so successfully. The nature of the problem is revealed in this example that stresses the meaning of medical terminology.

Suppose a patient is told that a potential side effect of a medication is impotence. The meaning of the word "impotence" is not universally understood, and a physician may be unwilling to define it explicitly because the power of suggestion may increase the probability that the effect will take place. But if we assume that the patient does not understand the meaning of this term, then mere verbal agreement to the above medication may not be consent. Indeed, one can imagine the surprise and anger that a person might feel if he discovers the real meaning of the term after the medication has produced the effect.

The problems associated with achieving genuine understanding are difficult to resolve. Many critics of the principle of informed consent have argued that informed consent must be limited precisely because it is so difficult to achieve full understanding of complex medical procedures, especially those associated with medical experimentation. For example, Franz Ingelfinger has claimed that "the chances are remote that the subject really understands what he has consented to."[14] There is little doubt that if informed consent requires a very high degree of understanding, it is likely to be impossible to achieve. In short, as with the problem of competence, the crucial factor is how we should define our terms. It is very easy, for example, to say that full understanding is required and therefore informed consent is impractical or impossible within medicine, but if a lower but still reasonable standard is acceptable, then informed consent can survive this criticism.

This lower standard of understanding may be approached by disclosing the relevant information and then asking patients some questions to determine whether they have grasped the material. Such informal tests are especially important when the information presented is complex or if there is a large amount of it. Furthermore, the fact that the patient is in pain or depressed or anxious about his health can obviously affect his capacity to appreciate the implications of what is disclosed. Effective illustrations and analogies can often aid in communicating. Frequently, video or audio tapes increase understanding because patients can take these items home and return with questions. These considerations were at the root of Community Hospital's policy requirement regarding "information rich" consent documents. Perhaps the strongest tool for achieving understanding is the power of time. When the caregiver suspects that the patient does not fully understand, she should consider setting another appointment so that the patient can further explore the meaning of specific disclosures.

## Waivers

Perhaps the most common problem with informed consent involves patients who wish to relinquish or waive their right to informed consent. "Doc, whatever you say is fine with me. You don't have to tell me anything about it! I trust you!" These are not uncommon remarks in the physician's office. Such remarks indicate the patient does not wish to be an active partner in the healing process. How does the health care professional concerned with communication deal with such disclaimers? One solution is simply to note them in the patient's chart, thereby recognizing the patient's right to refuse information. One might then proceed with the treatment. A second approach involves asking the patient to formally relinquish her right to information in a written document. The formality of such an response may cause a change of opinion in the patient. In a third approach, the physician says, "No, there are important decisions that need to be made and I need your input!"

   With medications and procedures that have a low risk of harm, the first approach may be acceptable, but as the possible consequences become more life-threatening, the second and third approaches become more reasonable. For example, the first approach seems inappropriate for deciding whether to withhold or withdraw life-sustaining treatment. Serious surgeries such as a pancreatic resection also seem to require the second or third approach. The first two approaches accord well with the tradition of paternalism in which patients trust health care professionals to secure their welfare. The third approach, which is especially relevant for human subject research and other inherently risky therapies, involves telling the patient that because he is needed as a partner in the healing process, it is essential to give him information so that the partnership between patient and physician can produce its most effective results.

## Voluntary Consent

The last element that needs to be satisfied is that the consent must be genuinely voluntary. A voluntary action is one that is self-initiated rather than unduly governed or controlled by another person or institution. However, because the concept of a "self-initiated" act is somewhat abstract, it is frequently difficult to determine when an act is genuinely voluntary. The health care provider, at the very least, must take reasonable means to avoid unjustifiably controlling the patient's actions. This caution does not involve refusing to influence the behavior of a patient. Advice can influence behavior, and surely it does not destroy genuine voluntariness. Furthermore, expressions of approval and disapproval at a patient's choice often influence behavior. When a physician creatively demonstrates disapproval of a patient's smoking and recommends quitting, she is clearly trying to influence the patient's behavior. But these influences are not coercive because they do not involve threats.[15] An example of how health care professionals can exercise coercive control over a patient is by threatening to abandon a patient who does not comply with the professional's recommendations.

With human experimentation the problem of exercising controlling influence over subjects is especially problematic. Two ways in which the value of voluntariness is undermined in such research involves the use of poor people and the use of prisoners as subjects. The Tuskegee syphilis studies involved offering to poor black males such benefits as death insurance that they could never dream of securing without participating in the experiments. These studies were aimed at determining the long-term effects of syphilis on men. What made these studies especially unethical was the fact that effective treatment was withheld from these men in order to determine the exact course of the disease. In effect, the poverty of these men made them especially vulnerable to being exploited for medical purposes.[16]

Prisoners also offer a special problem associated with voluntary consent. Prisoners are often used as research subjects. According to Henry Beecher, it is difficult to imagine how the prisoner can be a genuinely voluntary subject if he is being offered the benefit of freedom or reduced incarceration for participating in research.[17] These offers are similar to financial offers made to desperately poor people. There is no explicit coercion present, but they are potentially exploitative because frequently prisoners have little or no opportunity to secure early release except by participating in a research.

However, this general reminder that the imprisoned lack the freedom to genuinely volunteer for research may motivate us to exclude the prisoner from participating in any biomedical research whatsoever. This motive can lead to denying the prisoner the benefits associated with research. For example, AIDS is a serious health problem for prisoners. Our desire to protect prisoners against violations of their freedom may inhibit researchers from offering to prisoners the opportunity to participate in AIDS-related research that may prove beneficial.

## The Case of Warren Hayes[18]

Warren Hayes was admitted to Community Hospital for surgical treatment of a duodenal ulcer. He signed the attached informed consent document prior to surgery by Dr. Andrew Stiles. His attending physician, Dr. Henry Smith, described Mr. Hayes as a "very excitable and occasionally irrational man." He warned Dr. Stiles not to excite him because under pressure he sometimes becomes very muddled and even unstable. Ten days after the surgery, complications developed. Mr. Hayes began to experience severe pain, and, when he went into shock, he was brought back to the hospital. Emergency surgery was performed and internal bleeding was discovered at the base of the spleen. The spleen was removed in this surgery. For about six weeks Mr. Hayes seemed to be doing quite well. However, in the eighth week after the first surgery, Mr. Hayes began to experience severe gastric pains that were diagnosed as being caused by a gastric ulcer. A third surgery was performed involving the removal of 50 percent of Mr. Hayes's stomach in order to reduce the stomach's ability to produce acid.

While hospitalized for his third surgery, he became aware of the existence of the ethics committee and called the chair, Dr. Collins. He was angry because he was not told about these possible consequences of the surgery. He said that Dr. Stiles had merely said that "there might be some problems with surgery, but that given my condition, it was best to have the surgery immediately." According to Mr. Hayes, Dr. Stiles had said that if problems did arise, that he (Dr. Stiles) and the staff could "take care of them." Mr. Hayes did admit to signing the attached informed consent document but said that he really did not understand what he was getting himself into. He requested that the committee review the case and make some recommendations. He said that he was not interested in suing anyone but he was angry with Dr. Stiles.

The consent form on page 126 was signed by Mr. Hayes.

### Committee Discussion of the Case

| | |
|---|---|
| Dr. Mary Collins: (Chair) | I like to open with each of us asking questions about the case. I have asked Dr. Warren, the chairperson of our surgery department, who has become familiar with the case, to respond to our concerns. |

---

## Consent to Operation or Other Procedure

Patient **Warren Hayes**    Date **January 15, 1993**    Time **1 PM**

I, <u>Warren Hayes</u>, hereby authorize <u>Dr. Andrew Stiles</u> (and whomever he may designate as his assistants) to perform the following operation:

**Surgical Treatment for Duodenal Ulcer**

and such additional operations or procedures as are considered necessary and/or advisable on the basis of findings during the course of such operation. I also consent to the administration of such anesthetics as are necessary, with the exception of

_____

(None, Spinal Anesthesia, or Other (specify)

<u>NONE    x   </u>

2.  Any tissue or parts surgically removed may be retained, preserved, used, or disposed of in accordance with accustomed practice.

3.  I am aware that the practice of medicine and surgery is not an exact science and I acknowledge that no guarantees have been made to me concerning the results of the operation or procedure(s).

4.  I hereby certify that I have read and fully understand the above CONSENT TO OPERATION OR OTHER PROCEDURE. I further certify that <u>Dr. Stiles</u> has explained to me the reasons the above-named surgery or procedure(s) is (are) considered necessary, the advantages, risks, and possible complications, if any, and possible alternative modes of treatment.

Signature of Patient/Guardian_____

WITNESS_____    SIGNATURE_____

WITNESS_____    SIGNATURE_____

| | |
|---|---|
| Dr. Philip Davis: | Can we get a clear picture of what Dr. Stiles told Mr. Hayes about this surgery? Perhaps a better way of putting this is, can we hear Dr. Stiles's side of the story? |
| Marian Rhodes: | This document that Stiles used as a means for securing Mr. Hayes's informed consent is the one that our committee is all too well aware of, and it is the one that we specifically rejected as an instrument for securing consent. Was Dr. Stiles aware of the committee's views on this kind of document? And, if so, why did he choose to use this document that we rejected? |
| Atty. John Quinn: | Has Mr. Hayes hired counsel to represent him? |
| Mary Quigley: | As a lay person, I am not sure whether surgeons usually provide this kind of information regarding possible repercussions of this surgery. Just how likely are these side effects? |
| Prof. Martin Fisk: | I am concerned about Mr. Hayes's competence. Was he interviewed by a psychologist to verify that he was irrational and unstable? Is there any evidence that the patient's judgment and rationality were impaired? |
| Dr. Collins: | Are there any other questions? I will entertain more questions as we go on, but, for now, let us turn the discussion over to Dr. Warren. |
| Dr. Warren: | I spoke to Dr. Stiles and to the primary care physician during the last three days, and I will transmit their views as best I can. To begin with, Stiles kept it very general with this patient because he was concerned about Dr. Smith's (Mr. Hayes's primary care physician) psychological evaluation. He felt that he was acting in the best interest of the patient because discussing all the possible complications could emotion- |

ally undermine the patient. According to
Dr. Stiles, Mr. Hayes was in severe gastric
distress and, without this surgery, he may
well have died. It was not, however, an
emergency case because he did have time to
secure the informed consent of the patient.

Regarding the question of the policy,
you folks on this committee have passed
this policy but you haven't submitted an
alternative form that can be used by the
surgeons. More fundamentally, you haven't
faced the problem of how to construct these
informed consent documents. Such informed consent documents would all be
very different from one another because all
the patients are so different and all the
problems are so different. I think that a
surgeon, for example, would have to spend
hours creating just one of these first-class
documents, which would contain every
possible alternative and every potential
risk. After constructing such a form she
would probably be too tired to perform the
surgery. In short, there are tremendous
practical difficulties associated with this
informed consent requirement. You seem to
be imposing on the medical staff obligations that are, if not impossible, then at least
very burdensome.  To answer Nurse
Rhodes's question directly, therefore, Dr.
Stiles was aware of the committee's guidelines, but he could not follow them.

Regarding the issue of whether Mr.
Hayes has secured legal counsel, I do not
think so. I think that he wants to see if he
can get some resolution of this problem at
this level.

Regarding the question of whether
surgeons routinely reveal this kind of
information prior to surgery, I think that
you will find a mixed bag of views on this
matter. If it were me, I would reveal that
this surgery is associated with a low

probability of internal bleeding and a recurrence of the ulcer problem. Surgery is a good treatment for this problem, but it is not risk free. I would feel that the surgeon is better off, for his own sake, to provide this information. For if the side effects happen, no one is shocked. It is when they are not informed that patients get angry.

Prof. Carla Thomas: But, Dr. Warren, do you think that it is a requirement to specifically reveal that internal bleeding may occur and that an additional ulcer may develop from this surgery? Do good physicians disagree about whether revealing this kind of information is an obligation? Or do you feel that surgeons have the right to withhold this information in certain circumstances?

Dr. Warren: If you are asking me whether surgeons *do* disagree as to what to tell their patients regarding the side effects of this surgery, my view is yes! There are plenty of surgeons who would support Dr. Stiles's decision to "keep it general" in order to secure the best interests of the patient. It is not my approach, but his strategy is one that is quite common.

Dr. Collins: But "keeping it general" means withholding relevant information.

Dr. Warren: Yes.

Prof. Thomas: There is a principle in medicine that is called "therapeutic privilege." It grants to health care providers the right to withhold medical information if divulging that information would probably be harmful to an emotionally depressed or unstable patient. Does this rule come into play here, Dr. Warren?

Dr. Warren: I think that it is terribly relevant here. Dr. Stiles made a good faith judgment involving the conflict that frequently emerges in medicine. The conflict is between the patient's right to make a decision based on all the relevant information and the best interests of the patient. Based on the attending physician's recommendation, Dr. Stiles exercised his therapeutic privilege. I think the phrase "therapeutic privilege" is a good one because I strongly believe that physicians should be able to have different attitudes concerning informed consent. This means that it is ethically perilous (and I am borrowing that stunning phrase that appears in your policy) to obligate physicians or health care providers to act in the same way toward all patients. These kinds of obligations tend to produce mechanical, unthinking doctors who do not have the ability to think for themselves and take responsibility for their own actions. I worry a lot about the "mental mechanization" that is taking place in medicine.

Dr. Collins:

Can you tell us what you mean by "mental mechanization"?

Dr. Warren:

When physicians are all placed under the same obligations and they are given little or no latitude in the application of those obligations, then we get mechanized physicians. We eliminate differences among physicians and suppress their individuality. Stiles exerted his therapeutic privilege in a situation where I would not have exercised mine.

Regarding the suggestions by the patient's primary care physician that we needed to keep him calm, I cannot speak to it. I have spoken to Mr. Hayes on three separate occasions and he seems psychologically sound to me. I would hesitate before I withheld information from him because I simply do not see sufficient emotional instability. However, I am not his primary care physician and I am not a psychiatrist. It is possible that I am not well informed about Mr. Hayes's history. I have not called for a psychological consultation on him because I do not see any initial symptoms that would cause me to call for such a consult. He was treated for depression following a divorce three years ago, but that is not enough for me to question his competence.

Prof. Fisk:

I agree with Dr. Warren that it is not wise to make judgments that a patient has an impaired emotional status without some symptoms or evidence of significant cognitive dysfunction or impairment. But specialists are traditionally very dependent on primary care physicians, and, when the primary care physician informs a surgeon that a patient is unstable, I think that it is proper to treat this as evidence. I am leaning toward interpreting this as falling within the category of therapeutic privilege.

Atty. Quinn:

Can I suggest that we slow down and start rethinking what we are doing here! This committee meeting is sounding a great deal like a trial in which we are discussing whether a particular physician violated the rule of informed consent. Is that what we are supposed to be doing here? It is certainly not what I signed on to do. Furthermore, we are in no way equipped to gather the relevant information upon which to make significant decisions. For example, a trial lawyer would call a lot of what is going on here "hearsay." In addition, we do not have an adversarial mechanism in which reputed evidence can be challenged and criticized. I signed on to this committee to assist at the level of ethics policy development and consultation. I did not wish to get involved in evaluating specific people.

Let me summarize my concerns by saying that we are not in any way a judicial body. We are advisory in nature. We should advise the hospital on ethics guidelines. Perhaps we can consult on particular cases with the aim of providing advice to the crucial decision makers. But we should not constitute ourselves as the hospital ethics police. This is counterproductive!

Prof. Thomas:

I think Mr. Quinn's advice is sound, and I too would caution us to avoid making ethical judgments concerning particular health care professionals who serve the hospital. Professionals have rights to fair treatment, and there is no way that this committee has the resources to guarantee that we are fairly treating the accused physician. The purpose of this committee is advisory and consultative, and we should avoid the business of evaluating particular physicians.

Vivian Harris:

How then should we approach this case?

Rev. Richard Marcus:

At the least, we should avoid the trap of becoming a pawn in Mr. Hayes's conflict with Dr. Stiles. Mr. Hayes is angry with Dr. Stiles and he wants us to become his agent in some sense. It is not our function to secure justice or revenge for anyone, and I do not recommend that we enter into this personal conflict. By the way, I do not want to imply that Mr. Hayes is right or wrong, but merely to suggest that we avoid becoming involved in deciding whether his anger toward Dr. Stiles is or is not legitimate.

Dr. Collins:

Can I take as the sentiment of the committee that we do not wish to get involved in particular positive or negative judgments about particular physicians or other health care providers? And that whatever recommendations we make be kept at the level of hospital policy?

There is general agreement on this issue.

| | |
|---|---|
| Ms. Harris: | Well, I still have my question, namely, what do you want to do with this case? |
| Atty. Quinn: | My recommendation is to remove it from discussion and let Mr. Hayes deal with Dr. Stiles by himself. If Dr. Stiles asked us to consult on this matter, I would have no objection if the committee offered him some very private and very confidential advice based on our understanding of medical ethics. But I feel that we may be intruding on the patient-doctor relationship without the consent of both parties in the relationship. It is also possible that although we try to keep this information private and confidential, this report may be subpoenaed by a court at some future date. |
| Prof. Fisk: | Perhaps we can treat this as an anonymous case and remove all the names and other identifying information. It will remain, therefore, an educational exercise that is used as a tool for educating the staff about the problems of informed consent. |
| Dr. Collins: | I think a better approach is to ask Dr. Stiles if he would consent to our acting as a consultant on the case. |
| Dr. Warren: | I am not a member of this committee, but I have spoken to Dr. Stiles and I believe that he would have no problem with the committee discussing the case. He believes that this case indicates the need for the committee to rethink its policy on informed consent, and I think that he would welcome the opportunity to discuss the issue with the committee. |
| Dr. Collins: | I am going to direct Martin Fisk to call Dr. Stiles and ask him whether he will consent to our participation in this case as a consultative body. Martin, would you mind making the call? |

Martin Fisk leaves and returns in ten minutes.

| | |
|---|---|
| Prof. Fisk: | I called his office and the secretary put me through right away. He has consented to being reviewed by the committee. He also expressed the feeling that we have passed a very impractical policy and he hopes that this case will show that this committee should not get involved in informed consent matters. I offered him the opportunity to come and make a statement to the committee. I also told him what Dr. Warren has said, and he feels that we have all the relevant information. |
| Dr. Davis: | Well, that settles it for me. If both parties have agreed that this case can be discussed, then as long as we maintain strict privacy in our deliberation and recommendations, I see no problem with continuing. |
| Atty. Quinn: | This relieves a lot of my anxieties, but there is still the possibility of litigation in this case, so let's walk very carefully. Also, it is more than slightly dangerous to enter between parties in conflict. Our treatment of this case may not resolve the conflict. Indeed, it may increase the level of conflict. I am sorry to be so pessimistic, but ethics committees should not expect that they can function as resolvers of conflict. Frequently, conflict cannot be satisfactorily resolved. |
| Prof. Fisk: | Let's get back to the case! We left with Dr. Warren asserting that there is room for disagreement on this case and that good faith physicians could disagree about whether to withhold information based on therapeutic privilege. I tend to agree with this assessment. |
| Prof. Thomas: | I do not agree with this assessment. Mr. Hayes was not incompetent. It was not an emergency. He did not waive his right to informed consent. All that happened was that the primary care doctor characterized the patient as unstable. This judgment was |

not made by or verified by a psychiatrist or other mental health care provider. More importantly, Dr. Stiles did nothing to substantiate his "feeling" that therapeutic privilege could be invoked. If the last 20 years of advocacy on the issue of patient rights means anything, it means that invoking therapeutic privilege is a serious matter and should not be done without going through a well-thought-out process. From what I can see, no such well-thought-out process was followed by Dr. Stiles. He simply went on his gut feeling and the primary care physician's characterization.

Ms. Quigley:    But what about Dr. Stiles's contention that he could not secure Mr. Hayes's informed consent?

Ms. Harris:    Society requires this, not the committee. I think that professionals have the responsibility to secure the informed consent of their clients, and I think that the hospital should not take on itself this responsibility. The hospital is the site at which many patient-professional relationships take place, but that doesn't mean that the hospital has the duty to secure informed consent. This is a physician's duty! Furthermore, the hospital is not imposing this obligation on Dr. Stiles. Our society has granted Dr. Stiles the right to practice medicine, and, in return, the society expects that he will respect his patient's right to be informed. It is his duty, not the hospital's, to secure informed consent. Our policy is serving to remind the professionals at the hospital that this obligation is one that cannot be fulfilled by very general descriptions of procedures that do not contain the relevant information.

Rev. Marcus:    This is a matter that we talked about at length while we were discussing and constructing the informed consent policy. And I think that there was widespread agreement that informed consent was the responsibility of the attending physician and that, if the attending physician was an employee of the hospital, then the hospital would become at least partially responsible for securing informed consent. One of the reasons we pressed forward with this policy was that many of the physicians providing care are employees of the hospital, and therefore in these cases the hospital may become partially responsible for making sure that our employees secure the informed consent of the patients. We are setting goals for our staff and the attending physicians who practice in this hospital.

Atty. Quinn:     My major problem with this policy is that it places an additional burden on physicians. It requires them to secure written rather than verbal informed consent. Why should we demand this?

Prof. Thomas:    This is not exactly true. Physicians always had to provide written documents that had to be filled out prior to surgery, but they were vague. They affirmed that the physician had communicated the relevant information. They were not explicit with respect to the relevant information. The choice, therefore, is not between verbal and written consent but between written documents that contain specific information and written documents that do not contain this information. Furthermore, I think our case gives us an excellent answer to why specific rather than vague documents are preferable. Dr. Stiles, by his own admission, did not meet the standards of the policy. He withheld crucial information that Dr. Warren considers "relevant information." It was easy for Stiles to withhold the information because nothing needed to be stated in writing. His exercise of therapeutic privilege did not have to stand up to critical review. As long as the informed consent process remains informal and merely verbal, abuse will continue.

Dr. Davis:

Carla, you are assuming that there was abuse in this case.

Prof. Thomas:

I think that is more than a mere assumption. He withheld relevant information without solid evidence that significant harm would follow from disclosure. He did nothing to verify the incompetence hypothesis. Nevertheless, he acted on it. Furthermore, as far as I can see, he did not contact Mr. Hayes's family. Surely if Mr. Hayes were incompetent, Dr. Stiles should have contacted someone who could speak and act for Mr. Hayes. Finally, Dr. Davis is ready to excuse his behavior as a legitimate exercise of therapeutic privilege. I am not so convinced that the principle of therapeutic privilege, which Dr. Stiles used to justify his withholding relevant information, is an acceptable principle. This is a principle that was used for thousands of years as a basis for physicians acting in a paternalist fashion. Physicians used it to withhold terminal illness information. They used it to withhold information concerning options in the treatment of cancer. It is a principle that has been very much used to undermine patient autonomy, and I am extremely skeptical of it.

Dr. Davis:

Are you suggesting that medicine can do without this principle?

Prof. Thomas:

I would not endorse this principle without first demanding some general conditions for when it can be used. For example, I think that it should only be invoked with

|              | consent of a surrogate. Furthermore, I think that review processes have to be instituted for exercising the privilege. |
|---|---|
| Prof. Fisk: | Carla raises some important objections to the principle of therapeutic privilege, but I think that an attending physician who describes his patient as "unstable" is sufficient to warrant the exercise of the privilege. |
| Rev. Marcus: | I am surprised by your support for the privilege, Martin, since consequentialists usually argue that the principle of autonomy is so vital for securing human welfare, and it seems that an unrestricted principle of therapeutic privilege threatens patient autonomy. |
| Prof. Fisk: | The issue in this case is not my support for informed consent. Rather, it is the matter of whether Stiles had sufficient evidence to override the autonomy rule. I agree that we might want to increase the requirements for exercising the privilege, and that by tomorrow's standards, we might find that Stiles falls short, but by today's standards, I think he had enough justification to invoke his authority to withhold information. I would trust the attending physician's advice. |
| Ms. Quigley: | We need to address another issue in this case. Doesn't this discussion assume that professionals determine what constitutes adequate disclosure? If professionals in the field reveal the information, then the information needs to be revealed. But in our policy didn't we explicitly reject this professional standard because it placed too much authority in the hands of the professional? I thought that we had adopted a standard of "adequate disclosure" that was oriented toward the rights of the patient. |

Isn't that why we affirmed principle 3D, which asserts that adequate information is defined in terms of what a reasonable person would want to know? What matters for informed consent is not what professionals typically tell patients. What matters is that the professional provide information that a reasonable patient would want to know. What matters in terms of adequate disclosure is whether a reasonable person would want this information, and I think there is little doubt about this. A reasonable person would want to have this information. I certainly would want to be told this information in this situation.

Dr. Davis:

I do not agree that issues surrounding principle 3D are the main considerations in this case. First, I had a great deal of difficulty accepting 3D during our original meetings on the policy. I finally accepted it because Atty. Quinn maintained that it was the standard used by most courts in dealing with informed consent issues. I accept his opinion on the legal question, but it is a very vague standard, and it does not give the professional a practical guideline for achieving informed consent. In short, I accepted 3D because of its legal status, not because it was, in my opinion, an ethically solid definition. Secondly, I am not so sure that a reasonable man would never want information withheld.

Let me explain what I mean. If I were perfectly rational today and knew that tomorrow I was going to be unstable and that certain information if revealed would harm me, then I might authorize the withholding of that information. In short, a rational person might consent to what Dr. Stiles did if we assume that he was as emotionally unstable as his primary care physician believed.

| | |
|---|---|
| Prof. Thomas: | Health care providers spend a lot of time distinguishing competent persons from incompetent persons. It makes all the sense to treat these types of people differently. But Mr. Hayes was not incompetent. He had cognitive functioning. There is nothing in the case to indicate that he could not understand the consequences of refusing surgery. He may well have accepted the surgery even if he were informed. Notice that the primary care physician never said that Hayes was incompetent, and yet Dr. Stiles treated Hayes as an incompetent. |
| Prof. Fisk: | Prof. Thomas thinks that incompetence is necessary to invoke therapeutic privilege, but this is false. Something weaker is required, namely, diminished competence. In our case I agree that Mr. Hayes was not incompetent, but I think that it is reasonable to say that his competence was diminished. Even though this concept of diminished competence is legally vague, physicians know that many patients have diminished competence and frequently health care providers tailor information in accordance with a patient's capacities. I want to be faithful to this reality even though competence seems to be a black and white matter in law. |
| Ms. Quigley: | But, Martin, what does our policy say? Does it say that information can be tailored to fit individuals with diminished competence? Does it say that if an attending physician calls a patient "unstable," then the patient is unstable? Does it say that being called unstable is sufficient to mean that a patient has diminished competence? Does it say that having diminished competence makes you incompetent? It does not say any of these things. It merely says that health care providers should disclose the relevant evidence that a reasonable person would want. I think that if you look at the |

|  | policy and then ask the simple question, "Did Dr. Stiles follow the policy?" the answer is a simple and straightforward "no!" |
|---|---|
| Prof. Fisk: | I think that Mary is making this issue far too black and white. There are shades of gray here, and I do not think the intent of our policy was to gloss over these shades. |
| Ms. Quigley: | Martin is right and he is also wrong. He is right in the sense that revealing the relevant information to Mr. Hayes may have led Mr. Hayes to refuse permission to operate. He may not have been able to emotionally deal with a tough choice. But Martin is wrong in assuming that the mere possibility that he might have done something imprudent justifies overriding his right. His instability makes the job of securing consent more complex, but it does not remove the obligation from the health care provider. I think Hayes was a tough case and Dr. Stiles did not want to spend extra time with him in order to secure his consent. Time is money. |
| Rev. Marcus: | It is important to remind everyone here that these issues were discussed frequently when we were designing this policy. We expected that there were going to be problems like this. We agreed that we wanted to influence the behavior of health care providers with respect to informed consent, and that changing this behavior was not going to be easy. I think that we should see this case as the first of many and that we need to take seriously Dr. Warren's recommendation that we get about the business of preparing better informed consent documents for the health care providers who use this facility. |

Isn't there something that we can do in terms of computerizing a host of similar forms that serve to really inform our patients? It seems to me that a standard form for Mr. Hayes's operation could be constructed with enough room for the doctor to insert any individualized information about specific procedures. Is this so impossible?

Atty. Quinn:    I want to emphasize that we avoid making the hospital responsible for the quality of informed consent. I have no problem with the idea in general, but it is a physician's responsibility, not the hospital's responsibility.

Dr. Collins:    I think that we have covered this aspect of the case. Are there other areas that need to be discussed?

Ms. Rhodes:    I too think that we have covered the relevant issues in this case and that we should now turn to the issue of making a recommendation. Should we issue a statement to the parties or should we make a recommendation in our minutes or what? What are we to do with this case?

Atty. Quinn:    My answer is that we should reach agreement on whether Dr. Stiles should have informed Mr. Hayes and that we should privately inform Dr. Stiles of that judgment. Furthermore, we should inform Mr. Hayes that the committee has discussed the case with Dr. Stiles and that dealing with this case has improved the quality of care at the hospital. I do not think that we should reveal our private communications with Dr. Stiles to Mr. Hayes.

Dr. Collins:    Do we have a strong consensus on this matter? Dr. Davis and Prof. Fisk seem to think that withholding the information was justified by therapeutic privilege. Is there anyone else that sides with withholding the information? John Quinn has given us a number of judicial warnings, but he has not given us an opinion. John, what do you think?

| | |
|---|---|
| Atty: Quinn: | I have mixed feelings. I sympathize with the plight of the professional. I am in similar situations very often in legal practice, and I respect the difficulties faced by Dr. Stiles. However, our policy is quite clear. Hayes was not incompetent, and, therefore, he needed to be informed. Malpractice lawyers get rich with cases like this. Withholding the information was improper. But let's be careful with respect to how we address this matter. |
| Dr. Collins: | This is very difficult for me because I know Dr. Stiles very well. We went to medical school together and he was very instrumental in bringing me here as medical director. He is a first-rate surgeon and I think that he was acting in good faith when he withheld the information. |
| Prof. Thomas: | I know that you are struggling with this one because of your friendship with Dr. Stiles, but let me remind you that there is an ancient and very venerable distinction between evaluating actions and evaluating persons. Good persons often commit bad actions. Bad actions are often initiated by individuals with motives that are often not only good but also praiseworthy. We are not evaluating Dr. Stiles as a person. In fact, based on the evidence that I have heard, he was probably acting from a caring and concerned motive. What we are evaluating is the action of withholding information in this case. |
| Dr. Collins: | Thank you, Carla, for understanding my dilemma. My sense is to follow Carla's lead and develop a recommendation criticizing the action, despite the fact that it was based on the best of medical motives. Carla, do you want to take a shot at developing a recommendation? |
| Prof. Thomas: | How does this sound? |

Based on a review of the case involving Mr. Warren Hayes and Dr. Andrew Stiles, it is the opinion of this ethics committee that Dr. Stiles should have informed Mr. Hayes about the possible side effects of gastric surgery. The committee also believes that, while there was an error of action committed, there is every reason to believe that it was an error based on concern for the patient's well-being. We further recommend that Martin Fisk communicate these findings to both parties.

| | |
|---|---|
| Dr. Collins: | Is there discussion of the recommendation? |
| Dr. Davis: | From the point of the medical staff, I think that this is a very unbalanced recommendation. It does not address the practical problem faced by health care providers. How do you provide Mercedes Benz–quality informed consent in a hospital that runs on a Chevrolet budget? It is a very big job that will require a substantial change in the behavior of our staff. Furthermore, this kind of a demand has the potential of being ignored by health care providers, especially if preparing these forms will take us away from patient care. Let me be brutal about this. We have trouble keeping staff, and I think that this recommendation will create a thunderstorm of resentment throughout the hospital. And do not delude yourself about privacy or confidentiality! This news will be public within 24 hours. |
| Dr. Collins: | We are going to have to address Dr. Davis's concerns. I know that when I was in private practice I did not spend a great deal of time on informed consent. Informed consent has been on everyone's lips in the past 20 years, but now we are going to obligate the staff to alter their behavior in a significant way. We risk being ignored. |
| Prof. Thomas: | Dr. Davis is raising a red herring. The issue here is not about complex documents. Stiles never even verbally communicated with Hayes about the potential side effects. This is the central issue. |

| | |
|---|---|
| Ms. Rhodes: | I know that the nursing staff is going to flip if we start obligating them to spend a lot of time on informed consent. Every nursing unit could stand a substantial increase in staff, and, realistically, that is not going to happen in the short term. They are swamped with patient care concerns and they're not going to forsake patient care in order to increase the quality of informed consent. I agree that these are important matters, but we are already short-handed. |
| Prof. Fisk: | May I suggest an addition to the recommendation that addresses this issue? |
| Dr. Collins: | By all means, Martin. |
| Prof. Fisk: | I suggest that we add the following sentence to the recommendation: "The hospital is currently studying ways to improve the quality of informed consent documents that are used at the hospital." |
| Atty. Quinn: | This is a difficult sentence because the hospital does not want to be responsible for informed consent. We have enough responsibilities and liabilities. This sentence seems to indicate that we are taking the responsibility for this very difficult task when it should be the responsibility of individual practitioners. |
| Prof. Thomas: | I agree with Atty. Quinn that we are going on record as taking some responsibility for those who practice here, but it is a partial responsibility. It is the responsibility of constructing better informed consent documents. Let me illustrate what I mean. I think that Mr. Hayes should have been given a general informed consent document for intractable duodenal ulcer surgery. It would contain some information that perhaps was irrelevant to his particular case, but it could be used as a basis for the surgeon and Mr. Hayes to really enter into |

a solid discussion on the risks and benefits associated with the surgery. The job of the practitioner is then to tailor the general form to the patient and also answer questions regarding the general form. This would give the surgeon a way out of designing the entire form and yet would improve the quality of informed consent.

Dr. Collins:    Let's not forget that we are an advisory committee and that these recommendations are going to have to be reviewed by the chief executive officer of the hospital. He has vowed to keep the hospital in the black this year. In short, it is a time of scarce resources here at Community Hospital, and if this suggestion is going to increase our costs of operation, I doubt whether he will approve it. Are we ready to consider Martin's addition to the recommendation?

The committee agrees to bring the matter to a vote, and Martin Fisk's addition is approved by a margin of 8 to 1.

*Committee Recommendations*    Based on review of the case involving Mr. Warren Hayes and Dr. Andrew Stiles, it is the opinion of this ethics committee that Dr. Stiles should have informed Mr. Hayes concerning the possible side effects of gastric surgery. The committee also believes that, while there was an error of action committed, there is every reason to believe that it was an error based on concern for the patient's well-being. We further recommend that Martin Fisk communicate these findings to both parties. The hospital is currently studying ways to improve the quality of informed consent documents that are used at the hospital.

### Questions for Further Discussion

1. Has the committee given adequate consideration to the problem of communicating complex and possibly frightening information to uneducated patients?
2. Have they overly tied the hands of health care providers by overrestricting their right to exercise therapeutic privilege?

3. Has the committee given too much weight to individual autonomy and thus underemphasized the importance of patient welfare?
4. Imagine that you are Martin Fisk and that you have just informed Mr. Hayes of the committee's recommendation. Assume that Mr. Hayes is unsatisfied and then construct a list of reasons for this dissatisfaction. Respond to this dissatisfaction.
5. Imagine that you are Martin Fisk and that you have just informed Dr. Stiles of the committee's recommendation. Assume that he too is dissatisfied. Construct a list of reasons for this dissatisfaction. Respond to this dissatisfaction.
6. The committee did not seem to give a great deal of support to the notion that professionals should determine what constitutes adequate disclosure. What are some of the strengths and weaknesses of the professional standard of disclosure?
7. Suppose another patient in the exact some circumstances as Mr. Hayes presented himself to another surgeon on the staff of Community Hospital within a week after the committee's recommendation became widely known. Assume further that he, unlike Mr. Hayes, was fully informed. Suppose further that, due to the somewhat frightening information that was contained in the informed consent procedure, he refused surgery and died within one month. How might some of the committee members respond?
8. How would you respond to the case mentioned in question 7?
9. Are the administrative problems mentioned in the Hayes's case relevant to the ethical consideration? Why? Why not?
10. Atty. Quinn insists that informed consent should be the responsibility of the physician and that the hospital should not get involved in this aspect of patient care. Is he right? Why? Why not? What level of responsibility should the hospital take with respect to informed consent?

## More Cases Involving the Policy

### Muscular Dystrophy and the Adolescent

Warren Smith is 15 years old. In addition to having muscular dystrophy, he is also an Eagle Scout who has received over 15 Boy Scout badges for community service. Much of this service has been related to speaking that he has done before public meetings on the subject of his disease. His doctors consider this young man a full partner in his treatment because he is so well informed. His parents have also been model parents in terms of cooperating in the management of his disease. They love their son and he has been a genuine joy to them.

However, for the last few months his disease has grown steadily worse. He has been hospitalized and his breathing has deteriorated. He has been intubated, and his physicians have told both Warren and his parents that they cannot stop the decline that the disease is producing. Warren's knowledge of the disease has prepared him for this eventuality, and he has informed the doctors that he does not wish to be ventilated any further. He wants to die. His physicians believe that this decision is a reasonable one, but Warren's parents refuse to consent. They want their son maintained on the ventilator in the hope that he will recover.

### Transplantation and Informed Consent

The need for organs for transplantation far outreaches their availability. One main cause for this shortage is that physicians must secure individuals' informed consent to remove their organs after their death. In the absence of the dead person's consent, the physician must secure the consent of the appropriate guardian. Without consent no organ can be removed from a dead person for transplantation. One week ago a surgeon at Community Hospital removed two kidneys, a liver, and a heart and in the process saved four lives. No guardian was available and the dead man did not carry a uniform donor card. The surgeon argued that he had "presumed consent" to do so because he talked to the man's friend, who thought that the man would approve. No other formal guardian was available. How should the hospital ethics committee manage this case?

### Depression and Informed Consent

One month ago John Peterson, a 47-year-old man, was admitted to Community Hospital's adult psychiatric ward with severe depression following the death of his wife and child in a car accident. He was the driver of the car and he blames himself for the accident. He seems unresponsive to counseling and is being treated with antidepressants. He began to refuse food and water two weeks ago, and he is now being force-fed with a great deal of difficulty. He claims that he wants to be left alone so that he can die. He is quite articulate about this desire and maintains that he has no reason to continue living. The staff responsible for forcing food on him find this activity repulsive. They have injured him and the bruises on his face are now quite severe. The physician in charge of his care is considering having a naso-gastric tube inserted and restraining Mr. Peterson so that he cannot remove the tube. The head nurse within the unit has brought the case before the committee and states that Mr. Peterson is being harmed by the coercive treatment. She also thinks that the treatment is "brutalizing" her staff nurses. How should the committee manage this case?

## The Drunk and Informed Consent

"Jim" came into the emergency room of Community Hospital. He gave no last name. He lived on the streets and he said that he drank quite a bit of wine every day. He gave off a strong odor of alcohol, but he was answering questions and talking with the staff. He was experiencing a good deal of gastric discomfort and was coughing up a brownish colored blood. The staff was concerned that he might have a gastric bleed, and they wanted to insert a scope down his throat in order to make a diagnosis. Jim did not want anything sent down his throat. He said that he hated anything being put down his throat. The doctor did everything possible to convince him that it necessary to do this, but Jim refused.

The doctor in charge then called two orderlies. He ordered them to restrain Jim. The doctor then "scoped" Jim against his will. He discovered a severe bleed. Emergency surgery was performed. The emergency room doctor claims that this action probably saved Jim's life.

The case was brought to the committee by an emergency room resident who felt that Jim's right to informed consent was violated.

## Further Reading

Brody, H., *Ethical Decisions in Medicine*, 2nd ed. (Boston: Little, Brown, 1981).

Capron, Alexander, "Informed Consent in Catastrophic Disease Research and Treatment," *University of Pennsylvania Law Review* 123 (December 1974): 340–438.

Dworkin, Gerald, "Autonomy and Informed Consent," in President's Commission for the Study of Ethical Problems in Medicine and Biomedical and Behavioral Research, *Making Health Care Decisions: The Ethical and Legal Implications of Informed Consent in the Patient-Practitioner Relationship*, vol. 3: Appendices, Studies on the Foundations of Informed Consent (Washington, D.C.: U.S. Government Printing Office, 1982).

Engelhardt, H. Tristram, Jr., *The Foundations of Bioethics* (New York: Oxford University Press, 1986).

Faden, Ruth R., and Tom L. Beauchamp, *A History and Theory of Informed Consent* (New York: Oxford University Press, 1986).

Freedman, Benjamin, "A Moral Theory of Informed Consent," *Hastings Center Report* 5 (August 1975): 32–39.

Meisel, Alan, Loren H. Roth, and Charles W. Lidz, "Toward a Model of the Legal Doctrine of Informed Consent," *American Journal of Psychiatry* 134 (1977): 285–289.

President's Commission for the Study of Ethical Problems in Medicine and Biomedical and Behavioral Research, *Making Health Care Decisions: The Ethical and Legal Implications of Informed Consent in the Patient-Practitioner Relationship*, vols. 1–3 (Washington, D.C.: U.S. Government Printing Office, 1982).

Pelligrino, E. O., and D. C. Thomasma, *A Philosophical Basis of Medical Ethics*, (New York: Oxford University Press, 1981).

Veatch, Robert M., *A Theory of Medical Ethics* (New York: Basic Books, 1981).

Veatch, Robert M., "Three Theories of Informed Consent: Philosophical Foundations and Policy Implications," *The Belmont Report: Ethical Principles and Guidelines for the Protection of Human Subjects of Research*, in Appendix B, DHEW Publication No. (OS) 78-0014 (Washington, D.C.: U.S. Government Printing Office, 1978). Vol. II, (26-I)-(26-66).

## Notes

1. *Schloendorff v. Society of New York Hospital*, 211 NY 125, 105 NE 92, 95 (1914).
2. *Salgo v. Leland Stanford Jr. University Board of Trustees*. 154 Cal. App. 2d. 560, 317 p. 2d 170 (1957).
3. Herbert Benson, and Mark Epstein, "The Placebo Effect: A Neglected Aspect in the Care of Patients," *Journal of the American Medical Association* 232 (1975):1225.
4. Eugene G. Laforet, "The Fiction of Informed Consent," *Journal of the American Medical Association* 235 (April 12, 1976): 1579–1585.
5. Jay Katz, *The Silent World of Doctor and Patient* (New York: The Free Press, 1984).
6. Hippocrates, "Decorum," in *Hippocrates*, vol. 2, trans. W. H. Jones, 4 vols., The Loeb Classical Library (New York: G. P. Putnam's Sons, 1923), pp. 296–299.
7. The major exception to this rule involves incompetent patients in emergencies.
8. Tom Beauchamp, "Informed Consent," in *Medical Ethics*, ed. Robert Veatch (Boston: Jones and Bartlett Publishers, 1989), pp. 173–200.
9. This claim is emphasized in the important case of *Canterbury v. Spense*.
10. The Hippocratic tradition in medicine represents this paternalistic model.
11. Contracts are written between insurance companies, who represent classes of patients, and health care–providing institutions. This is the basis for saying that the contractual model is still present within medicine.
12. William F. May, "Code, Covenant Contract, or Philanthropy?" *Hastings Center Report* 5 (December 1975): 24–28.

13. Allan Buchanan, and Dan Brock, "Deciding for Others: Competency," *The Millbank Quarterly* 64 (Supp. 2) (1986).
14. Franz Ingelfinger, "Informed (but Uneducated) Consent," *New England Journal of Medicine* 287 (1972): 455–56.
15. Bernard Gert has argued that coercion requires threats and that in the absence of threats we cannot speak of a person being coerced. See Bernard Gert, "Coercion and Freedom," *Coercion: Nomos XIV*, ed. J. Pennock and John Chapman (New York: Aldine, 1972).
16. For a thorough discussion of the ethical issues that were involved in the Tuskegee studies, see James Jones' *Bad Blood* (New York: Free Press, 1981).
17. Henry K. Beecher, *Research and the Individual: Human Studies* (Boston: Little, Brown, 1970).
18. This case is adapted from *Cobbs v. Grant*, 8 Cal. 3d 229, 104 Cal. Rptr. 505, 502 p.2d 1 (1972).

# 5

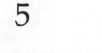

# Reproductive Rights: Surrogacy

## Introduction to the Problem Area

Despite the fact that we often fantasize about medicine's "good old days" when ethical problems were few and far between, the history of medicine shows us quite clearly that the "good old days" never existed. Reproduction illustrates this point. Conflict about procreation among mothers, fathers, fetuses, society, religions, and others often took place against a medical background. Questions concerning sterilization, contraception, and abortion have been treated as "medical-ethical" problems. However, during the last 30 years, the truism that medicine, reproduction, and ethics are vitally linked has been demonstrated beyond any doubt. Developments in reproductive technology have precipitated new ethical challenges. New terms like *in vitro fertilization, fetal tissue transplants, embryo micromanipulation, gamete intrafallopian transfer, surrogate gestation, cryopreservation,* and *DNA sampling* have been introduced. Once again the "miracles" of modern technology force us to reconsider our values regarding reproduction. While these technologies provide immense benefits for thousands of human beings, they also threaten us with images from Aldous Huxley's famous novel *Brave New World*.

In the future of Huxley's novel, reproduction is completely dehumanized and mechanized by a dictatorial government. This "new order" treats children as manufactured objects who are little more than commodities. If the product does not come up to "someone's" standards, it is rejected. "Quality control" is finally achieved in reproduction. The heart of this dehumanization of reproduction is not just the "loss of reproductive rights" but the removal of the family "as a way of life." Families become useless. Individual men and women no longer control their own reproductive lives. Birthing is a centrally controlled manufactured process. Once the society gains the power to perform technological "miracles," it uses this power to

reduce persons to things. In the process something of indescribable value is
lost.

## Two Attitudes toward Technology

The power of *Brave New World* is connected to the growth of reproductive
technology and the inevitable expansion of human control over reproduction.
However, there are at least two different attitudes toward this inevitability.
First, human beings can just adapt to the novel technology, and if we must
sacrifice some values to accommodate this adaptation, then so be it! In the
context of Huxley's novel, the values associated with family, gestation,
birthing, and child rearing seem to have been completely sacrificed in order
to accommodate the new technology. This represents the *technological
determinist attitude* because values are created or destroyed not by human
choice but by technology. From the viewpoint of the technological
determinist, technology is the mother of all human values.

By contrast, *the autonomous attitude* assumes that values associated with
gestation, birthing, and child rearing can be retained and preserved despite
the development of new reproductive technology. Indeed, these values can
determine how the new technology is used. In the autonomous view our
values can survive a technological transformation and can control how the
technology affects humanity. A person with an autonomous attitude assumes
that our technology can and should be adapted to our values.

## The Basis of the Surrogacy Conflict

Surrogacy is a recent social practice that involves the conception, gestation,
and transfer of a child from a woman who gestates a child for another person
or couple who raises the child. Members of the Community Hospital ethics
committee have ethical differences play a very large role in the committee's
discussion. These differences flow from opposing interpretations of the
three principles that dominate bioethics: the "do no harm" rule, the "respect
autonomy" rule, and the "benefit the patient" rule. Some members of the
committee believe that surrogacy arrangements will harm the parties
involved. For example, protracted custody battles over children may occur.
Some believe that surrogacy will harm society as a whole by exploiting
women. Furthermore, the debate about surrogacy is so strong because
autonomy plays a vital role in reproduction and surrogacy.

Many members of the committee believe that individuals have the
right, based on autonomy, to decide for themselves whether to engage in
surrogacy arrangements. However, some members think that society must
restrict this right in order to prevent potential harms associated with

surrogacy. Others believe that medicine has a long tradition of respect for different value systems, so if an individual competently chooses to enter a surrogacy arrangement, then the hospital should refuse to interfere. Finally, the hospital is committed to securing the benefit of patients, and there is some hope that surrogacy may reduce the problems associated with infertility. The committee will decide the question of surrogacy by "balancing" these conflicting values.

## Surrogacy and the Women's Movement

But attitudinal differences toward technology and disagreements over the application of fundamental values are not the only sources for debate in the area of reproduction. The social relations between adult women and men have changed more in the past 30 years than they did in the previous 300. For example, most married women now work outside the home. The single parent family is commonplace. The number of women who earn a college degree has skyrocketed in the last 30 years. The number of women in powerful political positions throughout the world has also burgeoned. Women are beginning to realize their political, economic, and social potentiality. The women's movement continues to influence this transformation.

The women's movement has not only altered our economic, political, and social landscape, it has altered the philosophical landscape as well. Feminist approaches to ethics are developing and influencing our understanding of surrogacy. Women now seek all the rights that Thomas Paine once referred to as the "Rights of Man," and one of the most important rights that women demand is the right to control their own reproductive lives. Many women now insist that they control their reproductive lives, by having not only the right to abortion but the right to enter into surrogacy arrangements.

But the feminist movement is not altogether unified over the question of surrogacy. While many feminists view surrogacy as a means of enhancing a woman's control over her body, others view surrogacy contracts as a threat to feminist values. These opponents view surrogacy as another opportunity for "exploiting women," especially poor women. In most cases of surrogacy, they argue that upper-middle-class couples are buying the bodies of poor women. Rather than enhancing the lives of women in general, surrogacy merely creates a new way to "use" women for the convenience of the wealthy.

The presence of significant debate over the surrogacy issue among feminists is another indication that a social revolution is taking place in conjunction with a technological revolution, and both are happening in the context of conflict over basic values. The surrogacy issue, therefore, will call upon all the collective wisdom of our hospital ethics committee because its members must manage a technological, a social, and an ethical revolution. You can decide how well they cope with this challenge.

## Background on the Surrogacy Policy

Most hospitals do not have surrogacy policies. Two factors motivated Community Hospital to develop one. First, since the 1960s the technology involved in artificially uniting human sperm and eggs has developed at a very fast rate. The ovum can be fertilized artificially through insemination (in vivo) or outside the womb (in vitro). In the former case, the ovum is fertilized without being removed from the woman. In the latter case, the ovum is removed from a woman's body and fertilized "in a dish," then after fertilization, the embryo is transferred either into the woman from whom it was removed or into another woman. This sometimes produces some strange new relationships: for instance, a child has already been born to a gestational mother who is also the child's genetic grandmother. Embryos can also be united in vitro (outside the womb) and transferred to a gestational mother who is completely unrelated genetically to the embryo. These are but two of the possibilities that have emerged from this technological development. These new options clearly have created new challenges for physicians, philosophers, jurists, and society as a whole.

Many terms may be used to describe the parties involved in the surrogacy context. In this text, we will refer to the woman who gestates the embryo as the *surrogate mother* or the *gestational mother*. The individuals who supply the ova and sperm are the *genetic parents*, the individuals who plan to raise the child are the *environmental parents*. Frequently, through not necessarily, the environmental parents are the genetic parents. Most frequently, the genetic or environmental parents contract with the surrogate or gestational mother to provide the needed service.

The second factor that caused the Community Hospital to act was that two members of its ob-gyn department, Drs. King and Brewster, are vitally interested in providing services to infertile individuals. At first these physicians initiated action independently of the committee. However, when legal as well as political problems confronted both the hospital and the physicians, the Board of Trustees asked the committee to carry out a thorough review of the issues. Furthermore, the board requested that the committee develop some guidelines on surrogacy, which were then approved by a majority of committee members. To respect the dissenting viewpoints, reasons for and against the policy are presented.

## Community Hospital's Surrogacy Policy

*Definition:*    Surrogacy will stand for the activity of artificially inseminating or transferring an embryo into a woman who will gestate the fetus and then transfer the infant after birth to another person or couple. The goal of surrogacy is to provide an infertile couple or person with the opportunity to have a child that is genetically related to them.

This procedure is medically indicated for women who are incapable of supplying an ovum or who are incapable of providing the gestational aspect of reproduction. As such, it is a tool in treating some forms of infertility. For example, a woman may have functioning ovaries but lack a uterus. Or she may have another disease that mitigates against her becoming pregnant.

*Principles:*

1. Under limited circumstances, it is ethically permitted to employ the surrogacy procedure within this hospital. The committee recommends that it be initiated for medically indicated reasons. If medical indications are not present, the procedure is not recommended.
2. The procedure should be treated as a scientific protocol or experiment that is being used for investigational reasons. One cannot determine whether any harms will actually occur without employing the technique of the clinical experiment. Another reason for treating surrogate arrangements in this fashion is that such arrangements will require the hospital to make sure that the involved parties are well informed about the risks they are undertaking and that their actions may generate some harmful consequences to themselves. All parties to the arrangement are to be treated as research subjects and, thus, as having all the rights associated with that position. [See Chapter 9 for a more detailed discussion of the ethical issues involved in human subject research.]
3. All contracts that are involved in the procedure will be approved by the legal department of the hospital. If the legal department does not approve the contracts, no procedure will take place at the hospital. The hospital has a prudential duty to the community to avoid placing itself at unjustified levels of risk, hence, the law department of the hospital should be apprised of all agreements surrounding the procedure.
4. No conditions of the contract will interfere with the gestational mother's right to abort the fetus subject to the limitations set forth in *Roe* v. *Wade*. Nor will any provision of the contract limit any other rights of control that the gestational mother exercises over her body.

5. Every participant will voluntarily sign an informed consent document that fully discloses all the relevant risks and benefits involved in the procedure. This informed consent document will outline not only the risks but also the alternatives that may be open to the parties. This document will emphasize that all parties are free to withdraw from the protocol at any time.
6. Appropriate investigational follow-up will be required of all participants so that an adequate data base for evaluating the harms and benefits of the procedure can be compiled. This data base should involve both the physical and psychosocial effects on the parties involved.
7. No procedure will be permitted without a thorough medical screening of all the parties including the gestational mother, the genetic mother, and the genetic father. If any of the relevant parties have genetic diseases or disorders that may harm the offspring, the procedure is not recommended.
8. Payments of any kind to the surrogate are not recommended. If "brokers" are involved, it is recommended that their services be provided without monetary compensation.
9. It is recommended that all parties agree that, at the time of the birth, the child will be transferred to the appropriate probate court, where all matters concerning custody will be decided. The court will authorize any transfer of custody to the genetic parent. All parties should agree, therefore, prior to the implantation, that the custody of the child is a somewhat undecided matter and that the court will make these determinations.
10. The committee believes that state control over surrogacy is required so as to minimize the harms that are associated with the procedure. In this respect, just as states regulate adoption through licensed "adoption agencies," so too the state ought to create "surrogacy agencies" to regulate surrogacy.

### Reasons for Policy:

The major reasons for our support of this novel procedure are as follows:

1. We believe that for many individuals infertility is a medical problem. Medical science can and indeed has developed the novel technologies and procedures involved in surrogacy as a response to this medical problem. Physicians and hospitals have the right to provide these procedures under the following conditions:
   A. The procedure does not clearly violate any rights of the parties involved. Most importantly, the individuals must enter into the arrangements freely.

B.  There is no compelling state interest that overrides the rights of the individuals to engage in this activity.
C.  The benefits of the procedure for the relevant parties outweigh the harms and risks associated with it.

It is our opinion that the recommendations outlined in the policy secure these conditions. In effect, these recommendations provide the parties with *adequate protection* against harm, but by no means ensure *full protection* against harm. Medical experimentation is, by definition, a risky affair, and those who wish to secure the benefits associated with experimentation take on associated risks.

2.  Surrogacy is clearly a technology and procedure that offers substantial benefits, but it also involves considerable risk. The primary risk to the offspring is that the child may be reduced to property that is bought and sold. The primary risk to the genetic or environmental parents is that the gestational mother will not relinquish the child to them at the time specified in the agreement. The primary risk to the gestational mother is the danger associated with pregnancy and the possibility that she will suffer psychologically after the child is transferred. These risks are by no means the only risks that are possible within this context, but they do represent crucial points that must be addressed by the policy.

Principle 9 responds to the question of treating the child as a piece of property by affirming the traditional notion that women who give birth to children are the mothers of those children. The gestational mother is *presumed* to have custody rights over the child. The committee recognizes that this last claim is open to debate, but in order to maximally safeguard all parties, the committee believes that this is the safest assumption to make. Custody rights belong to the gestational mother and these rights are not to be confused with property rights. Unlike property rights, custody rights cannot be transferred merely by the consent of the relevant parties. A mother may wish to give up her child, but she does not have the authority to transfer her rights to anyone she chooses. The courts must become involved in order to protect the interests of the child. There is no compelling reason to change this approach. Gestational mothers may thus give up their children, but they may not transfer them to anyone for monetary gain.

The courts may then decide to allow the genetic parents to adopt the child, subject to a complete inquiry that all such adoptive parents must submit to.

The committee recognizes that courts have not affirmed this policy. This policy does not have the force of law. It is an ethical requirement that the hospital imposes on those who wish to use the hospital's services. Furthermore, although this policy is not a judicially dictated policy, its value is that it puts all parties "on notice" that the process of surrogacy will involve substantial court action "after the birth of the child." Also, this court action may be extended, and it may involve substantial costs and suffering on the part of the relevant parties.

The concern for the welfare of both the genetic and environmental parents was significant. Principles 1, 2, 7, and 8 were written to address this concern. Under our policy, the genetic parents have no legally rigid guarantees that the child will be relinquished by the gestational mother, or that the court will transfer custody rights to them. These uncertainties can be minimized but not eliminated without undermining the state's authority to control the transference of custody rights of children. To make the transference of custody rights a private affair is the primary way that children are transformed into property, and the committee wished to establish significant roadblocks against this possibility.

### Reasons against Policy:

The major reasons why we dissented from the above surrogacy policy are the following:

1. This procedure is filled with legal complexity and, therefore, we believe that it is impractical for the hospital to become involved in the use of surrogacy arrangements. Fundamental legal and social questions must be answered before we can endorse this procedure. For example, the question of custody of the child is still a matter that we consider unsettled. It is our belief that it is beyond the legal authority of the hospital to settle these questions.
2. While all of us have knowledge of clinical research, this kind of experiment seems more like a social engineering experiment rather than a clinical experiment. We believe that the above policy merely masks a social experiment as a medical experiment. We are, in principle, against confusing the two activities.
3. We maintain that this policy fails to guarantee that gestational mothers will not be exploited by those who use their bodies. Most surrogacy arrangements in the past have involved the transfer of funds from the genetic parents to the gestational parent. In the past, brokers have been involved, and it is unlikely that their continued presence in the arrangements can be prevented merely by hospital fiat. Finally, we believe that once money is involved, the specter of "child selling" is before us. We are opposed to opening the door to this possibility, and

we believe that the near-universal opposition to using money as an incentive in the context of transplantation is an excellent rule to follow in reproduction ethics.

4. Finally, we maintain that one important principle of human subject research is that the individuals affected by the experiment have the right to refuse this treatment. This principle is violated by surrogacy arrangements since the child has no say in the arrangement. In short, we believe that this experiment threatens the welfare of the unborn child to such a degree that its benefits to the genetic parents and gestational mothers do not outweigh these threats.

In the light of these concerns, we recommend that the hospital table this policy and that surrogacy arrangements be prohibited at Community Hospital.

---

## Commentary on the Philosophical and Ethical Aspects of the Policy

The major philosophical issues presented by surrogacy are as follows:

1. Unjustified paternalism directed toward those who wish to engage in surrogacy relationships.
2. Exploitation of those who contract to gestate children.
3. Commercialization or commodification of women and babies.
4. Imposition of private visions of the good life on those who wish to engage in surrogacy.

### Paternalism and Surrogacy

Proponents of surrogacy argue that to prohibit surrogacy amounts to unjustified paternalism toward those who wish to avail themselves of the "prima facie" benefits of surrogacy contracts. Proponents of the procedure maintain that criminalizing surrogacy is motivated by the paternalistic desire to protect those who would enter these surrogacy arrangements from potential harm as well as to protect society from the potential social evils associated with surrogacy.

Paternalism is therefore at the heart of the surrogacy debate, so we need to explore this philosophical concept. Few philosophers have had more influence on the topic of paternalism than John Stuart Mill. In his essay "On Liberty," Mill expressed what he called his "very simple principle that the sole end for which mankind is warranted individually or collectively in interfering with the liberty of action of any of their number, is self-protection. That only purpose for which power can be rightfully exercised over any member of a civilized community against his will is to prevent harm to others. He cannot rightfully be compelled to do or forebear because it will be better for him."

At first glance, this antipaternalism principle applies to laws mandating seat belts, possible laws against smoking, or actual laws against using recreational drugs such as marijuana. But how does this principle apply to the surrogacy case? The similarity is this. One has the physical power to use recreational drugs, but states have passed laws against using it. One has the power, but not the right, to use these substances. One reason that is often mentioned to justify these laws against using recreational drugs is that they are harmful to those who use them.

Some philosophers think of surrogacy along similar lines. If the state has the right to criminalize drug use because it is harmful, then the state has the right to criminalize surrogacy because it too is presumably harmful. In this line of reasoning, surrogacy is harmful to the people who engage in it. These contracts, as a matter of fact, will harm the parties involved. This seems to be Rosemarie Tong's position when she claims that "since there is evidence that surrogacy arrangements harm contracted mothers, a ban on commercial surrogacy needs only to rely on the harm principle (as opposed to legal moralism)."[1] This view treats surrogacy not as if it were a dangerous activity like mountain climbing that *might* cause harm to an individual, but as a more substantively dangerous activity. As a result of this danger, society is justified in restricting it.

There is some evidence for Tong's view. For example, surrogate mothers such as Mary Beth Whitehead, in the "Baby M" case, have claimed that they were harmed by engaging in such contracts. The "do no harm" rule is thus at the heart of the surrogacy debate. All the parties involved, including the child, are at risk. The Baby M case illustrates this concern regarding harm to the participants, but is also important for understanding the philosophical problems associated with surrogacy in general. The following is a review of the case.

Through a surrogate broker, Mr. and Mrs. William Stern in February 1985 contracted with Mary Beth Whitehead to act as a surrogate. The contract had many stipulations. For example, Mrs. Whitehead was forbidden to form any maternal attachments with the child. She was paid $10,000 plus medical expenses to deliver this child. She was required to surrender the child to the genetic father, William Stern, at the time of birth. The Infertility Center of New York, a private company, acted as a broker in the deal and was paid $10,000 for its services. Mrs. Whitehead was artificially inseminated with Mr. Stern's sperm, and she delivered a child known in the courts as Baby M. After the delivery, Mrs. Whitehead took the child, whom she called Sarah, home and then delivered the child to the Stern's family. However, after transferring the child to the Stern family, Mrs. Whitehead changed her mind and wanted the baby returned. Mrs. Whitehead managed to convince Mr. and Mrs. Stern to let her have the baby for a short time. Mrs. Whitehead took the baby home and then informed them that she and her husband wished to retain custody of the baby.

Based on the surrogacy contract, the Sterns received a court order from Judge Harvey Sorkow mandating that Mrs. Whitehead return Baby M to them. At this point, Mrs. Whitehead escaped judicial jurisdiction and fled to Florida in order to keep her baby. Mr. and Mrs. Whitehead were finally apprehended after three months of flight. The baby was temporarily placed in the custody of the Stern family. A court battle then began.

Two conflicting court actions then took place. A lower New Jersey court, presided over by Judge Sorkow, ruled that the surrogacy contract was valid and it was in the best interest of the child to be transferred into the hands of Mr. and Mrs. Stern. Immediately following the ruling, Judge Sorkow brought Mr. and Mrs. Stern into his chambers and ordered that adoption proceedings take place so that Elizabeth Stern could become the legally adopted mother of Baby M.

This ruling was immediately appealed to a higher court, the New Jersey Supreme Court. The lower court's decision was reversed by the higher court. The New Jersey Supreme Court declared that the surrogacy contract was "invalid" and could not be enforced. The court held that the provision of money and the loss of autonomy made the contract invalid. Because the contract was invalid, the adoption that was based on the contract was also ruled invalid. Therefore, Mrs. Whitehead was ruled the legal mother of Baby M.

The court also declared that the use of money as an incentive in the surrogacy context violated New Jersey law prohibiting the use of money in connection with adoptions. Finally, custody rights were settled in New Jersey according to what the court considered the best interests of the child. The contract was not the primary basis for determining who would have custody of Baby M. The contract was viewed by the court as fundamentally at odds with law and social policy. The court did rule that Mr. Stern should have custody based on what it considered the best interests of Baby M, but it also affirmed Mrs. Whitehead's claim to be "the natural mother" and, furthermore, granted her visitation rights.[2]

If the Baby M case reveals anything, it is that people may be harmed when they choose to enter into surrogacy arrangements. But whether surrogacy can harm those who freely engage in it is only one issue in the debate. The question that we face is whether the potential harm to those who engage in a possibly dangerous activity is sufficient grounds for using the coercive power of the state to outlaw this activity. At first glance, Mill's principle of liberty, which amounts to the claim that liberty can only be restricted in cases where the exercise of the liberty is harmful to others, would seem to require us to explicitly reject the idea that the state has the right to force people to do what is in their own self-interest or to avoid doing what is harmful to them. One can agree that exercising daily is generally in one's interest without believing that we should pass laws mandating exercise programs for everyone. Similarly, one can believe that smoking is harmful without holding that the state ought to coerce everyone to quit smoking or to penalize people for smoking in areas where smoking is permitted. Thus, many supporters of surrogacy agree that harm may result from engaging in surrogacy contracts, but they appeal to Mill's principle of liberty as a basis for establishing the right of individuals to engage in surrogacy despite the potential or actual harm that may accrue to surrogate mothers or genetic parents.

Also, proponents of surrogacy often claim that, although the Baby M case illustrates the potential for harm, many surrogates claim they were not harmed by engaging in surrogacy. Mill's principle requires more than proving that the exercise of a liberty produces harm for some limited number of people. To outlaw the surrogacy contract one must prove that, all things considered, it produces more harm than benefit *to everyone*. We can outlaw surrogacy only when we establish that the exercise of the liberty to enter into a surrogacy arrangement produces more overall harm than good. This interpretation of Mill's paternalism principle makes some sense because most contracts do indeed produce some level of harm to the people who sign them. Think of the last car you purchased. Weren't you partially harmed as a result of paying the monthly installments? According to Mill, the mere production of some harm is not sufficient to justify the exercise of the coercive power of the state.

But the issue of producing overall harm is not the only relevant issue in the debate. Many legislators might assume that currently illegal drugs like marijuana produce more harm than good to those who use them. But opponents of these laws often argue that such antidrug laws are still inconsistent with Mill's paternalism principle because there is a sense in which drug use does not harm anyone but the users. For example, the neighbor of the drug user does not suffer the physical harms associated with drug addiction. The neighbor will never have withdrawal pains or risk acquiring a disease associated with drug use. Nor will the neighbor lose his ability to work as a result of his neighbor's addiction. Drug laws and laws mandating motorcycle helmets should be stricken not because recreational drugs cause no harm to the users or because motorcycle helmets cannot provide genuine safety benefits. Rather, these laws are illegitimate because proponents of them cannot prove that they produce more overall good than harm.

The issue here is who bears the burden of proof of establishing overall social harm or overall social benefit? This is an important question because judgments of this sort are riddled with difficulties. Furthermore, it is easy to argue that either party bears the burden of proof. For example, one might assume that anyone who would restrict a liberty must bear the burden of proof of establishing that the restriction produces overall social welfare. If paternalistic laws were already in force, then one might assume that anyone who would repeal a current law bears the burden of proof of establishing that the change would secure more overall social welfare.

But there is another problem with Mill's liberty principle. How does one define harm? And how does one calculate, measure, or weigh social harm? We can illustrate the problem in the context of surrogacy in the following way. One may feel that the suffering experienced by Mary Beth Whitehead, when her baby was forcibly taken from her, was so great that it overwhelms all the potential good that might be produced by surrogacy. But how would one prove this feeling? Others might feel that Mrs. Whitehead's suffering is outweighed by all the potential benefits of surrogacy. But how would one prove that feeling? The suspicion underlying these questions is that Mill's "social welfare judgments" are really difficult or impossible to make. One might be able to determine what the citizenry prefers with respect to surrogacy, but it is more difficult to prove that actual social welfare is identical to the preferences of citizens.

Mill's principle regarding the limits of state authority to coerce self-interested behavior aims at enacting laws exclusively on the basis of overall social utility. In this view, the main task of any government regarding surrogacy is simply to determine whether, as a matter of fact, more social harm or benefit will be produced by admitting surrogacy contracts. But many philosophers have argued that surrogacy presents a problem of a deeper sort. We can approach this deeper problem through the following example. Suppose we did develop a series of restrictions on surrogacy contracts that produced more benefit than harm. Suppose we found out that most surrogates, unlike Mary Beth Whitehead, were satisfied with the surrogacy arrangement. Does Mill's principle of liberty allow the state to interfere in these cases. Presumably not!

## The Validity of Surrogacy Contracts

Surprisingly enough, however, many philosophers believe that Mill's principle is compatible with laws that outlaw some self-regarding behavior. Ronald Dworkin's famous analysis of Mill's liberty principle suggests that there is another understanding of Mill's rule deeper than the one involving the calculation of social harms and social benefits.[3] There is, according to

Dworkin, a "principled aspect" to Mill's liberty principle. Mill admits that his rule applies to and regulates the kind of contracts that will be upheld as valid. But Dworkin asks whether there are any contracts that are invalid, i.e., that are ruled out in principle. Mill says "yes!" The example used by Mill is that no person may agree to become a slave. According to Dworkin, Mill's objections to slavery contracts are independent of any utilitarian calculations of social welfare. Rather, Mill objects to slavery contracts because the person who chose to enter into a slavery contract would lose his future choices. Mill wants to outlaw this possibility in principle. For Mill an individual is not at liberty to make his own calculation of pleasures and pains regarding slavery. Furthermore, even if one could benefit from becoming a slave, one cannot do so. Persons "ought to reign" over themselves and, therefore, they cannot make calculations in this regard.

For Mill, some contracts may be ruled invalid as a matter of principle. But Dworkin suggests that this limitation is restricted to cases in which the person's liberty to make future decisions is involved. In this analysis, antidrug laws are permitted because the decision to use heroin destroys one's future ability to cease using heroin. One is addicted to heroin and, therefore, its slave. Opponents of surrogacy can use this qualification of Mill's liberty rule as a basis for objecting to surrogacy, but for Dworkin Mill's exception is limited to cases in which the activity destroys the autonomy of the person who enters the contract. And since surrogacy does not seem to involve any addictions that would make someone a slave, it seems as if this aspect of Mill's rule cannot be used to justify antisurrogacy laws.

### Surrogacy and Exploitation

However, opponents of surrogacy may appeal to another principle that surrogacy contracts violate. What is this principle?

One common answer is that surrogacy contracts should be ruled invalid because they "exploit" the women who enter these contracts as surrogate mothers. Peter Singer, a well-known consequentialist utilitarian, has claimed that "Once money enters into the [surrogacy] arrangement, the possibilities of exploitation are everywhere."[5] This notion can also be found in the Warnock Report, which was an official report to the British government regarding surrogacy.[4] The report claimed that surrogacy was inconsistent with human dignity because it involved child selling. The report also suggested that surrogacy was similar to selling kidneys. In short, the poor might be exploited by surrogacy contracts, and this should be outlawed. This view of surrogacy admits that the parties to a surrogacy arrangement occasionally benefit from it but that the arrangement is essentially exploitative. Furthermore, if we assume that exploitation harms society, we can give a consequentialist argument against surrogacy. Such contracts are socially harmful because of their exploitative character.

However, one major difficulty with this involves the meaning of "exploitation." The difficulty especially affects consequentialists for it is no small problem to provide an analysis of exploitation in purely consequentialist terms. Most such analyses involve nonconsequentialist concepts. For example, Stephen Munzer defines exploitation in the following way. He claims that X exploits Y by doing Z if

a. X benefits from Y by doing Z,
b. doing Z involves using Y as a tool or a resource,
c. doing Z causes Y serious harm.[6]

Opponents of surrogacy argue that in the case of Baby M, Mrs. Whitehead meets these conditions. She was harmed by the contract in that her baby was forcibly taken from her against her wishes. Second, the Sterns benefitted from the contract because they got a baby. And, finally, Mrs. Whitehead was used as a tool or resource.

Although Munzer's theory of exploitation has many virtues, it is obviously not a consequentialist vision of exploitation. It clearly employs the notion of using a person, a prohibition associated with non-consequentialist theories like Immanuel Kant's. As such, it is difficult to analyze in terms of the consequences of specific actions. But more importantly, Munzer's theory is also an incomplete analysis of exploitation. It fails to emphasize that voluntary consent and genuine alternatives must be structurally excluded from the definition of exploitative relationships. The surrogate is exploited because she does not have any other genuine alternatives but to sell her baby. As a result of this absence of alternatives, she is not able to give her voluntary consent to acting as a surrogate. The exploited surrogate is much like the exploited worker. She appears to give consent to a job that barely provides her and her children with enough to eat, but she is exploited because she has no other genuine alternative.

This dependence of the concept of exploitation on the economic status of the surrogate mother has suggested to Lori Andrews, a defender of commercial surrogacy, that the problem of exploitation can be resolved not by banning commercial surrogacy, but by paying the surrogates more.[7] If Mary Beth Whitehead had been paid $1,000,000 rather than $10,000, the harm to her would have been so meager relative to the benefits she received that she would have had no complaint against the Sterns. Critics respond, however, that markets do not allow setting fees at such high rates. If there is to be commercial or free-market surrogacy, then the government cannot coerce people to accept only high rates. Poor women, according to free-market perspective, need to be free to accept lower wages so that they can compete with richer women. Furthermore, even the Sterns, who were upper-middle-class professionals, could not afford such a high cost. In effect, setting the surrogacy fees at other than what the free market determines would exclude middle-class or lower economic groups from the benefits of commercial surrogacy.

But there is a deeper problem associated with the idea that increasing the amounts paid to surrogates can solve the exploitation problem. Some critics of commercial surrogacy such as Mary Gibson have argued that increasing the amount paid only increases the inability of the poor women to say "no!"[8] Increasing the amount paid to a surrogate is like increasing the amount that one offers to a person to become a slave. It only makes saying "no" to an immoral offer more difficult.

What is important to note is that explaining exploitation in purely consequentialist terms is difficult. More importantly, because a person consents to signing a contract, this does not say decisively that she was not exploited. Furthermore, the concept of exploitation takes us to the very heart of ethics because it attempts to define in more specific terms what it means to use a person in an unethical way. Finally, the concept of exploitation is itself closely connected to the economic and social conditions of the surrogate. It is poor women who are most in danger of being exploited.

### Surrogacy and Commodification

But there are other philosophical concepts at the heart of the surrogacy debate. One such notion is the idea of commodification. Critics of commercial surrogacy such as Elizabeth Anderson argue that the same reasons that justify outlawing the buying and selling of human organs in a free and open market can also be used to justify laws that outlaw commercial surrogacy.[9] The argument is that like human organs, women's reproductive abilities should not be viewed as commodities like sugar and timber. A woman's timber may be her property, but her reproductive abilities and the children produced by them are not. The claim is that a person's relationship to her body is so close and so intimate that the body cannot be viewed as property. Furthermore, the product of gestation is not like the products of a manufacturing plant. A factory produces objects. A woman gives birth to a person. And persons, even little persons, are qualitatively different from manufactured objects. The practical result of this view is that surrogacy should not be governed by the body of law that governs the transfer of commodities. Rather, family law, custody law, or probate law should be the set of operative legal principles. The concept of commodification, therefore, is philosophically vital because it determines what set of legal principles ought to operate in matters involving surrogacy.

The practical outcome of adopting this philosophical viewpoint is very substantial. Again according to Elizabeth Anderson, if commercial surrogacy involves treating women's bodies as property, then commercial surrogacy ought to be outlawed in the same way that commercial transfer of transplantable organs is outlawed. One should not buy and sell gestation abilities on the open market because the value of money is "incommensurable" or incomparable with the value of a person's body and the value of the persons produced by gestation. No amount of money would be "equal" to the value of a person, and because a person bears such a close relationship to his heart, no amount of money would be enough to compensate someone for selling his heart.

The issues involved in this debate concerning the role of commodification within surrogacy are profoundly philosophical; therefore, they are open to continued review and criticism. Alan Wertheimer has claimed that Anderson's view of commodification fails to recognize that contemporary society allows many forms of incommensurable values to be exchanged in a free market.[10] For example, one can agree that da Vinci's "Mona Lisa" is a priceless masterpiece in that no amount of money can actually represent its true value to humanity. The "monetary value" and the "artistic value" of the painting are so different that they cannot be compared. However, although it may be true that money and the "Mona Lisa" are valuable in very different ways, this still does not mean, according to Wertheimer, that a very rich consortium of people are forbidden or ought to be forbidden from making an offer to buy Picasso's "Guernica" or the "Mona Lisa" for money. According to Wertheimer the fact that we think that money and a painting are valuable in very different senses of "value," i.e., that they are incommensurable, does not preclude the possibility that money can be a basis for exchange. Wertheimer's analogy, however, does not establish that paying money for children should be permitted. The fact that some priceless objects, such as paintings, can be transferred for prices does not imply that all priceless beings, including babies, can be transferred for a price. What his analogy between surrogacy and paintings establishes is merely that the incommensurate nature of the things exchanged is not by itself a sufficient basis for outlawing commercial surrogacy.

We close this discussion of paternalism, exploitation, and commodification by noting that all of these ideas may be mutually dependent. This means that we may not be able to formulate an adequate definition of unjustified paternalism without first understanding what exploitation and commodification involve.

## A Religious Objection

Opposition to surrogacy also emerges from some religions. Roman Catholicism, for example, claims that it is immoral to separate reproduction from intercourse because reproduction by means of intercourse is the means that God intended to repopulate the earth. Many surrogacy cases involve reproduction by in vitro fertilization, in which conception occurs without intercourse. It also may involve inserting the embryo into the womb of a female other than the one who produced the ovum. The Roman Catholic Church considers this procedure "unnatural reproduction" and therefore immoral. Many other Christians also view surrogacy as fundamentally wrong because they claim that children should be viewed as "gifts from God" to whom the parents have profound and lasting duties. In commercial surrogacy the child is a means for securing money for the surrogate. The child is not treated as an end in itself. Surrogacy thus changes the meaning and purpose of reproduction and thereby threatens a way of life in which parents are obligated to protect children rather than manipulate them for financial gain.

But religious people are not the only ones who fear that technological developments, and especially technological advancements in reproductive technology, will have frightening consequences. The American College of Obstetricians and Gynecologists and the American Medical Association have argued that social interests will not be served by physicians becoming involved in surrogacy arrangements.[11] Ann Neale argues that responsible stewardship over a hospital requires that hospitals view surrogacy as something that violates "the meaning and purpose of parenting" and poses great danger to society.[12]

### The Public-Private Distinction and Surrogacy

The difficulty here is that questions concerning the meaning and purpose of parenting are viewed by many philosophers as private matters that should not influence our public life. This violates our society's attempt to separate private life from public life.

But how should we understand this distinction between private and public? H. Tristram Engelhardt has argued for an *individualist model* of the public-private distinction.[13] This view has been so widely adopted in contemporary culture that it requires substantial discussion. The individualist model is based on four assumptions.

First, ethics in a religiously pluralistic culture must be divided into two separate spheres: public and private. The public sphere is governed largely by formal principles that are justified as the necessary conditions for social collaboration in general. These principles are formal in three senses. First, they offer no specific prescriptions on what constitutes the "good life" for all individuals. For example, we can all have equal opportunity without determining what specific goals individuals should seek. The content of the moral life defines what is good for individuals, and questions concerning what is good for individuals must be relegated to the private domain.

Second, public sphere morality is best understood as "procedural" morality in that it spells out not how moral conflicts ought to be resolved, but merely defines the procedures that social groups ought to follow in reaching agreement concerning their moral conflicts. Finally, although it does not spell out a specific definition of the good life, the individualist model of the public-private distinction makes different definitions of the good life possible by permitting, and indeed encouraging, a high degree of personal autonomy within the pluralistic society. Thus, respecting the autonomy of individuals, avoiding harm to others, requiring peaceful rather than violent conflict resolution, and contractual faithfulness are the linchpins of this public morality. These principles constitute a *minimalist ethic* that can govern this realm. The key to this minimalist public ethic is the Kantian notion that others must be treated as ends, not as means.

The second characteristic of the individualist model is that questions concerning the good life are relevant only to the private sphere. The agnostic, the Jehovah's Witness, and the Catholic can each define the good or meaningful life in their own private communities. These groups can seek protection for their definitions of the good life as long as they are respectful of the rights of others. Religious values are not public matters. As private prerogatives, religious values deserve protection, but the public cannot impose them on the society as a whole.

Third, rational citizens within a pluralistic republic must avoid the temptation to transform private convictions into public requirements. Virtuous citizens in such a republic construe tolerance as the chief civil or public virtue, and such tolerance extends to that which they take to be immoral in the private sphere. In this individualist view, the good life is a private construction unfit for public determination.

Fourth, private ethics, like private opinions on dress, can be deeply idiosyncratic. This is because the private domain specifies the content of ethics while the rules of the public sphere merely contain the form of any possible social collaboration. The public ethic is minimalist but universal. It emphasizes a series of noninterference duties based on respect for individual autonomy and prevention of harm.

Let us now apply to surrogacy this individualist model of the relationship of private morality to public life. It is easy to imagine that all manner of private groups, from Catholics to feminists, would oppose surrogacy from their private perspectives. It is easy to imagine that many people view surrogacy as violating the meaning and purpose of parenting. But for the individualist, the crucial question is whether these private perspectives are part of the minimalist morality. The minimal morality required for the public secular state is just too limited to tell us the meaning and purpose of reproduction. To say that surrogacy violates the meaning and purpose of parenting, therefore, crosses the line that separates public from private morality. In this view of the public-private distinction, Catholics and feminists cannot call on the state to use its coercive power to inhibit surrogacy arrangements without imposing their private views regarding the meaning and purpose of human existence. To prohibit surrogacy violates the tolerance rule.

### The Hermeneutical Model

However, alternative models of the public-private distinction are available, and one of them suggests that the distinction between public and private is not as rigid as Engelhardt maintains. One such alternative view may be called the *hermeneutical model* of the public-private distinction.[14] Hermeneutics is the study of the general principles of interpretation and explanation. We call this model hermeneutic because it emphasizes that interpretation is essential in order to resolve debates involving the public-private aspects of society. This model begins with two criticisms of the individualist view.

First, religious and philosophical groups frequently defend positions on what most of us consider public matters. In short, there is a wide, significant, and very ambiguous borderline or gray area that separates public and private. There are theological justifications for a wide variety of public matters. The Ten Commandments forbid murder and stealing, yet these are classically public matters. Historically, religious arguments were very influential in the development of laws, and religious arguments continue to be influential in public debate. For example, religious groups frequently argue that the government should increase its commitment to the poor, and their arguments are frequently theologically based.

Second, guiding the individualist view is the assumption that if we allow the religious speaker into the public debate, then this necessarily interferes with the principle of church-state separation. The difficulty with this viewpoint is that it requires one to avoid speaking from religious conviction, which violates one's public right to speak as one chooses. The very essence of the Western public ethic is to allow individuals to speak as they see fit. While others are surely free to disregard such discussion, they are not at liberty to prevent individuals from interpreting and defining public issues from a private or theological perspective.

According to Engelhardt's minimalist vision of the public ethic, if one wishes to speak about a public matter, one must speak in a secular voice, for if a theological argument were relevant to an issue such as surrogacy or abortion, then that fact in conjunction with the individualist model would settle the question of whether surrogacy is a private or public matter. It is private, since according to the individualist model, the public sphere must be immune to theological infection. However, this result is paradoxical since all the relevant issues that affect public life can be addressed in theological discourse.

According to the hermeneutical model, history is the key to the reconstruction of the public-private distinction. In the history of social ethics there is no instance in which the form of ethical conflict is logically separable from its particular content. For the hermeneut, a universal minimal ethic is mythical. Rather, history provides a broad spectrum of relations between public and private affairs. At opposite ends of this spectrum are the individualist view—which holds that theology plays no legitimate role in public affairs—and theocracy—which holds that theology plays the only legitimate role in public affairs. The hermeneutical model attempts to develop a middle ground or compromise position.

This model is based on a new metaphor for understanding society. Instead of a structure resting on universal and minimal foundations, society can be represented as a conversation whose rules are flexible and variable. Unlike structures, conversations can proceed for very long periods of time without a firm and constant set of minimal rules to govern them. Ideal principles may exist within the conversation, but practical decisions such as those involving surrogacy require compromises among opposing ideals. Compromises often come by way of new interpretations of ideals. Later we will discuss the ways in which Community Hospital's surrogacy policy involves compromises among ideals.

According to this hermeneutic model, culture is an ongoing conversation, a conversation with a history but without a fixed foundation.[15] There are no minimalist foundations of modern society because society is not a building. This conversational picture of society offers three new ways of understanding public and private. First, it does not require a timeless unchanging litmus test to distinguish public affairs from private in the pluralistic society. The public matters of 1910 are the private matters of 1995. For example, consider the laws regarding observance of Sunday as a day of rest. Furthermore, the private matters of 1910 become the public matters of 1995. Consider contemporary environmental laws that make dumping toxic wastes unlawful. The border separating public from private is ambiguous. Surrogacy fits this aspect of the hermeneutic model because it is both a public and a private matter.

Second, we cannot decide in principle, prior to the actual presentation of arguments, what are the relevant issues in a public debate concerning an ethical matter such as surrogacy. Shared theological or political or economic conviction may influence the public debate, and in a democracy these public values need not be viewed as irrelevant.

Third, this hermeneutic model represents public ethics as a social conversation among a thoroughly divided citizenry rather than a conversation among people who agree about a formal minimal ethic but disagree about the good life. The ethical division within modern society is real and deep on both public and private levels. The conversation occurs without a fixed language in which the relevant ethical terms have the same meanings for all the citizens. This social conversation takes place in a language in which words like *good* and *right* and *obligatory* are governed by secular (philosophical), economic, and political, as well as religious, usage and meaning. Social conversationalists share a rough and ready language, not a common foundation.

Conversation among proponents of secular and religious analyses of moral discourse only seems impossible if we assume the foundationalist picture of society. When this image is scrapped, the historical fact of conversations among vastly different peoples with vastly different convictions emerges as not only possible but commonplace. History and politics are full of examples of groups that are ideologically opposed but that work together to achieve a common goal. In the surrogacy debate Catholics and certain feminists who disagree about fundamental ethical values can still communicate and form a common opposition to surrogacy. A common ethical language is not necessary for cooperation.

### Surrogacy and the Hermeneutic Model

Community Hospital's policy on surrogacy is hermeneutic because it emphasizes compromise among opposing values and no ethical viewpoint is minimally universal or foundational. The following examples illustrate this point. First, individual women are permitted to act as surrogate mothers but payment for their services, or commercial surrogacy, is forbidden. Second, contracts or agreements are permitted *but* these agreements are not presented as irrevocably binding on the gestational mother. All parties should be informed that this agreement is not legally valid, that it represents a mere understanding among the parties that may have little or no legally binding force. Third, the policy admits, for the sake of initial clarity among the parties, that the gestational mother should be assumed to be the mother of the child *but* it also recommends that all decisions on custody and legal adoption must be left to the discretion of the courts. Fourth, the policy addresses the question of the moral status of children by forbidding any transfer of funds to the surrogate mother, so that no hint of treating children as property will be present. But while money cannot be the basis of transfer, transfer itself is not forbidden, provided that it is carefully regulated by the legislature and monitored by the courts. Fifth, the policy does interpret surrogacy as exploitative and it also is profoundly concerned with potential commodification of persons. *But* the committee also took seriously the idea that forbidding all surrogacy arrangements would violate the liberty principle. The compromise thus involves permitting people to exercise their right to noncommercial surrogacy. Surrogacy remains a risky method for addressing infertility,*but* the hospital has left the door open for those who wish to accept that risk.

## The Case of Mr. and Mrs. Douglas and Harriet Neil

Robert and Martha Douglas want a child of their own, but as a result of Mrs. Douglas's diabetes, her physician has recommended that she avoid becoming pregnant. She does, however, have functioning ovaries and is anxious for her ovum to be fertilized in vitro with her husband's sperm. They then wish to implant this embryo into a surrogate mother who will gestate the fetus and subsequently transfer the child to them.

Harriet Neil is 21 years of age and a friend of the Douglases. She has never been pregnant. She has agreed to gestate the embryo and thereby act as a surrogate. The three individuals contact Dr. Mark King, director of Community Hospital's Department of Obstetrics and Gynecology. Dr. King has done substantial work in the area of artificial insemination and has artificially inseminated women at the hospital. These cases involved insemination of wives using their husband's sperm. During his residency, he assisted in two in vitro surrogacy arrangements, both of which were concluded without any medical or legal difficulty. Because the Douglases are his patients, Dr. King is anxious to help them. Furthermore, he has been supporting the development of the hospital's surrogacy policy and is anxious to proceed.

He comes to the committee with the following agreements signed by the three parties and requests that the committee approve of the arrangement.

---

### Agreement

I, Harriet Neil, agree to be the surrogate mother for the child of Robert and Martha Douglas. I have taken no money nor will I take any money from the Douglases except those involving my medical expenses associated with the embryo transfer and delivery. I have been informed by Dr. King of all possible health-related dangers involved in gestating this child for the Douglases. I have entered into this agreement solely in order to assist my friends, the Douglases, to have a child of their own. I agree that, at the time of delivery, I will relinquish any and all custody rights to the child's genetic father and mother, Robert and Martha Douglas. I recognize that this may involve court hearings and perhaps a trial, and I am fully willing to participate in these activities in order to assist Mr. and Mrs. Douglas in their goal of becoming parents.

## Agreement

We, Robert and Martha Douglas, agree to provide all medical expenses for the embryo transfer of our embryo into the womb of Harriet Neil. We also agree to pay for the prenatal care and all expenses related to the delivery of the child by Harriet Neil. We will not pay Ms. Neil any other funds. We have been informed by Dr. King of all the risks and harms associated with embryo transfer, and Dr. King has also informed us about the potential psychological harms associated with surrogacy. We agree that Ms. Neil has some custody rights over the child and that, at the time of birth, she may or may not choose to relinquish these rights. At the time that Ms. Neil relinquishes custody, we will seek custody of the child.

---

## Committee Discussion of the Case

Rev. Richard Marcus:
Well, as you know, Attorney Quinn and I continue to be opposed to this policy. I certainly had the opportunity to express my views in our endless meetings over this issue as well as in the minority report. But I feel myself in a strange dilemma right now. I can function as an obstructionist to any attempts to initiate surrogacy or I can attempt to abide by the committee's decision and apply the policy as fairly as I can. I plan to do the latter. These people have come before us seeking approval for their request, and it fits within our guidelines. Yet my misgivings toward the whole policy are still quite strong, not only because the policy still seems ethically mistaken, but because Mr. and Mrs. Douglas and Miss Neil are foolishly risking their welfare. I plan to evaluate each case on whether the applicants have complied with our policy. Let me close with the hope that we are going to have the opportunity to meet with and discuss these matters with the parties involved.

| | |
|---|---|
| Dr. Mary Collins: | Thank you, Richard. I am very glad that you are going to hang in with us. We need your good sense, and perhaps we need to hear more of your skepticism on the policy. With respect to meeting the Douglases and Harriet Neil, they have agreed to meet with us immediately. |

The chair introduces Robert and Martha Douglas and Harriet Neil as well as Dr. Mark King, the obstetrician, who has beenthe physicianto the parties.

| | |
|---|---|
| Marian Rhodes: | Mr. and Mrs. Douglas, we have the medical report from your physician regarding your infertility, and we would like to give you the opportunity to say anything you wish to the committee concerning your request to engage in this surrogacy arrangement. If you could, we would especially like to know why you have chosen surrogacy rather than adoption as your course of action. Likewise, Ms. Neil, we would like to know why you have chosen to assist them in surrogacy. |
| Mrs. Douglas: | We have thought a lot about this, and especially about adoption, but Robert and I would really like genetically related children. When we found out that we couldn't have children, we were devastated. Both of us looked into adoption, and it seems difficult to get a child. The waiting lists are so long and my health problems might count against us with the adoption agency. But when we found out about Dr. King, we went to see him, and when he told us about the possibility of surrogacy, we knew right away that it was something we wanted to do. We really do want a child, and we think that we would make great parents. |
| Ms. Neil: | I have known the Douglases for many years. I think they would make great parents and that I would really feel good about helping them. It is something that I |

|  | have thought a lot about and I really feel that I want to help them. |
|---|---|
| Rev. Marcus: | Do you realize, Mrs. Douglas, that many surrogacy arrangements have ended up with a great deal of bitterness and hostility between the genetic parents and the surrogate because they wind up disputing over the custody of the child? There is no reason to think that you will avoid this outcome. After all, it is very easy for Ms. Neil to bond with the child even though at this time she feels that this will not occur. She then could withdraw her consent to relinquish the child because these agreements that you have signed are probably not legally binding. It has happened before, and it may happen in your case. |
| Mr. Douglas: | We realize this but we both know Harriet and we have every confidence that she will give us *our* baby when it is born. |
| Atty. John Quinn: | Mr. Douglas, you say that it is your baby. Indeed, you emphasize this point, but this is the debatable issue, and I for one think that the child will no more be your baby than it will be Ms. Neil's. I know I am being blunt and, perhaps, insensitive, but it is crucial that you understand that custody of this child is in the hands of the courts to decide. You might lose, and you might be getting yourselves into a situation that is fraught with emotional and financial misery. |
| Mrs. Douglas: | We understand this and we are fully willing to take this chance to have our child. |
| Prof. Carla Thomas: | Ms. Neil, have you or do you intend to receive any compensation from the Douglases for being the surrogate mother of this child? |
| Ms. Neil: | No! I have no interest in surrogacy other than to help these people. |

| | |
|---|---|
| Atty. Quinn: | Mr. Douglas, allow me to pursue the matter of a potential court battle with you. You must be aware that Ms. Neil is a solid citizen in our community. She has no criminal record. She is employed. She has no past character flaws or behavioral problems that a court would find to be indicative of being a bad parent. In short, if she contested this matter in the courts, the courts may well find in her favor. Or they could also resort to some kind of divided custody. She is definitely not like Mrs. Whitehead in the celebrated "Baby M" case who exhibited some behavior that the courts found to be inconsistent with the interests of the child. But even in that case, the courts awarded the gestational mother, Mrs. Whitehead, visitation rights. I am not a psychologist, but I know that women cannot turn their bonding instincts on and off so easily, and it is very easy to imagine that Ms. Neil may bond with this child and want it desperately. |
| Mr. Douglas: | We both are aware of these potential problems, and we want to do this despite the inherent dangers. Dr. King spent many hours with us discussing just these concerns, and we understand that trouble might await us. |
| Dr. Philip Davis: | Ms. Neil, my wife described her pregnancies as nine-month wall-to-wall nausea experiences. She was sick and miserable a great deal of the time, and although she loves the end product, she hated the means. I notice by your medical record that this is the first time you will be pregnant. Do you understand what you might be getting yourself into? More importantly, at the end of my wife's "horror show" pregnancies, she had a wonderful child to hold and love. My wife said that holding and loving the baby made it all worthwhile. Do you realize |

how bad you might feel during and after the pregnancy, especially when you have to give this baby to someone else?

Ms. Neil:

I really feel that I can do this, and I think that I can be happy in knowing that I am assisting my friends.

Ms. Rhodes:

Dr. King, can you tell us a little about why you have supported these people in this surrogacy experiment? Many of us find your enthusiasm for this strategy curious.

Dr. King:

Look, it is as simple as this. These folks are my patients. They want children, and I think that as long as they know the risks involved with this procedure, they have the right to try it. I have informed them of the relevant risks, but I think that by focusing on a few surrogacy cases that have turned sour, you might be misleading them. Hundreds, perhaps thousands, of surrogacy arrangements have been concluded without serious harm to the parties involved. I respect your need to be frank with these people, but honesty should require you to present the positive evidence as well. Mrs. Douglas has a medical problem that is not, in my judgment, compatible with pregnancy. I think that surrogacy is a legitimate means for managing their problem.

Dr. Collins:

Dr. King, I think this committee is composed of honest people struggling to deal with a difficult issue, and I do not think that questioning our honesty is appropriate.

Dr. King:

I certainly do not wish to attack anyone, but I wanted to insert that there is plenty of evidence that these arrangements have yielded many beneficial outcomes.

Dr. Collins:

Mr. and Mrs. Douglas and Ms. Neil, are there any questions you wish to ask us?

| | |
|---|---|
| Mr. Douglas: | What authority do you folks actually have in this matter? If you do not approve of this, does that mean that we cannot have this procedure at this hospital? |
| Prof. Martin Fisk: | Our role, Mr. Douglas, is an advisory one. The final decisions belong to the physicians and the administration of the hospital. All of us hope that they give careful consideration to advice, but the decision is ultimately in the hands of the administration and the physicians who would provide this service. |
| Dr. King: | Let me add something, Mr. Douglas. I presented this option to you, but I made it quite clear that without the support from the ethics committee of the hospital, I would be unable to provide the service to you here at Community Hospital. I would be very reluctant to provide you the service without the committee's endorsement. |
| Mrs. Douglas: | In the light of Dr. King's remarks, my husband and I would plead with you to support our request. We have a great deal of respect for Dr. King and for the hospital. If we are going to do this, we want it done here at Community Hospital. I suspect that if you refused, we would go elsewhere, but we would very much like to avail ourselves of the service here at Community Hospital. |
| Dr. Collins: | Thank you, Mr. and Mrs. Douglas and Ms. Neil, for taking the time to come and speak to us. We will be in contact with you. |

The committee resumes discussion after the parties leave.

| | |
|---|---|
| Atty. Quinn: | I have problems with this one. As the attorney for the hospital, I think that supporting this surrogacy arrangement may place the hospital at significant risk of being sued, and I would not be doing my job if I did not recommend a lot of caution |

on this. Also, I think it may be a public relations fiasco and may earn us a lot of bad will in the community, especially among those who find surrogacy unnatural. I did not support this policy because it places the hospital at too much risk, and I am not going to support this request for precisely the same reason. We are sticking our necks out too far into legally uncharted territory, and I believe that it is imprudent.

Dr. Davis:

Let me ask, Attorney Quinn, are you playing the role of hospital attorney or the role of a member of the committee? I ask this because it seems to me that there is a possible conflict of interest here. What we are asked to do on this committee is offer medical-ethical advice, not to offer advice on how to keep the hospital out of harm's way. Offering advice on how to keep the hospital out of harm's way is not the same as offering advice on what is the ethically right thing to do. I mention this, John, because all of us respect your views. What I would like to hear from you is your considered ethical opinion rather than merely what the hospital pays you so much money to do, namely, to keep the institution out of liability trouble.

Atty. Quinn:

My expertise is in the area of law, risk management, and liability. That is what I know very well. I think surrogacy is still legally uncharted territory and poses possible risk to the hospital. I feel that we should avoid it.

Dr. Davis:

But is that your ethical recommendation or your recommendation as a risk manager? I still haven't heard that!

Atty. Quinn:

Phil, I have given you my expert opinion and that is all I can say!

Prof. Fisk:

Allow me to shift gears a little. I think we have to return to an idea that Rev. Marcus employed: that, despite our reservations, we have a policy that, in principle, supports the concept of surrogacy as a response to infertility. I think that we have a duty to this couple. We approved this policy, and they have in good faith come to us and have abided by our conditions. I think that it would be bad faith to turn them down because of our general reservations.

Ms. Rhodes:   Martin, that is not true. I approved the policy, but I did not mean that I would automatically approve every request that came in to us. Quite frankly, I have a lot of trouble with Ms. Neil. I know that she has reached the age of competence, but she has never had a child. She has never gone through the process of delivering and bonding with a child. Believe me, bonding begins long before the delivery. I think that she has very little knowledge of what is involved in surrogacy and that she may very well wind up bonding with this fetus and creating serious problems for everyone. In short, I have problems with approving her as a reliable surrogate. So I think it makes perfect sense to say that we can approve of the policy in general and nevertheless refuse to approve of a particular application.

Prof. Fisk:   On what basis do you justify your claim that she will not be a reliable surrogate? Is there any clinical evidence that supports this claim?

Ms. Rhodes:   There is not at this time a lot of clinical evidence on this subject in general. I simply feel that she is immature and unrealistic about how pregnancy can alter your feelings about the child. I think that she is setting herself up for a hard fall, and I do not want to participate in it.

Prof. Fisk:
I agree that we have a risk here, but I do not see that the risk is greater in Ms. Neil's case than in any other. Remember that Mary Beth Whitehead, the gestational mother of Baby M, had previously had three children. This did not prevent her from bonding with Baby M and refusing to relinquish her voluntarily. The fact that Ms. Neil has not had children does not seem sufficient to disqualify her as a surrogate. Also, remember that we are trying to gather information on surrogacy here. Part of the experiment may involve seeing whether there are any good predictors for what would make a successful surrogate.

Prof. Thomas:
Let me remind you that the consequences of a lot of our actions are often horrendous and that bad consequences or the possibility of bad consequences by themselves are not enough to make an action bad. Consider, for example, boxing or mountaineering or professional football. The list is practically endless. All these enterprises cause substantial risk to the participants. Many of the participants do get hurt, but all these actions are covered by the rule of autonomy because they do not violate anyone's rights. The harm they produce is real and it certainly is unfortunate, but it doesn't seem to me that we can dictate to people what is or is not good for them. We cannot force people to act in ways that maximally insure them against harm.

Prof. Fisk:
Carla, this issue divides us. I think that, although we agree on the policy, our reasons and our attitudes differ substantially. I think that surrogacy is a medical treatment, and that if it yields good responses to the problem of infertility, then it should be supported. The purpose of our policy is to gather the information that will

allow us to make a good clinical judgment on whether surrogacy is good treatment. If it leads to bad results, I would be the first to recommend that we cease the experiment and withdraw our tentative support of the policy. This is not your attitude, is it, Carla?

Prof. Thomas:

No! It seems to me that engaging in surrogacy is a matter of right. Individuals in the autonomous state have the right to act in self-regarding ways without interference from government. If the behavior is unjustifiably harmful to others or if it interferes with the rights of others, then I can support restricting a liberty, but where there is risk only to those who voluntarily engage in the behavior, then I think we had better restrain our tendency to interfere. To engage in surrogacy is to engage in a self-regarding behavior, so I resist restraining it just as I resist restraining football or boxing or smoking, even though I believe that all these behaviors are harmful to the people who engage in them.

Dr. Collins:

I am by no means a philosopher, Professor Thomas, but I am not sure that your approach is the only way to understand the phenomenon of surrogacy. Some feminist thinkers reject this "rights-based" understanding of surrogacy. Rights are based on the concept of what is just. While males may conceive justice as the basis of ethics, females tend to emphasize "caring" as the basis of their moral lives. Thinkers such as Carol Gilligan[16] have argued that the experience of oppression throughout their history has made women more open to the importance of caring as the most significant factor in our moral lives. Women do not exclude justice as an important consideration in ethics. It is just secondary to caring.

But there is another problem with your view of ethics as it relates to women. You keep talking about women as if they were really separated from all other women. You see them as fundamentally autonomous, isolated individuals who exist independent of communities. Carla, you seem to think of women as having their own isolated identities and projects, as being "moral strangers" to one another. In your account, these moral strangers appeal to ethics in order to secure protection against a threatening community. You keep talking about Ms. Neil as if she were in danger from the community.

But isn't there another way of picturing Ms. Neil? I can understand why a woman like Ms. Neil "cares" about her infertile friends who are suffering. I can also understand why she would choose to assist them without concentrating on all the possible social and individual harms that might accrue to her as a result.

Prof. Thomas:    Dr. Collins, it seems that you and I agree that Ms. Neil should be allowed to act as a surrogate, but we disagree about why she is entitled to do it. I think there are some feminists who view surrogacy as just another form of "female exploitation" by wealthy males. For example, some feminist thinkers want to caution women about this potential exploitation. Susan Sherwin's important work on "in vitro fertilization" and other reproductive technologies raises serious questions about surrogacy.[17] I believe that Sherwin would want to focus as much on Mrs. Douglas as on Harriet Neil. For example, is Mrs. Douglas under social pressure to have a child of her own? No one has inquired into why she has consented to a surgery to remove ova. Is her husband demanding this of her? Does she feel that she is incomplete if she does not reproduce? Does she feel unnatural, or selfish, if she does not fulfill what men might call her "reproductive role" as a woman? Does she feel that she is a disappointment to her husband because she cannot gestate children and therefore she wants to participate in a surrogacy arrangement? In short, Sherwin is deeply concerned that reproductive technology is assisting in the lingering oppression of women rather than contributing to the genuine interests of women.

Mary Quigley:

Would Sherwin forbid Mrs. Douglas from using a surrogacy arrangement based on these fears? Or should Mrs. Douglas have to pass some kind of test that proves that her decision to secure a surrogacy arrangement is really genuine?

Prof. Thomas:

My point is that we need to take some action to assure ourselves that her wishes and interests are not being disregarded.

Prof. Fisk:

But, Carla, you do not buy this viewpoint, do you? Your view of ethics is tied intimately to respect for the individual.

Prof. Thomas:

Yes. Mrs. Douglas and Harriet Neil may both be instruments in a vile plot by Mr. Douglas or the physicians or society. But you need some evidence to this effect. Speculation about the possibility that these women are being unethically manipulated is not evidence that they are, in fact, being harmed. I would have no part in cutting off their access to surrogacy even though it is clearly possible that they are being used. I tend to believe women when they tell me that they want something. It is not my job to validate their wishes or to show that their wishes are consistent with some feminist vision about what they should want.

And while I am at it, I might as well respond to Dr. Collins about the fact that I am an individualist. I certainly am an individualist. And I do not think that communities of men and/or women should define what is best for every individual in every situation. My emphasis on rights may be caused, as Dr. Collins suggests, by the overinfluence of male modes of conception on my way of thinking, but my practical concern is to grant Ms. Neil the power to act as a surrogate even though I may think that she is going to take a hard fall. Granting power to individual women doesn't liberate them from harm.

Ms. Quigley: There is something to what Professor Thomas is saying. We do not know what people are going to do if surrogacy becomes a genuine option. It might change the face of reproduction. This, quite frankly, frightens me because I am scared of the unknown. This fear motivates me to resist offering people the option, but I do not feel very good about restraining people from doing what might wind up giving them their heart's desire. I have children, and I know what they contribute to my life. If these people want to try this new procedure, and are willing to abide by our safeguards, then I support them. I think that they have a right to try this.

Prof. Fisk: I want to address Attorney Quinn's concerns. To my knowledge no hospital has been subjected to significant liability consequences because of its participation in a surrogacy arrangement. Before we act on your concerns, I think we need solid evidence that we are substantially increasing our risk. In other words, John, there is fear of risk but as yet no evidence of risk. Furthermore, 20 years ago lawyers were telling hospitals not to engage in withdrawing and withholding treatments because of the fear of liability. And today forgoing treatment is commonplace in the American hospital. We tested the practice of forgoing treatment, and it was beneficial to patients. I think that we should take the same approach to surrogacy. Let's not react on the basis of unwarranted fear. Rather, let's proceed cautiously and turn to experiment to see if patient benefit can be secured by this practice. Medicine has always entered into uncharted waters using the clinical experiment as its guide, and I think that this is a wise strategy within this area.

Prof. Thomas: I think that we need to address some concerns regarding the children. Many authors have expressed opposition to surrogacy based on the assumption that surrogacy opens the door to treating babies as property that can be bought and sold. Let me address a few remarks toward this concern. Adoption in the United States was at one time a private affair. Abuses occurred, and some of these abuses involved selling adoptable children to the highest bidder. It was a disgraceful practice and we put an end to it. States now outlaw the use of financial incentives to relinquish children. Using money as an incentive to a woman, especially a poor woman, to give up her child is, in my opinion, despicable and violates the rights of women. The same thing holds true of the surrogate, and I think that our policy goes on record as opposing this. However, we have no means of enforcing this part of the policy or guaranteeing that Mr. and Mrs. Douglas haven't privately agreed to pay Ms. Neil $20,000 at the successful transfer of the child. Not only can we not prevent it from happening but we certainly cannot penalize them if they do pay her. Our policy is a paper tiger that has no real teeth.

Dr. Collins: Carla, we are not in the enforcement business, and I see no reason for suggesting that we get into enforcement. That is a matter for the state. Just as the state enforces reasonable regulations on adoption, I think that the state ought to regulate surrogacy. But that is not and cannot be our responsibility.

Prof. Thomas:    That was not my point, Dr. Collins. I merely wanted to say that we cannot guarantee that our rules will be followed. They have no legal force nor do they have the force of contract, because I think that these agreements are not legally valid at this time. What I am saying is that there is genuine risk here, and we cannot go into this thinking that the parties will behave according to our rules.

Dr. Collins:    It seems that we have covered the relevant ground on this—or am I cutting off the conversation too quickly?

Vivian Harris:    Well, I have one further issue. Suppose the child that results from this surrogacy arrangement is handicapped. Let's suppose that neither Ms. Neil nor the Douglases want it. Who is going to be responsible for this child if it is not perfect? Are the parties just going to throw it away or trade it in for another model the way you would trade in a car that was a lemon? After all, they negotiated for the child; why not negotiate for a new and "better" child? Surrogacy seems to encourage an attitude toward children that they can be "arranged for." They can be contracted for and negotiated for. If the product doesn't fit our needs, then we can dispense with it. But kids frequently fail to meet our expectations. They require an enormous amount of adjustment on our parts.

Prof. Fisk:    Vivian, the principle that governs this arena is that restrictions on reproductive liberty need to justified. And the only way to justify such restrictions is to establish that unjustifiable harm will occur as a result of exercising the liberty or that the exercise of the liberty will lead to the violation of the rights of others. Your concern seems to be that unjustifiable harm will happen to the child.

Ms. Harris:    Martin, don't try to put philosophy in my mouth. I said that by allowing surrogacy, we may reinforce a questionable attitude toward children. Although children can and should be controlled to some degree, they also exist for themselves, and they frequently require us to radically alter our lives in response to their needs and demands. I am worried that surrogacy encourages parents to view children as things that exist to satisfy the parents' needs, and as such they can be produced to fit our needs like any product.

Prof. Fisk:    Vivian, I am glad that you have noticed that sometimes I try to categorize positions before I understand them. It is my way of attempting to understand complex issues. I hope that I did not offend you. Let me try again: is your concern a "slippery slope concern"? That is, are you concerned that small violations of traditional reproductive practices will lead to greater and greater violations of traditional reproductive practices?

Ms. Harris:    The practice I am concerned with is the practice of accepting your children as they are rather than attempting to completely control and manipulate them. The premise that we see here seems to give individuals unconditional reproductive rights. This principle seems to justify surrogacy, but I am worried about what else this kind of principle could justify. It scares me because it seems to allow parents to select and

|  | manipulate their children. If the selection process doesn't work out to the parents' satisfaction, then, presumably, they can discard children. |
|---|---|
| Prof. Thomas: | Vivian, it seems to me as if your remarks are aimed at a different topic, which is the genetic manipulation of children. I am not sure how they apply to this case. |
| Ms. Harris: | The connection is this: if the principle of autonomy confers on individuals unconditional authority to control their reproductive lives, then I think that we may face a very frightening future. Furthermore, surrogacy may be a significant legal and ethical precedent when the time comes to address the genetic questions. I think that we need to think about the implications of this principle of unconditional reproductive autonomy in relation to the new genetic technologies. |
| Dr. Collins: | I, too, share Vivian's concerns but think that we need to put these questions on another agenda. Not today's agenda. Does anyone wish to put forth a motion? |
| Prof. Fisk: | The motion that I would make would be in the form of a recommendation. |

*Committee Recommendations*    Because of the infertility of the Douglas family, and because all parties agree to abide by our surrogacy policy restrictions, I move that we approve the request to use the services and personnel of the hospital.

| Dr. Collins: | Discussion of the motion is in order. |
|---|---|
| Atty. Quinn: | I recommend that we table this motion until there is more legal clarity on the issues. |
| Dr. Davis: | These folks have postponed their family for a long time, and I think that it may be a long time before this is settled by the courts. I understand and applaud Dr. King's |

commitment to helping his patients. If I were in his shoes, I would do my best to address their infertility. The medical oath requires this. The oath does not require me to avoid legally uncharted areas. Furthermore, I think that it would be unfair to have passed this policy and then refuse to apply it. My vote is to support Martin's motion as it is.

Rev. Marcus: I do not accept the Catholic view that artificial insemination is against the will of God. Nor do I accept that artificial insemination is unnatural. But there is something in the Catholic position that a dyed-in-the-wool Lutheran like myself finds very attractive, which is that God intended that there be a close connection between sexual intercourse and reproduction. In this case, we are bypassing this connection for very serious medical reasons, but I would be very reluctant to support any plan that would allow techniques such as artificial insemination or surrogacy to be used in any but serious medical contexts. Furthermore, the suffering that is a part of pregnancy does unite the mother and the child. It is not completely meaningless, nor do I believe that we would be better off if it were completely eliminated. Surrogacy eliminates all the traditional sufferings associated with childbearing that mothers have experienced since the dawn of creation, and I fear that this suffering may not be all bad because what we suffer for becomes deeply and profoundly *ours* . I wonder what the elimination of this suffering is or might do to our families.

Dr. Collins: You know, Richard, many women have easy and very joyous pregnancies. Does that make them worse mothers? Is suffering necessary to being a good parent?

| | |
|---|---|
| Rev. Marcus: | No, but pregnancy is symbolic of the fact that you better be prepared to accept a lot of change, and perhaps suffering, when you become a parent. Let me close by saying that I intend to support this recommendation as one that fits within our guidelines, even though I am very suspicious of these very guidelines. |
| Prof. Fisk: | I want to go on record as saying that the symbolic significance of pregnancy is not a public matter. It belongs to what some people call the private sphere. I am sure that Richard is expressing a widely held religious view about pregnancy, but this committee is not empowered to endorse essentially private views about the will or intentions of God. I, for one, am suspicious that there is a God, so I am very suspicious about whether we can discover the will of a being that in my opinion does not exist. Furthermore, I am suspicious of any attempt to restrict the autonomy of adults based exclusively on private considerations. I would feel very uncomfortable if our committee decided to adopt a specific vision of what the good society or the good person is and then impose it on our patients. |

The committee approves the recommendation.

## Questions for Further Discussion

1. Is there a genuine conflict of interest involved when the hospital attorney, who is responsible for keeping the hospital out of litigation, serves on the ethics committee?
2. Is the hospital at legal risk in approving this policy? Research this question and offer an opinion.
3. Does the fact that there are no penalties for secretly violating the hospital's surrogacy policy transform the policy into a senseless set of rules? Are rules without enforcement meaningless?

4. Should the committee spend more time investigating whether the Douglases would be good parents?

5. Assume that the Douglases were poor and that they lived in a dangerous neighborhood and were also intermittent alcoholics. Given that these factors are not sufficient to restrict individuals from reproducing normally, should they be used as a basis for restricting surrogate reproduction?

6. Do we need the principle of unconditional reproductive freedom in order to support surrogacy?

7. Did the committee adequately discuss the possible harms that might happen to the child as a result of being produced via artificial insemination and surrogacy?

8. If Ms. Neil refuses to hand over the child, should she be allowed to keep it? If you need to make some assumptions in order to answer this question, be sure to make them explicit.

9. If the child is severely handicapped, who should bear the burden of caring for this child? Ms. Neil? The Douglases? Both parties? Furthermore, suppose Ms. Neil suffers a significant harm as a result of the pregnancy. Should the Douglases be responsible for caring for or supporting her?

10. Do the concerns expressed in questions 8 and 9 indicate that valid contracts are needed in this arena?

## More Cases for Examination

### The Single Parent and the New Partnership

Atty. John Martin and Dr. Harvey Finch have formed a new partnership in which they will work cooperatively to bring together surrogate mothers and infertile clients who wish to obtain surrogacy services. Dr. Finch is an obstetrician at Community Hospital. Through his contacts among other physicians he believes that he can obtain between 25 and 50 surrogacy referrals per year. Dr. Finch will be responsible for securing the clients and for all medical aspects of the procedure. Atty. Martin will be responsible for all the legal aspects. They expect to charge individuals $45,000 for their joint services. This does not include hospital or laboratory fees. The state in which Martin and Finch practice has no explicit legislative or judicial rulings that prohibit surrogacy.

Their first potential client is a wealthy single man named John Smith. He wants a biologically related child but has no interest in marriage. He says that he intends to raise the child as a single parent and openly asserts that he believes that traditional families are not necessary in order to raise healthy and happy children. Indeed, he claims that the traditional nuclear family is a harmful institution. He has given Finch and Martin a check for $10,000 and wants them to get going on the project immediately. Neither Finch nor Martin have any knowledge of this man except that he seemed to both of them to be quite reasonable during their one-hour interview. On the basis of this interview they have decided to accept him as a client.

Dr. Collins, the medical director of the hospital, learns of their decision and realizes that their actions violate the hospital's policy on surrogacy. Dr. Collins thinks that they need to do a background check on Mr. Smith in order to establish that he is free of any significant impediment such as mental illness. Dr. Finch and Mr. Martin believe that such checks are an invasion of their client's privacy. They argue that no one does a background check on married couples who conceive a child.

Finally, there is genuine concern both about the monetary aspects of the contract and about whether staff physicians are obligated to obey hospital ethics policy. How should the committee manage this case?

## Surrogacy and the Middle-Age Couple

Helen and Don Mathews are 53 and 54 years old respectively. Until recently both of them were so involved with their careers that they never felt the need to have children.

One year ago both of them changed their minds and their feelings. They now want their own children. They feel very deeply that they made a mistake by not having a family. They are both in sound health and are financially very well off. They do not wish to adopt. Helen has given up her lucrative law practice with the explicit aim of becoming pregnant, but with no success.

Like Helen, Don is very enthusiastic about starting a family. However, he has raised the possibility of securing a surrogate mother who would gestate one of Helen's eggs fertilized in vitro by Don's semen. Helen supports the idea.

They have contacted Community Hospital's surrogacy group and applied to participate in the surrogacy program. However, the Community Hospital's surrogacy group refuses to accept them on the grounds that they are too old. The physician argues that these arrangements occasionally wind up in the courts, if the surrogate mother bolts the agreement. He asserts that the agreement is not a legally binding document and that a custody fight in the courts might occur. He claims that their age would weigh against them in a custody battle and that they might not win custody. The Mathews respond that they will take their chances in a court fight. How should the committee manage this conflict?

## Further Reading

Andrews, Lori B, "The Aftermath of Baby M: Proposed State Laws on Surrogate Motherhood," *Hastings Center Report* (October/November 1987).
Annas, George J., "The Baby Broker Boom," *Hastings Center Report* (April 1986).
Cohen, Barbara, "Surrogate Mothers: Whose Baby Is It?" *American Journal of Law and Medicine* (Fall 1984).
Elias, Sherman, and George J. Annas, "Social Policy Considerations in Noncoital Reproduction," *Journal of the American Medical Association* (January 3, 1986): pp. 62–68.
Gilligan, Carol, *In a Different Voice* (Cambridge: Harvard University Press, 1982), p. 19.
Keane, Noel P., with Dennis L. Breo, *The Surrogate Mother* (Everest House, 1981).
McCormick, Richard, "Reproductive Technologies: Ethical Issues," in *Encyclopedia of Bioethics*, ed. Walter Reich, vol. 4 (New York: The Free Press, 1978), pp. 1454, 1459.
Meinke, Sue A., "Surrogate Motherhood: Ethical and Legal Issues" (Scope Note #7, Kennedy Institute of Ethics, 1987).
Wolf, Susan M., "Enforcing Surrogate Motherhood Agreements: The Trouble with Specific Performance," *Human Rights Annual* (Spring 1987).

## Notes

1. Rosemarie Tong, "The Overdue Death of a Feminist Chameleon: Taking a Stand on Surrogacy Arrangements," *Journal of Social Philosophy* 21 (1909): 47
2. For a more detailed analysis of the Baby M case, see George Annas, "Baby M: Babies (and Justice) for Sale," *Hastings Center Report* (3) (1987):15.
3. Ronald Dworkin, "Paternalism," in *Philosophy of Law*, by Conrad Johnson (New York: Macmillan, 1993), p. 241.
4. Peter Singer and Diane Wells, *The Reproductive Revolution* (New York: Oxford University Press, 1984), p. 125.
5. Mary Warnock, chair, *Report of the Committee of Inquiry into Human Fertilization and Embryology* (London: Her Majesty's Stationery Office, 1984).
6. Stephen Munzer, *A Theory of Property* (Cambridge: Cambridge University Press, 1990), p. 171.
7. Lori Andrews, "Alternative Modes of Reproduction," in Reproductive Laws for the 1990s, ed. Sherill Cohen and Nadine Taub (Clifton, N. J.: Humana Press, 1988), p. 371.
8. Mary Gibson, "The Moral and Legal Status of 'Surrogate' Motherhood," unpublished paper presented at the Eastern Division Meeting of the American Philosophical Association 1988.

9. Elizabeth Anderson, "Is Women's Labor a Commodity?" *Philosophy and Public Affairs* 19 (1) (1990): 71–92.

10. Allan Wertheimer, "Two Questions about Surrogacy and Exploitation," *Philosophy and Public Affairs* 21 (3) (Summer 1992): 211.

11. These views are reported in *Medical World News* (Jan. 9, 1984), p. 24.

12. Ann Neale, "Responsible Stewardship Requires Not Cooperating with Surrogacy," in *The Ethics of Reproductive Technology*, ed. Kenneth Alpern: (New York, Oxford University Press, 1992).

13. H. Tristram Engelhardt, *The Foundations of Bioethics.*

14. For a thorough discussion of this model, see Brendan Minogue, "The Exclusion of Theology from Public Policy: The Case for Euthanasia," *Second Opinion,*14 (July 1990): 85.

15. For a more detailed development of this conversational view of society, see Richard Rorty's *Philosophy and the Mirror of Nature* (Princeton, N.J.: Princeton University Press, 1979). Chapters 7 and 8 are especially relevant.

16. Carol Gilligan, *In a Different Voice* (Cambridge: Harvard University Press, 1982).

17. Susan Sherwin, *No Longer Patient: Feminist Ethics and Health Care* (Philadelphia: Temple University Press, 1992), esp. 132ff.

# 6

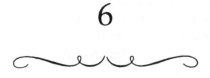

# Abortion

## Introduction to the Problem Area

In 1973 the United States Supreme Court affirmed in a decision called *Roe v.Wade* that there was a constitutional right to abortion.[1] Few judicial decisions have caused more conflict and controversy in the United States. *Abortion* is defined as the termination of pregnancy before the fetus is capable of independent life. Abortions are usually classified as either spontaneous or elective. A spontaneous abortion is one that occurs independent of deliberate choice. How often this happens is a subject of some controversy. An elective or induced abortion results from the deliberate choice of the individual woman to remove the fetus from the womb. Elective abortions may be further divided into either therapeutic or nontherapeutic procedures. In therapeutic abortions there is a medical reason related to the health and safety of the mother that motivates the abortive procedure; in nontherapeutic abortions the decision is based on personal, social, or economic reasons.

This distinction between therapeutic and nontherapeutic is not very precise because of the significant ambiguities surrounding the phrase "medical reason," but the distinction plays an important role in the abortion debate.

### Terminology and Fetal Development

There is a vast amount of complex biological information associated with abortion. Although no attempt will be made to offer a complete account of fetal development, no discussion of abortion can take place without some attention to biology.

During pregnancy change and development are continuous. Pregnancy typically begins with intercourse—artificial insemination and in vitro fertilization are important exceptions to this generalization—in which over 300 million sperm cells are deposited into the vagina. Sperm cells contain 23 chromosomes, or half the genetic information found in the nucleus of human cells. Following intercourse these sperm begin a journey upward through the uterus and into the tube leading to the ovary. It is important to note that this journey takes several hours, during which techniques employed to inhibit fertilization do not involve abortion since the ovum and the sperm have not yet united. Procedures designed to prevent fertilization are *contraceptive*.

The ovary is the source of the female germ cell called the *ovum*, which also contains 23 chromosomes. The ovum, deposited by the ovary, will fall into the same fallopian tube connecting the uterus with the ovary. The ovum will survive for approximately 24 hours. If no sperm unites with it during that time, it will die. If a sperm cell does unite with the ovum, then conception is said to occur.

The term *conception* refers to the process in which the male germ cell unites with the female germ cell or ovum to form a single cell called the *zygote*, or fertilized ovum or egg. The zygote contains all the genetic information (46 chromosomes) of the human being. These chromosomes will largely guide the biological development of the unborn being until its death. The zygote begins its developmental process almost immediately as it attempts to move through the fallopian tube toward the uterus. Cell division occurs while it is in the fallopian tube. After about seven days the zygote implants itself into the lining of the uterus. Implantation is critical, for at this point the zygote is renamed and referred to as an *embryo*. This embryonic stage lasts for approximately six weeks, during which many of the organ systems begin to form. From the end of the eighth week until the point of delivery, the entity is called a *fetus*. It is common for writers to blur these distinctions and refer to the unborn entity as a fetus from the moment of conception.

The stages of development are also marked in other ways. At some point after the 12th week of pregnancy and usually before the 16th week, the woman begins to feel the fetus moving within her. Traditionally, this is called *quickening*. It is important because in ancient times many authors held that it was at the point of quickening that the soul entered into the body. Another term that is widely used in the abortion debate is *viability*. This is the point at which the fetus is capable of living independently outside the body of the mother. Because of technological developments, the point of viability is continually changing. Forty years ago it was nearly impossible to save the life of a fetus that was born 28 weeks after conception. Today, with the help of neonatal technology, it is possible to maintain and sustain infants born even earlier. Indeed, premature infants have survived prior to this stage, but the number of viable fetuses drops off dramatically as we go back to the 20th week. At this point in scientific development, fetuses born prior to the 20th week are generally agreed to be nonviable. Perhaps the two most important factors in determining viability are the weight of the fetus and the length of the gestation period.

This issue of viability is, however, crucial in the discussion of the *Roe* v. *Wade* decision because the Supreme Court required that fetuses cannot be aborted after viability. However, the decision also permits abortions on demand until the end of the second trimester (the 24th week after conception). These two criteria may conflict since some fetuses are viable prior to the 24th week. In the future, viability may become common before the 24th week, especially if neonatal technology continues to develop. In short, the *Roe* v. *Wade* decision permits abortion until the beginning of the third trimester and yet forbids it after viability, and these criteria may conflict. This problem has motivated Supreme Court Justice Sandra Day O'Connor to recommend that the court surrender the trimester system as a basis for determining when abortion is permissible.[2]

Let us close this section on terminology and fetal development with some advice from Andre Hellegers, a widely respected professor of obstetrics and gynecology at Georgetown University, who is well known for his scientific descriptions of fetal development.[3] Hellegers warned participants in the abortion debate that the sciences of biology or obstetrics cannot prove or disprove opposing answers to the one crucial philosophical question within the debate, namely, at what point in the process of development does human life or personhood begin. He claims that "human life" is to be understood in terms of "human dignity," "human personhood," or "human inviolability." If human life is understood in these terms, then science cannot answer this question. Hellegers suggests that this is a "societal judgment," not a scientific question. Unfortunately, Hellegers does not explain what he means by societal judgment, but we shall return to this concept in more detail in our philosophical commentary.

## Abortion Methods

There are at least five methods used for elective abortions, and these vary with the time of gestation. During the first five weeks after conception a woman can take the drug RU 486. This drug will inhibit the implantation process from beginning or continuing. The drug works by blocking the action of the ovarian hormone progesterone, which is necessary for implantation. Earlier versions of RU 486 required women to return to a physician's office within two days to receive an injection of prostaglandin, which brings about the emission of the uterine contents. Recently, a new version of the procedure has been developed. Two days after taking RU 486, women can take pills containing prostaglandin. Proponents of abortion believe that this simplified procedure is the safest method of abortion and that it may significantly reduce the need for abortion center, which have become the site of conflict.

After the five-week period, another method, called suction or vacuum aspiration, is employed. This is usually performed on an outpatient basis in a clinic. It is a brief procedure in which the cervix is opened and a small tube connected to a vacuum pump is inserted. The contents of the uterus are then removed by vacuum pump.

Early in the second trimester, a method called dilation and evacuation (D&E) is used, in which suction curettage and forceps are utilized to terminate the pregnancy. This method can also be used in the clinic setting. After the 15th week, the method of saline infusion may be used. This involves the removal of some amniotic fluid. This fluid is then replaced by a salt solution, which produces contractions within 48 hours. Prostaglanden may be used instead of the saline solution, but this sometimes leads to live births.

In very late abortions, a procedure called brain suction abortion is common. The safety of these procedures is now widely accepted in the sense that they provide less risk to the patient than full-term delivery.

### History

The practice of abortion has been common throughout history. The Greek philosopher Aristotle maintained that the soul entered the male fetus at approximately 40 days after conception and the female fetus after 90 days.[4] Following Aristotle, St. Thomas Aquinas, the Catholic philosopher and theologian, maintained that there were three kinds of soul: vegetative, animal, and rational. The rational soul did not enter the body until the later stages of development. For Aquinas, abortion was a sin but a lesser sin than murder because there was significant debate over the point at which the rational soul, which distinguishes humans from animals or vegetables, enters into the body of the fetus. Many medieval Christian scholars classified abortion with contraception in seriousness. Abortion was widely forbidden for the same reasons that contraception was forbidden; both were seen to violate natural law, which was viewed as expressing God's will regarding reproduction.

Abortion was not made a secular or public crime throughout the West until the 19th century. Indeed, according to most scholars, it was easier for a woman to obtain an abortion during the early days of our republic than in 1950. The primary reason given for 19th century antiabortion legislation was that abortion practices at the time were viewed as dangerous to the health of women. Furthermore, even these laws stipulated an exception: elective abortion was permitted to save the life of the mother and, occasionally, to secure her health.

Following World War II, Japan and a host of European countries legalized elective abortion, and by 1970 liberalized abortion laws were commonplace throughout the world. In the United States, many states followed the trend of passing abortion laws that generally opposed abortion but widened the scope of exceptions. However, by 1972, Alaska, Hawaii, New York, and Washington had passed "abortion on demand" legislation. This set the scene for the *Roe* v. *Wade* decision in 1973.

The Supreme Court is empowered to determine whether state laws are consistent with the U.S. Constitution. The Constitution has priority over all state and federal laws. When *Roe* v. *Wade* asserted that there was a limited constitutional right to abortion on demand, this meant that state laws that prohibited abortion on demand were invalid.

## The Elements of *Roe* v. *Wade*

But what exactly was determined in *Roe* v. *Wade*? The decision had five elements. First, it noted that the safety arguments that were the original justifications for the antiabortion laws in the 19th century were no longer valid because safe abortion procedures were now technically available. But more importantly, the widespread practice of abortion at the time the Constitution was written indicates that the original writers of the Constitution did not intend to treat the fetus as a person. There were no laws outlawing abortion at the time, and the founders of the republic did not see fit to prohibit abortion in the Constitution itself.

Secondly, the Court claimed that the word "person," as it is used in the Constitution, "does not include the unborn." However, nowhere in the decision can we find systematic answers to the questions "what is a person?" and "when does the fetus attain the status of a person?"

Third, the decision derived the right to abortion from the right of privacy. "We therefore conclude that the right of personal privacy includes the abortion decision."[5] However, the decision does not treat the right of privacy as absolute.

Fourth, the Court recognized that the individual's right of privacy could be restricted if there was a state interest to do so. Furthermore, it affirmed that a state interest did exist with respect to protecting the health and safety of mothers. *Roe* permits states to regulate second trimester abortions "to the extent that the regulation reasonably related to the preservation and protection of maternal health." Though the expression "abortion on demand" does not appear in the decision, the effect of *Roe* was to grant the right of "abortion on demand" during the first and second trimesters.

Fifth, in order to secure the state interest with respect to protecting potential human life, the decision allows a state to prohibit "if it chooses" some later abortions. The abortions that states are permitted to prohibit are those that are "subsequent to viability." However, these prohibitions cannot interfere in cases where the health and safety of the mother are at risk, i.e., therapeutic abortions.

## The Ethical Aspects of Abortion

But the legal and political aspects of abortion are distinct, at least intellectually, from its ethical aspects. There are at least seven ethical considerations at the heart of the issue. The first is *the moral status of the fetus*. For if the fetus is considered a full and complete person, and if morality forbids any and all actions that would directly kill a person, then abortion may indeed be immoral.

There is a continuum of positions on this question. One can maintain that a fetus is a person from the very moment of conception, or one could argue that the fetus becomes a person at a later stage, for example, when it is able to experience pain and suffering, which is often called *sentience*. The appearance of electrical activity in the brain of the fetus may be taken as the criterion for personhood. Or one could argue that viability is the point at which the fetus should be considered a person. These criteria will be discussed in our philosophical commentary on the problem, but at this point it is important to note that it is difficult to prove scientifically that the fetus is or is not a person at any given point. This is because questions regarding the moral status of the fetus are ethical questions, not simply empirical ones. Although there are close connections between ethical and factual questions, there are also significant differences between ethics and science.

The second ethical issue is *privacy*. Many philosophers refer to the right of privacy as the right to be left alone. More specifically, this right is often construed as the right to be protected against public or private interference with family planning. In a very deep sense, the decision to reproduce is up to the individual. But privacy is notoriously hard to define, and it is even more difficult to determine what particular actions it applies to.

If privacy is understood by reference to "private property," then we can see that there are significant restrictions placed on the right of privacy because the value of private property can come into conflict with other important human values. One's property can be private in the sense that others cannot arbitrarily interfere with one's use of it. I cannot simply take your car without your permission. However, one simply cannot do anything one wishes with private property. I cannot, for example, use my privately owned knife to stab another person in the process of stealing his car, nor can I dump toxic wastes on my private property. An individual's rights with respect to private property are thus limited and restricted.

Many supporters of abortion have argued that a woman has the moral right to make her own reproductive decisions and that this right is tied to the right of privacy over her body. According to these "pro-choice" advocates, privacy requires not only that government avoid interfering with a woman's reproductive life but also that it has a duty to prevent others from interfering with a woman's autonomous choice to abort. The right to abortion is often pictured as a noninterference right. Just as the government is prohibited from interfering with a woman's choice to become pregnant, so, too, the government ought to be prohibited from interfering with the decision to end a pregnancy.

Opponents of the right to abortion on demand have argued, however, that although the right to control one's body is broad, it does not extend to ending the life of a person. These opponents assume that the fetus is a person. Critics of the pro-choice position argue that granting the woman the right to abort on demand is similar to granting the owner of the knife the right to use it to kill another person. Just as property rights are restricted when their exercise harms others, so the exercise of reproductive rights should be restricted when these rights violate the rights or welfare of other persons.

The third ethical issue at the heart of the abortion debate involves the notion of *potentiality*. It is clear to many that the fetus has the potential to become a full person. It is often argued that although the fetus is not a person in itself, it is a potential person. By virtue of this potentiality, critics of abortion argue, the fetus deserves to be respected as a person.

The fourth issue involves *slippery slope considerations*. Critics of abortion argue that once we permit it, terrible consequences will follow. The aim of this argument is to establish that once we give up our protection of the fetus, we can no longer *logically justify* our laws that protect the rights of the infant. Abortion, they argue, leads inevitably to infanticide, since if we permit it we cannot consistently justify our current opposition to infanticide.

A fifth ethical issue is the question of *harm*. Although many women have relatively easy pregnancies, being pregnant can clearly harm women in many ways. Among the numerous harmful side effects of pregnancy are nausea, severe backache, and tiredness. Anemia is not uncommon, and there are a host of complications associated with pre-existing conditions such as diabetes or kidney disease. If a woman is diabetic, for example, pregnancy can cause very serious complications. Although there are many psychological joys associated with pregnancy, many pregnant women experience significant negative psychological effects such as periods of depression and anxiety.

There are also powerful social and economic hardships that many pregnant women must endure. Jobs are often lost as a result of pregnancy, and opportunities are often sacrificed. We may call this defense of abortion the *self-defense argument* for it claims that one is entitled to abortion rights for the same reason that one is entitled to the right to protect one's body or one's property from harm.

The sixth issue involves the motives or reasons that cause and/or justify an abortion decision. These reasons may be viewed as forming a continuum. At one end are reasons that are widely accepted as legitimate. At the other end there are reasons that are not so accepted. For example, nearly all opponents of elective abortion will admit that abortions to save the life of the mother are legitimate. Many will also accept abortions of pregnancies that result from rape or incest or abortions that protect the health and not the life of the mother. At the other end of the continuum are those who argue that there are other legitimate reasons that justify abortion, such as family planning or financial or psychological considerations. *Roe* v. *Wade* has attempted to bypass these considerations by dispensing with any "good reasons" test prior to viability. After viability, the "good reasons" test reappears and becomes critical since the only good reasons for abortion after viability are those involving the life or health of the mother.

A seventh issue involves the *duty to help others*. Our society does not generally accept any broad and sweeping duty to save the lives of other people. Thousands of people die every day because of lack of food or shelter or medical care, yet we do not obligate individuals to save these people. The society may praise an individual for saving the lives of others but we do not ordinarily condemn an individual for failing to do so. For example, a homeless person may solicit money from a Mr. Smith. Let us assume that the money is needed to save the life of the homeless person. We may praise Mr. Smith for assisting the homeless person if he chooses to, but we do not generally obligate Mr. Smith to provide what the homeless person needs in order to survive.

Some pro-choice advocates appeal to this principle and assume for the sake of argument that the fetus, like the homeless individual, *is* a person. However, just as we cannot obligate Smith to provide what the homeless person needs, we cannot obligate the pregnant woman to provide what the fetus needs in order to live. These defenders of abortion argue that our society does not accept any general obligation to bring aid to others and therefore we cannot obligate the unwilling woman to save the life of the fetus. Furthermore, if we did obligate the woman to do so we would be forced to obligate Smith to save the life of the homeless person. The issues surrounding our duties to assist others are essential in the abortion debate because critics of this argument often argue that the analogy between the pregnant woman and Mr. Smith is too weak to support the conclusion.

## Abortion and the Hospital

Hospitals are unavoidably involved in the abortion debate for at least four reasons. First, when *Roe* v. *Wade* was first written in 1973, it was the opinion of many health officials that second trimester abortions required, for the woman's safety, a hospital setting. However, in the late 1970s, the American College of Obstetricians and Gynecologists recommended that because the safety of second trimester abortions had greatly increased, such abortions could be safely performed in nonhospital settings. Hospitals breathed a sigh of relief, for if hospital settings were required, then hospitals would have been forced to take a position on abortion. At present many hospitals, including Community Hospital, simply refuse to offer elective abortion services because these services are offered in private clinics. Hospitals are thus able to avoid common and direct involvement in abortion services, Most importantly, they are able to avoid the protests and social unrest that are common at abortion sites.

The second reason involves bioethics education, which is common in the hospital. The ethics committee faced the challenge of making recommendations about how the abortion issue should be raised within ethics education sessions. One approach was to advise those who teach bioethics in the hospital to avoid the subject. Others were to recommend defending one side of the issue, or presenting a balanced position in which the conflicting positions and various compromises could be presented and explained, leaving the students to develop their own views on this controversial issue.

Third, hospitals are involved in the abortion controversy because many community hospitals have family practice clinics associated with them and abortion questions come up in this setting. Pregnant women often need abortion information. As a result, the hospital must determine policy for dispensing abortion information in these clinics. One can choose to allow physicians to treat abortion information as a private matter between patient and physician, or one can develop hospital policies that prohibit providing abortion information to patients. One can also affirm that patients have a right to abortion information and require that if they want it, the physician must either provide it or transfer the patient to a physician who will do so. Public hospitals like Community Hospital must face this information issue.

Fourth, hospitals must face the issue of therapeutic abortion. Some opponents of abortion believe that one should not abort a fetus even to secure the health of the mother. For example, a pregnant woman may be severely diabetic. To abort her fetus would involve, according to some opponents of abortion, an unjustified killing of an innocent person in order to protect the health of another person.[6]

## Community Hospital's Policy on Abortion

*Purpose:*    The purpose of this policy is to clarify the position of the hospital on abortion.

*Definition:* Elective abortion is the deliberate termination of pregnancy before the fetus is viable or capable of independent life. Therapeutic abortions are those aimed at securing the life, health, or safety of the mother.

*Preamble:*

The hospital recognizes that the issue of abortion raises fundamental ethical problems. It is the aim of this policy not to resolve all the ethical issues involved in the abortion debate but to effectively manage the problems relating to abortion that emerge within the hospital.

*Principles:*

1. The hospital will not generally provide elective nontherapeutic abortion. These services are currently being provided at local clinics. However, the hospital stands ready to admit patients who develop complications arising from elective abortions.
2. Some nontherapeutic abortions, especially those near the end of the second trimester, require hospital facilities. Patients who request these services will be directed to other hospitals within the region that provide this service. If these services become scarce and the safety of pregnant women is at risk, then the hospital will reconsider this policy.
3. The hospital continues to accept the trimester system as a basis for deciding when abortions are permissible. It is the view of the committee that because the right to abortion during the first and second trimester is a legal right, all women should have access to abortion information. The family practice clinic will offer abortion information to patients who seek it. This information will be provided upon request. If a physician or nurse is ethically opposed to providing this information, this staff person is not required to provide it. The medical director of the hospital will appoint another physician to provide such information.

4. The hospital will perform therapeutic abortions. If a pregnancy is a genuine threat to a woman's health and/or safety, then the intent of the abortion is to protect the mother from this danger. However, the committee will not attempt to offer any systematic and complete definition of all the situations that medically justify an abortion. Questions as to what constitutes the health and safety of the mother will be answered by the attending physician who is responsible for the case. The committee will periodically review therapeutic abortions performed at the hospital with the aim of verifying that a legitimate medical reason is present in all cases.

5. Therapeutic abortions may be performed at any stage in the gestation process.

6. If the fetus is delivered alive, every effort will be made to preserve its life.

7. No hospital employee will be required to participate in an abortion that violates their convictions. The hospital will make every reasonable effort to find substitutes for staff if they refuse to participate in an abortive procedure.

8. There will be no interference with physicians and patients if they jointly decide to use the drug RU 486. However, if RU 486 continues to be an "experimental drug," it is expected that physicians will follow rules spelled out in the human subject research guidelines of Community Hospital.

9. All issues regarding abortive methods will be left to the discretion of the physician and the patient.

10. The method used in therapeutic abortions is viewed as a matter that should be decided by the patient and the physician. If both parties agree that the fetus might be sentient, then some anesthetic may be employed.

---

## Commentary on the Philosophical and Ethical Aspects of the Policy

The approach of this philosophical commentary is to provide a continuum of positions representing at least three approaches to abortion. We shall call these positions the orthodox, the radical, and the moderate views. Our goal is to present the main arguments for and against these positions in order to enhance the reader's appreciation of the conflicting issues within the debate. As the reader will see, many of the issues mentioned in our introduction will play a vital role in these arguments.

## The Orthodox View

The orthodox view asserts that all elective abortions, except those aimed at saving the life of the mother, are immoral. Some adherents of this view consider such abortions the moral equivalent of murder and thereby deserving of the punishments associated with murder. Others consider abortion less evil than first-degree murder. In effect, holders of the orthodox view do not agree on the degree of evil that is involved in abortion, but they do agree that abortion is immoral.

One of the clearest defenders of this orthodox view is a law professor at the University of California at Berkeley, John Noonan, Jr. Although he is anxious to represent the theological position of the Roman Catholic Church, Noonan does not hold that opposition to abortion rests exclusively on any theological claims that are unique to Roman Catholics. The official teaching of the Roman Catholic Church is that abortion is immoral and those who participate in abortion are committing a grave sin. But according to Noonan, the immorality of abortion can be demonstrated by appeal to reason alone and is, therefore, independent of the religious commitments of the church. Noonan has defended this position in a number of places, but his best known book on the subject is *The Morality of Abortion: Legal and Historical Perspectives.*[7]

In this book he argues that the distinctions used as a basis for separating the fetus from the rest of the human community are flawed and, if the fetus cannot be separated, then it must be granted the same rights as any person. In short, for Noonan, the morality of abortion is determined by the moral status of the fetus. Specifically, the attempt to exclude the fetus from protection based on its nonviability or its time of gestation cannot withstand critical evaluation. Noonan grants that the fetus is surely nonviable at two weeks or twelve weeks but with the development of new neonatal technologies this is changing. Therefore, an exact timetable of viability cannot be given.

But even if we had a very clear picture of when the fetus becomes capable of living independent of the mother, it does not solve the philosophical problem that infants, children, and many full-grown adults present to us. It is perfectly clear to Noonan that many persons remain profoundly dependent on others for their existence. Merely because infants lack viability does not mean that their parents, on whom they are dependent, can ethically choose to end their lives. The same is true for dependent adults. For example, thousands of adults are acutely dependent on other persons for physical or emotional reasons, and yet we do not allow these dependent people to be killed. In short, the concept of viability that the *Roe* v. *Wade* decision used to separate infants from fetuses is too strong. For Noonan if we accept *Roe* v. *Wade* then we endanger persons.

Noonan also criticizes other strategies for separating the fetus from the rest of the moral community. For example, many defenders of abortion often argue that the fetus is not sentient until the second trimester and that the absence of sentience indicates that the fetus will not suffer as a result of the abortive procedure.[8] But Noonan writes that if sentience were necessary for being a person, we could justifiably kill anyone as long as they were anesthetized. Sentience, for Noonan, is just as irrelevant as viability for determining whether someone is a human being endowed with human dignity. If we accepted these criteria, we would be forced to withdraw our protection from defenseless and dependent people.

The last criterion we will discuss is what Noonan calls the criterion of "social recognition." The defender of abortion can claim that the fetus can be destroyed because society does not recognize it as human and, therefore, society can refuse to punish women who do not want to gestate. This, too, suffers from the problem of being an overly strong criterion in that it will eliminate individuals that we do not wish to exclude from protection. The Roman Empire did not recognize Christians as human beings and, therefore, opened the door to making them slaves. The United States did not recognize black people as fully human at the time the Constitution was written. Germany did not recognize that Jews were human beings during the Nazi period. In short, social recognition is a flawed criterion that has enormous potential for abuse, and it is especially harmful if one is interested in protecting individuals or groups that are viewed as socially unacceptable.

But Noonan does more than critcize the right to choose abortion. He also offers a positive account of the fetus as a person. For Noonan, the fetus has something that makes anyone a person: " . . . if you are conceived by human parents, you are human." The fetus, from the moment of conception, contains the complete genetic information of a human being. This genetic information contains a set of directions that will guide the fetus's development throughout the life of the person; therefore, Noonan maintains that we must speak of the fetus as a human being from the moment of conception.

This point is critical. At the moment of conception the fetus cannot do any of the acts that typical humans do. But for Noonan, this is irrelevant since it has the potential to perform these acts and this potentiality requires us to treat the fetus as a person. This is the potentiality argument discussed earlier: if the fertilized egg has the potential for developing into a person, then it ought to be treated as a person. Noonan attempts to differentiate the unfertilized egg or the sperm from the fertilized egg. All three have a "potentiality" in some sense to become a person, but the potentialities are vastly different. The sperm by itself has only a small potentiality, but for Noonan, a fertilized egg has a very high chance of developing into a person. The challenges to this potentiality argument will be raised by the critics of Noonan's pro-life position.

Noonan does admit that there is one reason that justifies abortion.[9] If the pregnancy is a direct threat to the life of the mother, then it is permissible to abort. For example, if a pregnant woman is diagnosed as having a cancerous uterus, then even the official teaching of the Catholic Church would permit the surgical removal of the uterus. Another example involves an ectopic pregnancy, in which the zygote begins to develop in the fallopian tube, thereby threatening the life of the mother. The surgical removal of the cancerous uterus and the surgical removal of the fallopian tube is justified by what Catholics have called the "principle of the double effect."

What distinguishes these cases from ordinary elective abortions is that the intent is not to abort or kill the fetus. Rather, the intent is to save the life of the mother by removing the cancerous uterus or the fallopian tube. The principle of the double effect asserts that it is ethically permissible to take an action such as removing the uterus even if it produces an unintended but foreseen result (the death of the fetus).

There are, however, some conditions that need to be satisfied in order to apply the principle to any concrete case. First, the action taken, such as removing the uterus, is the only way that the good result can be achieved. There must be no other way to save the life of the mother. Second, the death of the fetus must be viewed as the unintended and indirect effect of the action. The death of the fetus must be unintended even though it is foreseen. On the other hand, the good effect is seen as the intended and direct result of the surgery. Third, the act that produces the double effect must not be an evil act in itself, such as murder. Fourth, the bad effect is not the means to the end. For example, if we were to save the life of the mother by directly killing the fetus, then the good effect would be brought about by the evil means. However, if we merely remove the uterus to save the woman's life and the child dies as a result, then nothing immoral has occurred. Finally, the good result, saving the mother's life, must outweigh the evil that is permitted.

## A New Version of the Orthodox View

An updated version of this orthodox view is contained in a recent essay by Don Marquis entitled "Why Abortion Is Immoral."[10] In this essay Marquis develops what he believes to be a sufficient condition for why "it is wrong to kill us" (meaning persons). This may be called a theory of wrongful death. For Marquis "killing us" is wrong not because we are human, or because we are persons, or because we were conceived by humans, or because we have the human genetic structure, or because of the sanctity of human life; rather, killing us is wrong because it deprives us of "valuable future experiences." Marquis then generalizes this claim and asserts that the reason it is wrong to kill anyone is that it deprives them of future experiences such as pleasure, joy, and love. Killing the fetus deprives it of these valuable future experiences; therefore, killing the fetus is wrong.

Marquis maintains that this argument has a number of virtues. First, it bypasses the issue of whether the fetus is or is not a person. One may fight interminably over this issue, but for Marquis these debates are irrelevant. As long as we are confident that abortion deprives the fetus of valuable future experiences, then it does not matter whether the fetus is a person, a human being, an angel, or a robot. Killing any of these things would be wrong if it deprived them of valuable future experiences. The central question is not the moral status of the fetus but whether they are robbed of a valuable future.

Second, Marquis claims that those who justify abortion on the ground that the fetus is not a person face the problem of having to introduce ad hoc conditions to prevent justifying the killing of infants. He believes that his theory of wrongful death avoids this issue. Killing infants is wrong because infants are deprived of future experiences, and no ad hoc conditions are needed.

Third, Marquis thinks that this theory also has the virtue of possibly allowing active voluntary euthanasia of those who are suffering from a terminal illness. It may not be wrong to kill people when death does not mean depriving them of valuable future experiences, if the only future they face is bleak.

## Criticisms of the Orthodox View

A number of criticisms can be offered of this orthodox view. The first hinges on the question of potentiality, since the potentiality of the fetus is why many people consider it valuable. Noonan seems to think that the probability that the fetus will develop into a human being indicates that it is a human being. However, the principle that takes us from the claim that something is a potential X to the claim that the potential X is as valuable as X is dubious at best. Indeed, we do not assume, as a general rule, that something is valuable merely because it has the potentiality to become something valuable. For example, an oak tree may be potentially very valuable. It may be worth thousands of dollars at the lumber mill. But this does not mean that the owner of the lumber mill will give you thousands of dollars for an acorn. The seed is simply not considered as valuable as what it might become. There seems to be a value difference between mature oak trees and seeds. This is not to say that the acorn is without value—merely that the value of the tree and the acorn are not identical. This refusal to identify the value of something with that which makes it possible influences the abortion debate in that we need not assume that because the fetus is a potential human being, that it is as valuable as an actual human being.

Second, the defender of abortion rights can respond that the question of the status of the fetus deals with borderline cases and thus cannot be answered in a purely objective fashion. In effect, the abortion rights advocate can respond that there is a subjective aspect to the viability criterion, as there is to all criteria that attempt to separate persons from nonpersons. We can illustrate this idea of borderline cases by analogy to colors.

Colors run in shades. Although our language favors the idea that the colors are qualitatively different from one another, there is really a continuum of shades from the deepest reds to the deepest violets. Furthermore, where colors intersect there are often borderline cases where it is hard to tell whether a shade is actually, say, red or orange. Indeed, there may be no objective answer in such borderline cases, and yet we still may need to make a decision whether to call a given shade red or orange. In these cases we are forced to depend on some agreed-upon criterion rather than an objective fact that will distinguish the colors from one another. Indeed, even if we used a scientific instrument to detect the exact wavelength of the shade, we would still need to depend on a convention that determines that one wavelength is to be called red and the next higher one is to be called orange.

Humans need conventions in order to solve real problems in many different areas of human interest. One of the primary purposes of the law is to provide us with a fair procedure for developing these conventions, which we need in order to live together peacefully. When we follow fair procedures for answering these borderline questions, we sometimes refer to our answers as objective.

The fetus may indeed be a borderline case because we cannot develop an absolutely sharp biological or empirical criterion that would separate it from those who are normally protected by the law. This need to make tough choices by developing "precise" but conventional definitions appears also at the end of life since there may be no objective basis for saying that total absence of electrical activity in the brain is an acceptable definition of death.[11] The concept of death had to be made more precise, and legislative bodies developed conventions or laws that met this requirement for precision.

Viability may thus be treated as a chosen or conventional criterion because it depends on a choice by legislatures and courts. Surely Noonan is right in saying that there are many nonviable individuals being treated as persons, but that does not mean that nonviability in the context of gestation cannot be treated as a precising criterion that allows us to distinguish fetuses from persons. Just as the legislative bodies chose to make the absence of electrical activity in the brain a criterion of being dead, so too the Supreme Court was empowered to determine whether the protections of the state should be extended to fetuses. This is not a purely objective matter, but to say that the Court created a new convention is not to say that it acted in a completely arbitrary or irrational manner. The *Roe* decision did what many court decisions do: it constructed a precise and exact, yet conventional, definition of whom the state is obligated to protect.

Marquis's updated version of the orthodox position also has some difficulties. One involves his attempt to define wrongful killing in quantitative rather than qualitative terms. Wrongful killing deprives one of a valuable future, but how much value must someone lose before we say that killing them is wrongful? In Marquis's theory, in order to determine that a killing is wrong, one must calculate that future good experiences outweigh future bad experiences. If your future life lacks sufficient good experiences based on some standard, which Marquis never defines, then presumably Marquis must permit us to kill you. But this is counterintuitive. When we accuse Smith of killing Jones, we never allow Smith to defend himself by doing complex calculations that prove that the negative value of Jones's future experiences outweighed their positive value. The difficulties surrounding the quantitative aspect of Marquis's theory of wrongful death make it unlikely that this theory can determine the course of the abortion debate.

### The Radical View

The second position on the abortion question is the extreme opposite of the orthodox view. In the radical view, a pregnant woman's right to abort should be respected throughout the pregnancy. This view is most clearly represented in the philosophical work of Mary Ann Warren. In her essay "On the Moral and Legal Status of Abortion,"[12] she argues for three central claims.

First, like Noonan, Warren argues that the moral status of the fetus is the central question in the abortion debate. For Warren, this question cannot be answered until we notice that the word "human" is used with two different meanings. She refers to an argument that expresses an antiabortion position: because it is wrong to kill innocent human beings and because the fetus is a human being, it follows that it is wrong to kill the fetus. She claims that the fallacy of equivocation occurs within the argument because the word "human" has two different meanings and these different meanings can produce fallacious reasoning.[13] In the first sense, "human" means "genetically human," and in the second, human means "person." She claims that the class of persons is not identical to the class of genetic humans. There may be persons in other galaxies who can think and feel as we do but who have vastly different biologies. They may not be human but they may be persons. The term "human" is descriptive in that it describes a specific species. On the other hand, the term "person" is prescriptive rather than descriptive. It stands for those individuals who are said to be morally valuable and entitled to all the rights, privileges, and protections accorded to persons. Furthermore, breathing individuals who have lost all electrical activity in the brain may be construed as humans, but there was serious debate during the past few decades about whether they were persons. State legislatures have determined that the set of brain-dead humans does not belong to the set of persons. For Warren, whether someone is a human is a scientific question, but whether a human is a person or a member of the moral community is a moral question. She states that the strongest argument for the orthodox view rests on an equivocation fallacy that involves assuming that anything that is human, i.e., has the human genetic code, is a person in the moral sense. The issue cannot be settled by mere science; it must be settled through philosophical, legislative, and judicial activity.

For Warren, being human is not sufficient for being a person. The reader may return to the chapter on life-sustaining services for an eloquent example of this matter. In that chapter the ethics committee affirmed that there was no obligation to provide life-sustaining treatment to humans who were in a persistent vegetative state (PVS). Such individuals are surely human beings, but the question that faced us was whether PVS victims have the rights and privileges accorded to persons. Many would argue that because these individuals have permanently lost any power to think, feel, make moral evaluations, or interact as persons, they are no longer persons.

Second, Warren offers a positive account of what conditions are required in order to be treated as a person, i.e., as worthy of being protected. She identifies five relevant conditions. First, an individual must be conscious, especially in the sense that she can experience pain. Second, the individual must have the "developed capacity to reason." Third, the individual must be self-motivated in the sense that her actions are not controlled by genetic or environmental forces. Fourth, the individual must be able to communicate. Finally, the individual has some level of self-awareness. For Warren, the strength of an individual's claim to be a person varies according to its resemblance to these conditions. If an individual exhibits all these traits, then its claim to be a person is strong. If it exhibits only one trait or none at all, its claim is very weak or nonexistent.

However, Warren does not present these conditions as requirements for being a person. For example, an individual may not have the capacity to communicate and still be a person. The individual with "locked in" syndrome is a tragic example of this state. This paralysis prevents a person from communicating with the outside world. Rather, Warren claims that the point of this list of conditions is to demonstrate that "any being which satisfies none [of these] is certainly not a person," and this is true of the fetus at any stage of its development. It fails to satisfy any of these conditions, and, therefore, although the fetus is a human in the sense of being genetically human, it is not human in the sense of being a person.

## Criticisms of the Radical View

The first criticism of Warren's view is that it settles questions by violating the basic moral intuitions of many people. For example, the theory that the fetus is not a person involves more than fetuses. It seems to imply that newborns and other infants are not persons either. Warren herself admits in the postscript to her essay that the fetus, during the last days of pregnancy, does resemble the infant in critically important ways. Warren's critics argue that this insensitivity to the importance of being human undermines her view. The President's Commission treats infants as having the same status as persons. This reflects a widespread conviction among U.S. citizens.

Warren's response to this criticism was to show that her view is consistent with the general rule against infanticide. She believes that her view is compatible with the idea that it is generally wrong to destroy infants, though she clearly does not claim that infanticide is absolutely ruled out. To establish this compatibility she must show that it is ethically permissible to treat the infant and the late-term fetus differently. She claims that the difference of treatment is justified on the grounds that the infant's "continued life cannot pose any serious threat to the woman's life or health,"[14] while the fetus does pose such a threat. The late-term fetus and the infant are different in morally relevant ways, and therefore it is morally permissible to treat them differently.

This response, however, suggests that Warren's view is unclear. In the radical view, abortion is permissible for any reason at any time during pregnancy precisely because the fetus is not a person. She now seems to believe that aborting to preserve the life of the mother has a special status.

With this concession, Warren now seems to require that the third trimester fetus be a threat to the woman before we may justify abortion. It would seem that a woman in the third trimester of pregnancy is not entitled to abortion on demand. She must pass a "good reasons" test. This is exactly what the radical position was intended to avoid.

Another criticism of this radical view is that Warren's criteria for being a person are vague. Warren maintains that precise criteria are not necessary. But the critic argues that a great deal hangs on the definition of "person." If it is not precise, then a great many innocent persons may be denied the protection that they deserve. For example, it is easy to imagine that many elderly people with memory and reasoning deficits could not pass Warren's rationality criterion. They may lack a clear self-awareness or have a diminished capacity to communicate. Thus they might fail Warren's "personhood test" and yet still be persons.

## The Moderate View

This next view that we will discuss involves a compromise between the radical and the orthodox positions. The moderate view asserts that there is a determinable point at which the fetus becomes a person and, therefore, becomes entitled to the protections normally accorded to persons.

There are, of course, many types of moderate compromises. Some compromises may be described as liberal and some as conservative, depending on what point within gestation the fetus is protected. Perhaps the most widely known illustration of a liberal compromise is the view espoused by the *Roe* v. *Wade* decision. It is a liberal compromise because it accepts abortion on demand during the first trimester and only restricts abortion during the second trimester by stipulating that the abortion be done in accordance with the health and safety of the woman. In *Roe* v. *Wade*, the fetus has no moral standing until the third trimester, at which point abortion is generally forbidden except when the fetus represents a threat to the mother. *Roe* rejects both the orthodox and the radical view but is liberal in that it places no restrictions on abortion during the first two trimesters except those involving the woman's health and safety.

*Roe* v. *Wade*, however, does not offer any philosophical arguments for this liberal version of the moderate view. For that, we can turn to an essay by the philosopher Jane English entitled "Abortion and the Concept of a Person."[15] Like many authors, English maintains that "a conclusive answer to the question whether a fetus is a person is unattainable." She admits that being alive is necessary for being a person and being a U.S. senator is sufficient for being a person, but *between* being alive and being a U.S. senator there is a "penumbra region where our concept of a person is not so simple." Rather than defending the view that the second-trimester fetus is not a person, English chooses to focus on the question of harm.

The fetus in the first trimester has such little resemblance to the infant that abortion is permissible whenever it serves the best interests of the pregnant woman. However, English grants that there is sufficient resemblance between the fetus and the infant to require that, in the middle months, abortion be permissible only when the continuation of the pregnancy would cause harm to the mother. However, she offers a broad definition of harm that includes physical, psychological, economic, and social factors. In the late months, she claims, the resemblance is so great that abortion is permissible only "to save a woman from significant injury or death."

She defends her position on second-trimester abortion by appeal to a number of creative analogies. One of these philosophically ingenious analogies involves comparing abortion to being kidnapped by an innocent person who has been hypnotized by a mad scientist. The mad scientist wants the innocent hypnotic to bring you to him not in order to kill you, but in order to prevent you from achieving your life plans. English claims that if killing the innocent kidnapper is the only way that you can free yourself, then this is morally permissible—though, of course, it is also tragic precisely because the kidnapper is innocent.

The analogy with abortion proceeds in the following way. The innocent hypnotized person is comparable to the fetus in that the fetus is innocent. Second, killing is involved in both cases, and, according to English, it is justified not because the individual is not a person, but because the innocent person is unknowingly doing harm and there is no way to avoid the harm without causing the death of the innocent person. The death of the fetus, like the death of the innocent hypnotic, is tragic but not immoral. Third, in both cases, the harm done by the innocent kidnapper and the harm done by the fetus is real but it is not life-threatening. It involves loss of control over one's life.

Another, more conservative, compromise is found in the work of Ernest van den Haag.[16] Like moderates in general, van den Haag argues that it is impossible to empirically determine that the fetus is a human being. He claims that during the first weeks the fetus has little resemblance to a human being. Furthermore, he claims that the potentiality argument cannot work because a potential tree is not the same as an actual tree. But although it is impossible to determine that the fetus is a human being, it is possible to determine that a fetus is insentient. Van den Haag argues that sentience is not a metaphysical matter like humanity or personhood. It is possible to determine when sentience is present and when it is absent. Therefore, it is a more "stringent" or demanding criterion than personhood because it is possible to determine its absence. He claims that to be sentient requires an elementary nervous system and a functioning cortex, and these are not fully present until the end of the first 12 weeks. After the first 12 weeks the moral situation changes in the sense that the fetus has developed sufficient brain cortex and a sufficiently complex neural system that it can experience pain. This resemblance is the basis for opposing abortion after the twelfth week.

This moderate view is conservative because it forbids abortion after the first trimester. In addition, van den Haag holds that genetic abnormalities cannot be the basis for a second-trimester abortion. Amniocentesis, which is a test for genetic abnormality, is currently possible only during the second trimester. His position is conservative because it forbids abortions based on genetic testing. He argues that if we permitted such abortions, and if we assume that the second-trimester fetus is equal to the infant, then allowing abortion in the second trimester would permit us to kill infants with genetic defects.

### Criticisms of the Moderate View

These moderate views are very different from one another and it is difficult to offer generic criticisms of them; however, two lines of criticism are open to us. The first may be referred to as the problem of resemblance.

Moderates and radicals accept the notion that the lack of resemblance to persons constitutes sufficient evidence for permitting abortion on demand. But resemblance is a notoriously ambiguous concept, as the debate between radicals and liberal moderates illustrates. What must the fetus resemble in order to qualify as a person? If the radical is correct, the fetus must have the capacities of a full person. If the moderate is correct, then the fetus must resemble only the infant. But what is the standard against which we must compare the fetus? Selecting either the adult or the infant seems arbitrary. Therefore, the moderate view is as dependent on arbitrary assumptions as the radical view.

The second criticism involves the harm problem. The orthodox view claims that the harm caused by the fetus does not justify killing it. Many people harm other people, and the fact that one person named Smith harms another person named Jones is not by itself sufficient to establish that Jones can kill Smith or that Jones's right to avoid harm outweighs Smith's right to life. Smith might employ Jones and harm Jones by laying him off. Being laid off is a real harm, yet the mere fact that the company lays you off is not sufficient to assert that you can kill the owners of the company. Moderates appeal to the harm rule, then jump to the claim that harm or risk of harm is sufficient to kill the fetus. But this last claim is debatable.

## The Case of Delise Fortune

Delise Fortune is a 43-year-old mother of three who was admitted two days ago to Community Hospital by her gynecologist, Dr. Anna Bierce. She has been admitted for a therapeutic abortion. One of the nurses scheduled to assist in the abortion, Mr. Carter, refused to cooperate in the procedure and appealed to the hospital ethics committee to resolve the problem. The following account is based on his report.

Mrs. Fortune is not sure of the time of conception, but it looks to Mr. Carter that she is somewhere around 23 or 24 weeks pregnant. According to Mr. Carter, Mrs. Fortune did not receive adequate prenatal care and only recently saw a physician. She was informed that she was at risk of having a Down syndrome baby and she consented to amniocentesis. The test results confirmed that she is carrying a Down syndrome baby. She and her husband delayed making a decision because, according to Mr. Carter, her husband did not want the child and Mrs. Fortune did. Furthermore, even if it is a second-trimester fetus, the hospital's policy on abortion does not permit elective, nontherapeutic abortions. Mr. Carter says that this is a case of a nontherapeutic abortion.

In addition, the nurse is unwilling to participate in the abortion for a number of other reasons. First, he says that Mrs. Fortune is still ambivalent about the abortion. He claims that there is some reason to think that she is being pressured by her husband to have the abortion before she definitely enters the third trimester. Second, Mr. Carter is opposed to abortion on principle and rejects the idea that this is a therapeutic abortion. He claims that this is an abortion of convenience. Finally, he believes that the fetus has a chance to be born alive if proper precautions are taken, and he claims that Dr. Bierce has no interest in taking such precautions.

### Committee Discussion of the Case

| | |
|---|---|
| Dr. Mary Collins: (Chair) | Once again I would like to thank all of you for attending this meeting on such short notice. Medical-ethical problems are often like ordinary medical problems in that time plays a critical role. In this case, I think that time constraints are critical. Do you have some questions? |
| Dr. Philip Davis: | Why has Dr. Bierce classified this as a therapeutic abortion? Does the pregnancy constitute some threat to Ms. Fortune's health or safety? Is she a severe diabetic or does she have dangerously high blood pressure? For, if the fetus is a threat, then there is no time problem as far as the law is concerned, since third-trimester abortions are permissible in order to protect the patient. |
| Prof. Carla Thomas: | I am interested in this question of pressure to which Nurse Carter refers. I think someone from the committee needs to talk to Mrs. Fortune. If she doesn't want the abortion, then it should be pretty easy to decide this case. |
| Vivian Harris: | Is there any way we can determine the length of the gestation with exactitude? |

Atty. John Quinn:    Vivian, if it is a therapeutic abortion, then the gestation period is irrelevant. Our policy permits therapeutic abortions at any time. If it is nontherapeutic, then the gestation period is also irrelevant since we forbid nontherapeutic abortions at any time. However, I am concerned about the suggestion made by Nurse Carter that the fetus may be viable. Can we have some discussion of this matter? Furthermore, we need to find out what method of abortion Dr. Bierce is intending to employ. Some abortive methods may be more dangerous to a late fetus than others.

Rev. Richard Marcus:    Has Mrs. Fortune received abortion counseling? I know that the local abortion clinic offers counseling services prior to an abortion, and I think that the hospital needs to be ready to provide these services in cases like this. Are we able to provide such counseling services?

Mary Quigley:    If we do decide to allow the abortion, I suspect that we can make sure that Nurse Carter will not be required to participate. But I am wondering how much of a personnel problem we are facing. Are we going to have a serious problem with protests if we allow this abortion? The hospital has no interest in becoming a bomb target, and if we start to perform abortions, then we may become a target for the antiabortion squads.

Prof. Martin Fisk:    Let's not forget that this is a patient-doctor relationship that Nurse Carter is asking us to investigate. I think that we need to ask Dr. Bierce for her permission to speak to her patient before we take any action whatsoever. My reason for thinking this is that I view the committee as a consultative body. We advise the primary decision makers, i.e., the physician and the patient.

Dr. Collins:    If this is a third-trimester, nontherapeutic abortion, then we have no right to assist in the abortion because it violates the provisions of *Roe* v. *Wade*. However, I think we need to contact Dr. Bierce and speak with her regarding the case. I think it would be preferable to get Dr. Bierce's consent to consult with Mrs. Fortune. Martin, will you call Dr. Bierce and find out if she has any objections and, also, would you please ask her to come to tonight's meeting? I think that we need to have her respond to these questions. Mrs. Fortune and Mr. Carter also should be invited. He has made some accusations, and I think that we need to further appreciate his charges. I will call him and ask him to attend tonight's meeting.

Vivian, since you are the hospital's social worker, I would ask that you speak with Mrs. Fortune after we secure Dr. Bierce's consent.

The meeting adjourns and reconvenes at 8 P.M.

Dr. Collins:          Thanks again to all of you for coming to the meeting. I would also like to thank Dr. Bierce for coming and for giving us permission to consult on this case. Perhaps you would like to make an opening statement to the committee regarding Mrs. Fortune's case.

Dr. Bierce:          My first remarks have to do with my patient, Mrs. Fortune. She came to me three weeks ago for the first time. I examined her and estimated that she was about 20 weeks pregnant. I asked her why she had not consulted a physician earlier, and she told me that she had no health insurance and planned to do without medical treatment until she delivered. She already has three children and figured that she did not need any prenatal care. However, she complained about feeling depressed, and she was concerned that the pregnancy might be causing her real trouble. Because of her age, I thought that amniocentesis was a good idea. She agreed. She and Mr. Fortune came to my office, and I informed them about the Down syndrome. Mr. Fortune wanted her to get an abortion, but Mrs. Fortune said that she was not sure and that she wanted to think about it. I told them that she was very late in her pregnancy and that a decision would have to be made quickly if we were going to be consistent with the restrictions against third-trimester abortions.

Three days ago she returned to my office and requested that I set up an abortion. I told her that at this stage we needed to move quickly. I felt that I needed to come to the hospital to perform the abortion. The local clinic does a good job on abortions, but I felt at this late stage it would be safer to perform the abortion in the hospital.

Dr. Davis: What about other health considerations? Is she suffering from some disease that makes the child a threat to her health and safety?

Dr. Bierce: Mrs. Fortune is depressed and the continuation of this pregnancy is going to further exacerbate this condition. I see no point in forcing her to continue this pregnancy against her will.

Dr. Davis: Would you classify this as a therapeutic abortion?

Dr. Bierce: Yes! She is depressed and sees the fetus as the source of this depression.

Atty. Quinn: But other than the depression, are there other clinical indications that the pregnancy threatens her?

Dr. Bierce: The depression is a major problem. I believe that her overall welfare is endangered by continuing this pregnancy, especially in the light of genetic abnormality associated with the fetus.

Atty. Quinn: Dr. Bierce, I do not see why you brought this patient here. You know our policy on nontherapeutic abortion, and you know that depression is not a solid basis for therapeutic abortion.

Prof. Thomas: Hold on a minute, John! When did you get an MD? What gives you the right to say that depression is not a serious medical problem and that it cannot count as a basis for treating an abortion as therapeutic?

Atty. Quinn: The point is a lot simpler than you think, Carla. If anyone can get a "therapeutic abortion" because they say that they are depressed, then the distinction between therapeutic and nontherapeutic abortion is a distinction without a difference. If you allow depression as a basis for therapeutic abortion, then why not allow the common cold or a backache?

Dr. Davis: Dr. Bierce, are you a board-certified obstetrician, licensed to practice medicine in this state? And are you telling us that in your professional opinion, continuing this pregnancy endangers Mrs. Fortune's health?

Dr. Bierce: Of course I am board-certified. You have known me for ten years, Phil! And yes, I am telling you that she needs this abortion for her health.

Atty. Quinn: This is not good enough for me. I do not consider depression sufficient to justify an abortion, and, furthermore, I think the real reason that is motivating Mrs. Fortune to seek this abortion is the fact that the fetus has Down syndrome. Did she express any interest in an abortion prior to getting this information?

| | |
|---|---|
| Dr. Bierce: | We did not discuss the issue of abortion prior to the amniocentesis results. But she complained of depression prior to knowing the results of the amniocentesis. |
| Ms. Harris: | How long has she been pregnant? |
| Dr. Bierce: | I think about 23 weeks. |
| Ms. Harris: | So in your opinion this is still a legitimate abortion under the guidelines of *Roe* v. *Wade*. |
| Dr. Bierce: | Yes. But there are problems with making this judgment. There is a plus or minus factor in judging the gestation period, and I cannot say with certainty that we have not gone over the 24-week period. |
| Atty. Quinn: | Is there a chance that the child will be born viable? |
| Dr. Bierce: | I do not think so, but if it is delivered alive we will follow the protocol for managing severely handicapped children. |
| Atty. Quinn: | Doesn't it bother you, Dr. Bierce, that in one moment you are going to do everything that you can to kill this fetus and one moment after the child is born you are going to do everything that you can to save its life? In one second you are killing the fetus, and in the next second you might be trying to save it. Doesn't this bother you? |
| Dr. Bierce: | Abortion is full of these paradoxes. But it is not just in the context of abortion that this problem exists. For example, a job, like a womb, is sometimes necessary for a family to live. Yet we permit owners of companies to fire people even though this action is going to produce terrible consequences, even life-threatening consequences, for those who are dependent on this job. As soon as a family gets into a life-threatening position, we come to their aid even though |

we permit the actions that result in these life-threatening consequences. Abortion is similar. We are permitting something that is producing life-threatening results, and we must come to the aid of those who are threatened. We live with these paradoxes all the time.

Obviously, I would prefer that these abortions get handled as early as possible. But I support this woman's right to have an abortion at this period of her gestation. In fact, I think that she should have the right to abort at any stage of gestation. The right to bear children includes the right not to bear children. Given that Mrs. Fortune's womb belongs primarily to her and to no one else, it follows that Mrs. Fortune cannot be coerced to allow another being to use her womb against her will. Homeless people may need your house, Atty. Quinn, but we cannot obligate you to save their lives by giving them your house to live in.

Dr. Collins:    What about this claim by Nurse Carter that Mr. Fortune might be forcing his wife to have an abortion? Do you know anything about this?

Dr. Bierce:    This is the first time that I have heard about this. I know that Mr. Fortune did not want the child from the moment that I informed them about the genetic status of the child, but I am unaware of any pressure that he has imposed on his wife.

Atty. Quinn:    Wouldn't you say that the mere fact that he does not want the child constitutes undue pressure?

Dr. Bierce:    I agree that there is pressure, but I am not sure what is meant by "undue pressure." A lot of spouses disagree about children. Husbands often do not want children and wives often do not want children. I see this "give and take conflict" between spouses as a normal part of family planning decisions. I do not think that I would condemn him for expressing this feeling, because I think that it is sincere and that he has some decent reasons for not wanting another child. Furthermore, the pressures associated with raising a Down's child are profound, and I can understand why he would not want such a child.

Dr. Collins:

Vivian, you spoke with Mrs. Fortune this afternoon. Can you give us your opinion from a social work perspective?

Ms. Harris:

Yes, I spent about one hour with her this afternoon, and she agreed to come to the meeting. I will bring her in, in a moment. It is difficult to form a complete clinical impression of the patient in such a short time, but I will say that she is very upset about this "ethics committee investigation" and she has very strong feelings about Nurse Carter. I hope that all of us will remember that we are dealing with someone who is going through an emotional trauma right now and we need to get information from her, not threaten her.

Dr. Bierce:

Let me support Vivian's remarks. This is my patient and if I see any mistreatment of her, I will not hesitate to go to the Board of Trustees of this hospital and complain vigorously about it.

Atty. Quinn:

I am not sure what these warnings involve. If we are going to get information, then we need to ask sensitive questions. If we cannot ask tough questions, then we ought not to be consulting on this case. I plan to ask any pertinent question in a caring manner, but we need to get at the facts if we are going to offer advice.

Dr. Collins:

Vivian, can you ask Mrs. Fortune to come in?

Mrs. Fortune enters and sits at the table at which everyone is sitting.

| | |
|---|---|
| Dr. Collins: | Thank you for coming to our meeting. Do you understand who we are and the purpose of our meeting? |
| Mrs. Fortune: | Yes. Ms. Harris told me that you are the ethics committee of the hospital and that you are discussing whether I can get this abortion at this hospital. |
| Dr. Collins: | Do you wish to make a statement to the committee? |
| Mrs. Fortune: | My reason for coming here is to tell you that I want this abortion. Although I had some real doubts at first, I know that I could not raise a retarded child. Our family is struggling. My husband doesn't have a steady job and I need to work to keep food on the table. I don't know what I would do with a retarded child, and I don't feel that our family could withstand the pressures of having a retarded child. |
| Atty. Quinn: | We need to know what your reason for having the abortion is. Are you worried about your health? |
| Mrs. Fortune: | I sure am worried about my health. This pregnancy has been an unhappy situation from the beginning, and now when I finally make this decision, it winds up that I am being investigated by committees and made to feel as if I'm a bad person. I'm on the verge of a breakdown. |
| Dr. Collins: | What do you mean? |
| Mrs. Fortune: | Well, that Nurse Carter came to my room when I was first admitted to the hospital and asked me whether he could speak to me about my admission. He seemed to know that I was in for an abortion because he asked me questions about when did I decide to have the abortion? He asked if I knew anything about abortion and I said that I did get information from my doctor. |

He then gave me a lot of pamphlets that described how abortion was really killing an innocent baby. There were pictures of the fetus's fingers and its toes, and there was a picture of an aborted fetus that left me feeling that the fetus was very much like a little baby. He also told me that many women feel guilt-ridden after they have abortions because they come to feel that they committed murder. I have brought some of these pamphlets with me.

She hands the pamphlets to Dr. Collins.

He offered to help me save the baby and arrange an adoption. Well, I thought about adoption and I don't think anyone is going to adopt a retarded child. I do not want the baby kept in some state home for the rest of its life. The government says that it provides for these babies, but I think that they wind up in warehouses.

Dr. Bierce:          When you came to my office, Mrs. Fortune, what was your major complaint?

Mrs. Fortune:       Well, other than the discomforts of being pregnant, I was depressed. I had been feeling down for a number of weeks and I just couldn't pull myself together. I figured that it was because I was pregnant and because I did not want another child at this point in my life. I am too old to start this business again.

Dr. Bierce:          Could you be more specific about the depression? Can you tell us what you have been feeling?

Mrs. Fortune:       I felt as if I were trapped and could do nothing to get out of it. I had no energy and I was letting everything slide. I would just sit around all day and feel lousy. When I finally came to the decision to get the abortion, I felt that I was taking control of my life.

| | |
|---|---|
| Dr. Davis: | Now that you have made the decision to get the abortion, Mrs. Fortune, do you feel better? |
| Mrs. Fortune: | Well, I'm still very anxious, especially about this meeting. I don't know why you people can interrogate me like this. After all, I do have the right to obtain this abortion, and I don't see that you have any right to question me. |
| Dr. Collins: | Mrs. Fortune, our hospital has strict rules on abortions. We only do therapeutic abortions and we are trying to decide whether your abortion is therapeutic. I am sure you can understand our position. |
| Mrs. Fortune: | No, I do not understand your position. My doctor says I need an abortion and that the hospital is the safest place to have this abortion. I say that I need an abortion and that this hospital has the facilities that I need. To me you are violating my rights. You are interfering with my choices and that seems wrong to me. This is, after all, a public hospital. |
| Ms. Harris: | Mrs. Fortune, I wonder if you could say something about your husband? We have a memo from Nurse Carter that asserts that your husband is pressuring you to have this abortion against your will. |
| Mrs. Fortune: | No, that Carter is a "right-to-lifer" and he will do or say anything to prevent me from having this abortion. My husband did not want this child from the very moment that we found out that I was pregnant. At that time, I was unsure. We did have some big arguments about it, but when I found out that the baby was also retarded, I spent some time thinking about the abortion and I changed my mind. This child would be too much for our family, and, though it sounds insensitive, I think that it is a crime to allow this child to live. |

| | |
|---|---|
| Atty. Quinn: | What is your reason for having this abortion? Is it because the fetus has Down syndrome or are you concerned about your depression? |
| Mrs. Fortune: | I think both factors are part of my decision and I would not be honest if I lied to you. |
| Atty. Quinn: | Mrs. Fortune, if possible would you want the fetus to be born alive if we could preserve its life? |
| Dr. Bierce: | This committee is not authorized to enter into this subject. If you advised against the abortion, then I will take the matter to the next level, but I do not think that you are authorized to investigate what methods are appropriate. The manner in which I perform this abortion is something that lies within my professional prerogative, and that will be a judgment that I make in consultation with my patient. |
| Atty. Quinn: | I directed my question to Mrs. Fortune, not to you, Dr. Bierce. Can I have her answer? |
| Mrs. Fortune: | I was under the impression that the fetus is not able to live, so there is no reason to attempt to save its life. |
| Atty. Quinn: | I am under the impression, Doctor, that if you use a saline solution approach to this abortion, then the fetus will surely die, but if you used another method, perhaps inducing contractions with prostaglandin, then you may be able to save the fetus. Which method will you use? |
| Dr. Bierce: | Mrs. Fortune and I will make the decision regarding methods. I do not think that this is a matter for this committee to determine. |
| Atty. Quinn: | But the death of a possibly salvageable fetus is an ethical matter and we have the right to investigate what method you plan to use—especially if we have reason to think that your method will decrease the chances for delivering a viable newborn. |

| | |
|---|---|
| Dr. Bierce: | As of yet, I have not determined what procedure I will use, but I have no interest in spending millions of dollars to maintain a 450-gram baby. I will probably use a saline-induced approach. |
| Dr. Collins: | Mrs. Fortune, however we decide on this matter, we will inform you immediately so that you can take further action. Thank you for coming and speaking to us, Mrs. Fortune. Is Nurse Carter available? |

Mrs. Fortune leaves the room. Nurse Carter enters and takes a seat at the committee table.

| | |
|---|---|
| Dr. Collins: | Nurse Carter, you have written a memo that all of us have read. We would ask that you make a brief statement to the committee and then we would like to ask you some questions. Is this acceptable to you? |
| Mr. Carter: | Yes, this is fine with me. Thank you for inviting me to this meeting. My statement is brief. I spoke to Mrs. Fortune because I realized that I might be scheduled for the abortion procedure and I wanted to find out whether I could, in good conscience, participate. If Mrs. Fortune's life was at stake, I believe that an abortion would be tragic, but permissible. However, after my discussion with her, I believe that this is an elective, nontherapeutic abortion that is aimed at killing an innocent, handicapped person who cannot defend itself. I, therefore, cannot and will not participate in any procedure that involves the deliberate murder of another human being. Furthermore, I will do everything in my power to resist this murder. |
| Dr. Collins: | I will now ask the committee to raise any questions that they may have. |
| Marian Rhodes: | Nurse Carter, I checked the nursing schedule for last week and you are not assigned to work on the floor where Mrs. Fortune is |

staying. If you are not her nurse, then why did you go to speak to her regarding her decision?

Dr. Davis:

We spoke to Mrs. Fortune and she denied that there was undue pressure coming from her husband. I had no sense that she was being coerced to have this abortion. What led you to say that she was under pressure from her husband to have this abortion?

Ms. Quigley:

I am the patient advocate on this committee and I am concerned that you may have violated Mrs. Fortune's right to privacy. She referred to you as a "right-to-lifer." She claimed that you would do or say anything to prevent her from having this abortion. Was the purpose of your meeting to persuade her against having this abortion?

Dr. Collins:

In your memo you say that Mrs. Fortune is ambivalent about the abortion, and yet I detected no such ambivalence in our conversation. Why did you say this?

Atty. Quinn:

Can you tell us your reasons for opposing this abortion and why you refuse to participate in it?

Dr. Collins:

Our ethics policy permits abortions aimed at securing the health and safety of the pregnant woman. The same policy allows that you be excused from taking part in abortive procedures. I take it that your intent is to oppose this abortion.

Mr. Carter:

You have raised some important questions and I will do my best to answer them. Our local chapter of "right-to-life" will picket the hospital the minute this committee approves of the abortion. We also have plans to picket the offices of Dr. Bierce. There is no doubt that calling this a therapeutic abortion is just another name for murdering this child. We intend to resist it with all of our power.

Dr. Bierce:    He means business. My offices and my home have been picketed before, and my family and I have been harassed by these people. I am not used to it, but I have adapted to it. I think that the hospital better get prepared for some tough political times if you decide to go forth with this abortion.

Mr. Carter:    I was not finished responding to the questions. May I continue? I would like to say a few things about the role of the patient advocate. I know that Mary Quigley is the patient advocate and I cannot understand how she can stand by and let one of the patients be murdered. Don't you see that this baby is also a patient and that you have a duty to represent its interests?

Ms. Quigley:    In no uncertain terms, the Supreme Court has affirmed that the term "person," as it appears in the Constitution of the United States, does not apply to the fetus. Have you got information that the Supreme Court did not have?

Mr. Carter:    It is as clear as a bell to me that this fetus is a child. Denying the fetus the status of being a child is the same as what the slaveholders did prior to the Civil War. They had interests that motivated them to deny the obvious fact that slaves were persons. Many women have interests that conflict with the interests of the child and these interests motivate them to treat the child as a nonperson. But saying that the fetus is not a child does not make it a nonchild.

Ms. Quigley:    But saying that it is a child does not make it a child, either. You still have not proven your assumption.

Prof. Fisk:    Nurse Carter, I am one of those persons who think that the question of the moral status of the fetus is impossible to resolve. I think that there may be no fact of the matter

|  | that can resolve the problem, and so it appears as if you are forced into imposing your metaphysical or religious views on Mrs. Fortune. These views may be *your* views but I do not see why they have to be *everybody's* views. |
|---|---|
| Mr. Carter: | It was not everyone's view that blacks were human beings, but we fought a bloody Civil War to impose on everyone the value of a black person's life. The principle is the same. |
| Dr. Collins: | Does this mean that you countenance violence as a means of securing your goals? I wonder if you would support killing those who participate in abortion? |
| Mr. Carter: | No! I am nonviolent, but I understand those who support violent opposition to abortion. |
| Prof. Fisk: | I have another purpose in raising the metaphysical or religious nature of the definition of the word "person." I would like to suggest to you that it may be possible to permit abortion even if the fetus is a person. You admit that it is permissible to abort when the life of the mother is at stake, and I wonder if that principle can be further extended. Consider the $20 that I have in my pocket. I do not need it to live. I plan to use it to buy a crazy-looking shirt tonight. However, this money could save the lives of some people if I sent it to a relief organization that provided food for starving human beings. This $20 is like the womb of a woman. It can save the life of another human being. Now you will admit that I am not morally obligated to send this money to a relief organization? I have the right to send the money, but I do not have the obligation to send it. You do believe that I have the right to prefer a crazy-looking shirt to the life of a starving person? |

| | |
|---|---|
| Mr. Carter: | Yes, but I do not accept this comparison. |
| Prof. Fisk: | Please allow me to finish. If you do not obligate me to send my money to the relief organizations in order to save the lives of persons, you cannot obligate a woman to provide her womb to the fetus. In short, we can assume for the purposes of argument that the fetus is a person and we may therefore assume that it has a right to life, but it does not follow from the fact that something has a right to life that it also has a right to everything that is needed to support that life. If I need the $20 that you have in your pocket in order to live, I may have a right to life without also having a claim on your $20.[17] |
| Mr. Carter: | But the analogy breaks down because the person with the $20 is not responsible for the famine that is affecting the lives of starving people. The pregnant woman is responsible for bringing the fetus into existence. She caused the baby to exist and is therefore responsible for its vulnerable position. To use your example, if I stole the food of these starving people and was responsible for their starvation, then I would not merely have the right to send money, I would have the duty to send the money. And that is precisely the position that I think the pregnant woman is in. She is responsible for the infant and cannot kill it just to avoid the inconveniences of pregnancy. |
| Prof. Fisk: | But you will grant me that in the case of rape she is not responsible and, therefore, the abortion is permissible in that case. This extends your permission to abort beyond cases involving a direct threat to the life of the mother. To abort for rape is permissible because the woman is not in any way responsible for the life of the child. The rape |

victim's relation to the fetus is exactly like my relation to the starving people in foreign lands. Therefore, the rape victim is not obligated to save the life of this child.

Mr. Carter:

No, I simply do not see the point. Rape is a terrible thing, but it does not justify killing another human being. The child is not responsible for the rape. Why must the child die in order to redress the grievance that the mother has against the rapist?

Prof. Thomas:

I think you also miss another point. You simply assume that the woman is fully responsible for the fetus and so she bears all the burdens associated with the pregnancy. But most cases of unwanted pregnancy come about by way of an accident. Accidents happen and we do not always hold people responsible for the harms that result. For example, if the physician follows good medical practice and mistakenly diagnoses that you have a disease, and as a result of this mistake you suffer a harm, we do not always judge that the physician is responsible. We only hold him responsible if the diagnostic error was *negligent*.

Surely, if a woman takes proper birth control precautions, then we need not hold her responsible for the fetus any more than we hold the physician responsible for harm that resulted from following proper, though fallible, medical guidelines.

If we can hold the woman responsible for accidents, then it seems that we would have to be able to hold the doctor responsible for harmful, nonnegligent results of following good medical procedures.

Mr. Carter:

But when a woman chooses to have sex she knows that there is a small possibility that a fetus could result from intercourse. Therefore, she should be held responsible if she becomes pregnant.

| | |
|---|---|
| Ms. Harris: | That is simply not true. The amount of reproductive ignorance that exists among impoverished young women is far greater than you imagine. The misinformation about what can prevent conception is profound. More importantly, Nurse Carter, if you agree that reproductive ignorance weakens the responsibility of the pregnant woman to the fetus, then you have further extended the number of permissible abortions to include not only fetuses that result from rape, but those that result from reproductive ignorance. |
| Mr. Carter: | I do not accept any of these justifications except the one involving saving the mother's life. |
| Prof. Thomas: | Let me try another example to convince you that pregnant women need not be held completely responsible for the welfare of the fetus. I know that there is a small possibility that if I drive you home tonight we might have an accident that leads to your death. We can compute the probabilities based on the number of accidental deaths over a given period. If I decide to take that risk and drive you home and we do get into an accident that kills you, does this automatically imply that I am responsible for your death because I knew that there was a chance that you would die in my car? Surely not! If the police investigate and find that I followed safe driving procedures and did not violate any law, then the police will not file charges against me and I will not be held responsible for your death, even though I did know that there was a small possibility that driving you home would lead to your death. As long as I am not a negligent driver, I am not responsible for your death, even though I knew beforehand that there was a slight chance that you would die during the drive. |

| | |
|---|---|
| Mr. Carter: | Well, what is your point in this analogy? |
| Prof. Thomas: | It's a simple one. Just as we do not hold the safe, law-abiding driver criminally responsible for the harm done to the passenger, so we cannot hold the woman responsible for the fact that the fetus is in the vulnerable position of needing her womb. As long as she followed reasonable precautions to avoid pregnancy, she does not seem responsible for the life of the fetus. Just as the safe, law-abiding driver is not responsible for the death of the passenger so, the mother is not responsible for the death of the fetus if she took reasonable means to prevent the conception. |
| Dr. Collins: | I think that this conversation may last into the next decade, and I do not think that we can continue to discuss the merits and demerits of abortion indefinitely. If you have nothing further to say to the committee, I think that we need to conclude our meeting with you, Nurse Carter. |

Nurse Carter and Dr. Bierce leave the room.

| | |
|---|---|
| Dr. Collins: | Well, we obviously cannot solve the problem of abortion this evening. But we need to come to some resolution of this matter. |
| Atty. Quinn: | I think that it is fairly easy to resolve. It seems to me that Mrs. Fortune wants us to perform an elective, nontherapeutic abortion. Our hospital policy forbids these abortions. Therefore, we ought to refuse. |
| Dr. Davis: | Where is she going to get this abortion, John? I do not know of any hospital within a hundred miles that performs nontherapeutic elective abortions. They are all afraid of the right-to-life pickets, and as a consequence, many women are not being provided with the opportunity to receive safe and competent abortions. The problem |

is deeper than you think because hospitals are not even teaching residents how to perform abortions.[18] They are afraid of the right-to-life pickets. I asked two obstetrics and gynecology residents if they can train in abortion techniques here and they said "No!" Indeed, 38 percent of all obstetrics and gynecology residency programs do not offer any abortion training. If hospitals won't perform safe abortions or train doctors to perform safe abortions, then saying that a woman has a right to abortion is hollow.

Ms. Rhodes:    Atty. Quinn. . . I did not have the impression that you were given a medical degree along with that law degree. I think that if a respected obstetrician has judged that this depression is serious enough to warrant an abortion, then I am willing to call it therapeutic. I do know that depression is a serious mental illness and I have even been involved in the treatment of patients with depression. This is a serious dysfunction.

Atty. Quinn:    I think that a case could be made for depression if there was any history of the disease prior to the amniocentesis, but there is no such history. Therefore, I am skeptical that it is a genuine clinical depression. I think that she is just very unhappy about the results of the amniocentesis test.

Dr. Davis:    I am glad that you can judge this based on such a brief interview with her. Millions of patients report depression for the first time, and they have no history of it. Are you going to be just as skeptical of the millions of people who report depression and lack any prior history?

Dr. Collins:    Rev. Marcus, you have been very quiet about this case. Do you have any reactions?

Rev. Marcus:    I am pro-choice on abortion because there is nothing in the New Testament or the Old

Testament that explicitly tells us that the fetus is a human being from the time of conception. Theologians differ on this point, and I do not think that we can prove conclusively that the fetus is a human being. This is a matter where the individual's conscience must rule. Protestant Christians emphasize the supremacy of the individual's conscience. I believe that, on this matter, we must respect the right of the individual to decide.

Dr. Collins:

Marian Rhodes, you have been more than subdued in this conversation. Do you have any reactions to the issue?

Ms. Rhodes:

I have no answers on the question of the status of the fetus. I do, however, have strong feelings about how Nurse Carter tried to persuade a patient to follow pro-life moral convictions. I think that it is fine to do that on your own time, but to use your status as a nurse to manipulate a patient to follow your private morality is wrong. If Carter was on my unit, I would insert an official reprimand into his official personnel file. We need to keep politics out of this hospital.

Regarding the question of whether it is a therapeutic or nontherapeutic abortion, I think that we need to interpret that distinction broadly. I myself have been treated for depression and it is by no means a trivial disease. Furthermore, I have a great deal of respect for Dr. Bierce. If she calls the abortion therapeutic, then that is good enough for me.

Dr. Collins:

Then is there some consensus on the matter?

Atty. Quinn:

I am going to hang tough. There is no way that this counts as therapeutic. Merely because a respected physician calls it therapeutic does not make it so.

*Committee Recommendations*

| Dr. Collins: (Chair) | Then, except for Atty. Quinn, are we in agreement to recommend that this abortion be considered therapeutic and that it should be approved? |

Eight of the committee members approve of the decision.

| Ms. Quigley: | Allow me to ask what is your plan of action, Dr. Collins, when the pickets line up outside the hospital? |

| Dr. Collins: | That is their prerogative. We are simply going to have to respect their right to protest our decision. My guess and my hope is that this case will not have enough impact to produce that kind of result. |

## Questions for Further Discussion

1. Has the committee adequately resolved the question of whether the abortion is therapeutic? Have any relevant issues been left unaddressed?
2. How would you define the difference between a therapeutic and nontherapeutic abortion?
3. Does Community Hospital have any ethical duty to give this abortion based on the assumption that it is a second-trimester abortion and that typical abortion clinics are not equipped to handle this case?
4. Ernest van den Haag would probably argue that the fetus is sentient and, therefore, this abortion is not permitted. How would you respond to this claim?
5. Carla Thomas and Martin Fisk attempted to increase the number of exceptions to the orthodox prohibition against abortion. In doing so they employed analogies. Were these analogies effective? Why or why not?
6. If you were on the committee, how much would your judgment be influenced by the possibility of picketing by "right-to-life" organizations?
7. The committee discussed, but did not resolve, the issue of what method should be use in the abortion. Suppose Dr. Bierce and Mrs. Fortune agreed to used a saline solution method that would practically guarantee the death of the fetus. What would be your response to this decision?

8. If Dr. Bierce used another labor-inducing method that produced a severely premature but living baby, live birth weight 450 grams, would you let it die if Mr. and Mrs. Fortune said that they wanted no aggressive treatment applied?
9. Mrs. Fortune thinks that Down syndrome babies are not adoptable and that if she were to bring the baby to term and give it up for adoption, the baby would have a poor quality of life in a public orphanage. Is this true in your opinion? If it is true, does it justify the abortion?
10. Did Nurse Carter violate any professional principles by attempting to persuade Mrs. Fortune against the abortion? If you were his supervisor, how would you respond to his actions? Suppose he tells you that he intends to continue trying to discourage patients who are scheduled for therapeutic abortions?

## More Cases for Examination

### The Nurse and the Abortion Demand

Maggie Doe is a nurse in Community Hospital's family practice unit, and one of her tasks is to provide counseling to women who are pregnant. Her patient is a 14-year-old inner city prostitute who has been using cocaine for two years. She is about four weeks pregnant and she continues to use crack cocaine. Nurse Doe has advised the patient about the risks of cocaine to the fetus, but the woman admits to being severely dependent on the drug and it is unlikely that she can overcome her habit. The young woman also admits to being HIV positive. She then asks Nurse Doe about the possibility of getting an abortion. If you were Nurse Doe, what information would you provide this woman? Is the hospital's policy relevant to your management of this case?

### Abortion and the Mentally Handicapped

Ms. Smith is a 19-year-old woman with a diagnosis of chronic paranoid schizophrenia. She has been institutionalized with only intermittent attempts at independent living. Currently, she is in Community Hospital's long term care unit, which is attached to the hospital. Ms. Smith is now 14 weeks pregnant. She has firmly indicated her desire to continue the pregnancy and to keep the child. Abortion, she declares, "is evil." The father is unknown.

While Ms. Smith's psychiatrist does not consider her capable of responsible parenthood, he does think that she is capable, at times, of making meaningful moral decisions. Her schizophrenia and medication slightly increase the possibility of fetal defect.

Ms. Smith's mother wants her to have an abortion and has secured legal custody of her daughter in order to effect that result. She feels that the experience of pregnancy and the trauma of labor and delivery will harm her daughter. Moreover, she herself is unable to care for the child and fears that her daughter will suffer further if forced to give up the child.

Should the abortion be performed? Who should decide?

### The 15-Year-Old and RU 486

Dr. Harold Smith practices in Community Hospital's family practice unit. He has a 15-year-old patient, Mary Doe, who is about three weeks pregnant and is seeking an abortion. She does not want her parents to discover that she is pregnant. She asks Dr. Smith to prescribe RU 486. Dr. Smith states that the drug is available, but only on an experimental basis. However, Mary is very frightened to go to the abortion clinic and risk having her identity revealed. She feels that RU 486 would be perfect for her. What should Dr. Smith do?

### The Resident's Demand

Dr. Ronald Jones is doing a four-year obstetrics/gynecology residency at Community Hospital, and he is very concerned that he has not received any training in abortion procedures. He makes an appointment with Dr. Collins, the medical director, and complains that he needs to have these skills if he is going to be a minimally decent obstetrician. He claims that his right to a minimally decent education in this field is being violated by the hospital's refusal to provide him with abortion training. Throughout the conversation he repeats that without an opportunity to practice and develop the skills that are needed within his specialization, the hospital is failing him. If Dr. Collins brings this issue to the committee, how should they manage it?

### Further Reading

Aristotle, *The Complete Works of Aristotle* (Revised Oxford translation, ed. J. Barnes (Princeton, N.J.: Princeton University Press, 1984).

Augustine, St., *The Good of Marriage* (*De bono coniugali*), trans. Wilcox (New York: Fathers of the Church, 1955). Originally published in 401.

Brody, B. *Abortion and the Sanctity of Human Life: A Philosophical View*, (Cambridge: MIT Press, 1975).

Callahan, D., *Abortion: Law, Choice and Morality* (New York: Macmillan, 1970).

Cuomo, M. "Religious Belief and Public Morality: A Catholic Governor's Perspective," paper delivered at the University of Notre Dame, September 13, 1984.

Devine, P., *The Ethics of Homicide* (Ithaca, N.Y.: Cornell University Press, 1978).

Engelhart, H. T., "Medicine and the Concept of Person," in *Contemporary Issues in Bioethics*, 2nd ed., ed. T. Beauchamp and L. Walters (Belmont, Calif.: Wadsworth, 1982), pp. 94–101.

Feldman, D. M., *Marital Relations, Birth Control and Abortion in Jewish Law* (New York: Schocken, 1968).

Gordon, L., *Woman's Body, Woman's Right* (New York: Penguin, 1976).

MacKinnon, C., "Roe v. Wade: A Study in Male Ideology," in *Abortion: Moral and Legal Perspectives*, ed. J. Garfield and P. Hennessey (Amherst: University of Massachusetts Press, 1984).

Marquis, Donald, "Why Abortion Is Immoral" *Journal of Philosophy (April 1990)*.

Noonan, J., *Contraception: A History of Its Treatment by Catholic Theologians and Canonists* (Cambridge: Harvard University Press, 1966).

Noonan, J., *The Morality of Abortion: Legal and Historical Perspectives*, Cambridge: Harvard University Press, 1970).

Noonan, J. "Contraception," in *Encyclopedia of Bioethics*, ed. W. Reich (New York: Free Press, 1978), pp. 204–216.

Thomson, J., "A Defense of Abortion," *Philosophy and Public Affairs* (1971): 47–66.

Tooley, M., *Abortion and Infanticide* (Oxford: Clarendon, 1983).

## Notes

1. *Roe v. Wade*, U.S. Supreme Court, Jan. 22, 1973, 410 US 113, 93 S.Ct. 705.
2. Justice Sandra Day O'Connor, dissenting opinion, *Akron v. Akron Center for Reproductive Health* (51 LW 4767).
3. For a good discussion of the scientific aspects of fetal development, see Andre Hellegers, "Fetal Development," *Theological Studies* 31 (1) (March 1970): pp. 3–9.
4. Aristotle, *Politics*, 7.16.15.
5. Ibid., 706.
6. It should be noted that many of the strongest opponents of elective abortion argue that therapeutic abortion, which aims at preserving the life of the mother, is permissible.
7. John Noonan, *The Morality of Abortion: Legal and Historical Perspectives* Cambridge: Harvard University Press, 1970).
8. For a good discussion of this position, see Ernest van den Haag's brief note on abortion that appears in *The National Review*, September 26, 1985. We will discuss this further in the section on conservative moderate views.
9. For a thorough discussion of this issue, see David Granfield, *The Abortion Decision* (Garden City, N.Y.: Doubleday, 1969).

10. Don Marquis, "Why Abortion Is Immoral," *The Journal of Philosophy* (April 1989).

11. For a full discussion of precising definitions, see Irving Copi, *Introduction to Logic*, 7th ed. (New York: Macmillan, 1988), p. 144.

12. Mary Ann Warren, "On the Moral and Legal Status of Abortion," *The Monist* 57 (1): 55. A postscript to this essay, called "Postscript on Infanticide," appeared in *The Problem of Abortion*, 2nd ed., ed. Joel Feinberg (Belmont, Calif.: Wadsworth, 1984).

13. For a full discussion of the fallacy of equivocation, see Irving Copi's *Introduction to Logic*, op. cit., p. 113.

14. Warren, Mary Ann, "On The Moral and Legal Status of Abortion," op. cit.

15. Jane English, "Abortion and the Concept of a Person," *Canadian Journal of Philosophy* 5 (2) (October 1975).

16. Ernest van den Haag, *National Review*, Sept. 6, 1985.

17. This argument is similar to one developed by J. J. Thomson, "A Defense of Abortion," *Philosophy and Public Affairs*, 1 (1971): 47–66.

18. This issue is discussed at length in "Planned Parenthood Starting to Train Doctors in Abortion," *The New York Times* (June 19, 1993), p. 1.

# 7

# Rationing Health Care

## Introduction to the Problem Area

Since the end of World War II, the United States has perceived itself as a rich nation. This perception has profoundly affected our decisions in medicine. The history of renal dialysis, a technology that replaces part of the kidney's function, provides an excellent illustration. During the 1960s, when hemodialysis technology emerged, serious shortages developed because the technology was in short supply and expensive. Few hospitals were able to purchase the equipment and train the staff to operate it. These shortages were acute throughout the nation, but the administrators and physicians at the Northwest Kidney Center in Seattle, Washington, were the first to really face the scarcity problem. In order to do so, the center created an ethics committee. This committee's function was to decide who would live and who would die. Almost immediately the committee became known in the hospital as "the God Committee."

Northwest Kidney Center was not alone. Throughout the nation, hospitals faced the dilemma of allocating dialysis technology. To meet this challenge, hospitals imitated the Northwest Kidney Center and instituted ethics committees charged with answering two questions. First, what criteria should be used to select patients? Second, how should such criteria be applied?

The nation quickly discovered that these questions were easier to ask than to answer. This is because dialysis is much like a lifeboat. Lives can be saved using this technology, and nearly all who are threatened by kidney failure prefer this technology to death. But when the need for a life-saving service is greater than the ability to provide it, choices must be made. But if men and women are in some sense "fundamentally equal," as the Constitution seems to affirm, how can we make these choices? The problem, then, at the first stage is how do we reconcile our belief in human equality with the need to allocate a scarce resource?

## The Rich Man's Solution

The problems faced by hospitals were common enough to philosophers, who had been discussing the philosophical problem of dividing up scarce resources for centuries. But Americans were not accustomed to facing the challenge of scarce medical resources. A rich nation does not need to allocate. Consequently, when committees began distributing the dialysis resources, outcries of discontent erupted. What right do these committees have to make these decisions? They are not gods!

How did the nation respond to these outcries? It responded in accordance with its perception of itself as a rich country. In the early 1970s, the United States handled the problem of scarce hemodialysis services in the manner of a rich philanthropist. The government simply sidestepped all the difficulties inherent in rationing and covered all renal dialysis costs under the provisions of Social Security. The End Stage Renal Disease Amendments were added to the Social Security Act, creating a new social entitlement. The costs of dialysis and transplantation would be paid for by a rich nation.

The transformation came as fast as a bolt of lightning. Because government support meant a nearly limitless supply of funds, medical technology companies responded, and dialysis scarcity became history overnight. With government providing the funds, the medical marketplace immediately responded. Hospital-based renal dialysis centers sprang up throughout the nation. The big relief for hospitals was that now they could provide renal dialysis without appealing to ethics committees that rationed the service. All could live! We were rich!

This was the best of all possible solutions because it bypassed the claims of discrimination by minorities, women, the poor, the aged, and anyone else who was denied the service. Poor nations, perhaps even middle-income nations, might have an allocation problem—but not the United States. In addition to dissolving a vast amount of conflict among groups within society, this rich man's solution allowed a vast market to develop. Corporations began improving the technology because they were confident that the government would buy their expensive new machines. On the surface, government involvement not only solved the ethical and social problem of distributing a scarce resource, but also created a confident marketplace.

However, this solution also has a dark side. First, dialysis started out in 1973 covering approximately 11,000 people at a cost of about $280 million. Today nearly 60,000 patients are receiving hemodialysis at a cost of well over $2 billion. What started out as an affordable cost is now a major cost.

Second, relative to other nations, such as Japan, the wealth of the United States has changed. Banks illustrate this point. During the 1960s, most of the world's largest banks were located in the United States. Today most of the largest and richest banks are in Japan and Europe. Perhaps this will change in the future, but at this time the United States is no longer the unparalleled financial giant that it was following World War II. If we believe Willie Sutton, who said that he robbed banks because that was where the money was, and if the banks have left the United States, then perhaps the money has also left. It is also vital to note that in 1989 the United States became a debtor nation, meaning that we owe more money to foreign countries than we lend out. At present, no other nation comes even close to owing what the United States owes. The national debt is over three trillion dollars, which means that the government must pay vast amounts of its income merely for interest. When the wealth is lost, perceptions about what can be purchased often change. The United States is beginning this perceptual shift. Hemodialysis was the last catastrophic treatment that the government covered.

The third difficulty with the rich man's solution is that there is more than just one expensive life-saving technology now available. Heart and liver transplants are very costly. So are bypass surgery and AZT treatment for AIDS. Why should we cover dialysis and not these other treatments? If the government provides universal access to these technologies, it will likely be unable to pay for any other services. In short, to use the renal dialysis solution as the model for addressing all challenges posed by scarce medical resources would bankrupt the treasury.

### The Oregon Solution

But if the solution of the wealthy is no longer open to us, what other responses are available to addressing the problem of allocating scarce medical resources? The term *macroallocation* is used to describe the social policy that determines the allocation of limited resources. One approach is the public solution. In this public model, the state becomes the major provider of health care. In Oregon, the legislature passed a comprehensive health care insurance program that gives state government a key role in health care. In 1993 the federal government issued a Medicaid waiver that allowed Oregon to begin providing universal medical coverage to all Oregonians. But Oregon will be the first comprehensive health care system that contains a broad-based rationing plan in the United States.

Because the Oregon plan expands Medicaid coverage to all Oregonians who fall below the federal poverty line, the state had to make choices regarding what treatments or procedures it would cover. The Oregon Health Services Commission developed a definition of what counts as basic care and included in this definition 709 health services ranked by priority. These services included necessary care such as hospital care and medications. The ranking was developed not only by physicians and other health care professions but also by public debate at town hall meetings and public surveys. The legislature then determined how much money would be made available to cover these services. Not all 709 types of health care services could be funded. The basic package does not cover futile treatments such as severe brain injury, nor does it cover exotic life-sustaining services for babies who are born with extremely low birth weight. Cosmetic treatments are also excluded. Oregon's goal is to fund as many useful services as is practical within the context of scarce funding.

The Oregon plan also includes a number of provisions that involve inserting recipients into private managed care networks. These managed care systems operate within the private sector. These insurance systems set limits on the kinds of expensive care that a patient may receive. Thus they are able to stem the increasing costs of medical insurance. These systems have become the subject of a great deal of controversy throughout the nation. For although there is little doubt that they are economically efficient providers of health care services, they also ration and thereby restrict health care services to millions of consumers.

Although the Oregon solution and the host of private managed care systems have made significant advances in providing efficient health services to poor people and those with health care insurance, there still remains a significant problem in providing health care to Americans. The Oregon plan is needs-based in that it cuts off services to those whose income is greater than the federal government's definition of poverty. Private managed care systems provide health care to those who can afford health insurance. However, neither approach addresses the health care needs of the working poor. These are the nearly 45 million people in the United States whose family income is greater than the poverty limit. These are individuals and families who cannot afford private health care insurance or work for companies that do not provide such insurance. President Clinton's health care initiative, which was defeated in Congress in 1994, addressed the needs of these people. At this writing, no further federal initiatives have been proposed, though states such as Minnesota and Hawaii have developed public health care systems that have expanded basic health care to larger groups of citizens.

### Why Committees?

Some hospitals will choose to put allocation authority in the hands of physicians. Some will make administrators responsible. Others will introduce committees to serve a consulting role to the administrators who are responsible for making critical decisions. Community Hospital's approach involves the ethics committee. This committee includes men and women with medical and administrative expertise, but more than this is required. Consumers of medical care must be included. It is critically important that attention be paid to the ethical issues involved in rationing.

The need for such committees is illustrated by the Von Stetina case.[1] In this well-known case, a Florida court ruled that a hospital should have developed screening or allocation policies in order to avoid unnecessary harm to patients. The hospital had not created an ethics committee to develop these contingency plans and avoidable harm resulted. Susan Von Stetina was receiving treatment in an intensive care unit. She was, according to the plaintiff, severely injured because the nurses became very busy due to an emergency and did not provide adequate monitoring for her. The Florida court held for the plaintiff and the liability amounted to over $12 million. One of the court's reasons for penalizing the hospital was that the hospital had failed to develop a set of policies to ensure that patient care would remain at a minimally decent level even during periods of scarcity.

Many hospitals have begun to develop general guidelines for allocation. These guidelines often emerge from the hospital ethics committee. The ethics committee must spell out the values that it employs to determine who gets services and who does not. Because these ethical values affect patient care, they need to be explicit. For example, how much does "need for the service" affect who is entitled to receive it? How about the ability to pay? Should questions concerning the length of expected life, given the success of the treatment, be considered in determining the allocation strategy? Quality of life considerations? The value of a person to her family or to society?

## The President's Commission

Ethics committees do not have to create rationing policies without some general guidelines. Perhaps the most important nationwide attempt to address these questions was the President's Commission for the Study of Ethical Problems in Medicine and Biomedical and Behavioral Research: Securing Access to Health Care.[2] In this document the commission recommended that the provision of health care be treated as social obligation: "Society has an ethical obligation to ensure equitable access to an adequate level of health care without the imposition of excessive burdens."

This general principle has had a great influence on the development of Community Hospital's rationing policy, but as the reader will see, this principle is subject to many competing interpretations. For example, what kinds of treatments are included in "an adequate level of care"? What is the definition of "equitable access"? How does potential benefit to the patient determine whether a patient deserves the treatment? The president's commission presented a broad principle, but Community Hospital's ethics committee must transform it into a practical scheme for providing and refusing health care.

The focus of the committee's work will not involve large macroallocation issues since Community Hospital cannot directly determine how resources for medical care will be allocated at the national or state level. What falls directly within the scope of the committee's responsibility is *microallocation distribution*. If some intensive care resources are available, how should the committee and the administration of the hospital allocate them? Thus, the committee's task was to develop a policy regarding the distribution of scarce resources that are within the hospital's authority.

---

## Community Hospital's Policy on Rationing

*Purpose:*    The purpose of this policy is to set guidelines for distributing the intensive care unit (ICU) resources at Community Hospital. The ICU is currently a scarce resource of the hospital.

*Background:*    In a recent court case in Florida, the court ruled that hospitals ought to develop a plan for distributing scarce resources such as the hospital's beds. This plan would be acted on in the event that these resources are not sufficient to meet the needs of everyone. This policy sets guidelines for this allocation.

*Methodology:*    The committee assumes that often the number of those who would benefit from a scarce medical service such as the ICU exceeds the hospital's ability to provide that service. The hospital needs some principles to prioritize patients according to their need and their ability to benefit from the service.

*Principles:*

1. The hospital should assign an ICU triage officer who is authorized to allocate resources. This officer is encouraged to seek the advice of critical care committees of the hospital as well as the hospital ethics committee on all matters pertaining to resource allocation. Different units of the hospital such as the dialysis unit may appoint different officers.
2. Allocating decisions are not the prerogative of attending physicians who enjoy privileges at the hospital. The concept of the automatic admission by the attending physician is rejected. All decisions regarding admission, continuation, and termination of ICU service are the responsibility of the triage officer.

3. Attending physicians need to be consulted whenever a service is to be withheld or withdrawn, but the final decision on allocation is to be made by the triage officer. This is because the allocation decision must be made on the basis of the medical needs of all the patients who require the service, and the attending physician lacks access to this information.
4. Whenever a patient is discharged from a scarce resource such as the ICU, the attending physician is obligated to reassume responsibility for the care of the patient.
5. The following principles will govern the triage officer:
   A. All patients of the hospital will be viewed as equal with respect to their individual and social value. No discriminations will be made on the basis of race, creed, sex, sexual orientation, or profession. No one at the hospital will determine the value of patients with respect to their past contributions to society or the likelihood of future contributions to society. Although this may lead to providing service to socially disreputable individuals, the committee accepts this result as part of the price that we must pay for being fair.
   B. Patients who are to be "triaged" need to be separated according to the following broad categories:
      • Category 1 patients are those who are critically ill and who need intensive treatment such as ventilator support and technological monitoring. Category 1 patients are likely to benefit significantly from the ICU service.
      • Category 2 patients are not critically ill but need monitoring because they are at risk of needing intensive treatment.
      • Category 3 patients are those whose underlying disease processes make it unlikely that they will recover or benefit from ICU service.

      **Category 1 patients have priority over Category 2 patients and Category 2 patients have priority over Category 3 patients.**

   C. Age may be used as a basis for classifying patients if it affects the probability of medical outcome.
   D. The triage officer will allocate scarce resources on a "first come, first served" basis, but individuals who cannot medically benefit from a resource (Category 3 patients) will have no entitlement to the scarce ICU service, even if they are next in line for it. Judgments of medical futility will be made by the triage officer.
   E. Individuals who are currently receiving a scarce service of the hospital will be treated as being entitled to the service, subject to the following restrictions:

First, if a patient is currently receiving a service and the triage officer judges that the patient is no longer medically benefiting from the service (the patient falls from Category 1 to Category 3), then the triage officer may withdraw this individual from service. Examples: Patients with advanced age and three or more organ system failures who have not responded to treatment within 72 hours can be discharged, especially when beds are in demand. Patients who have permanently and completely lost neocortical function **can be discharged or refused admission.**

Second, the following factors are relevant to reclassifying a patient from Category 1 to Category 3:

The probability of survival given the service, the quality of life given the service, the length of survival given the service, and the cost of providing the service.

Individuals who score very low on all these factors may be reclassified and removed from the service. The committee recommends that, where possible, objective statistical techniques, such as the Apache scoring technique, should be employed in making these decisions.

6. It is the opinion of the ethics committee that, because triage decisions are the hospital's duty, the triage officer need not secure the consent of the individual or his guardian in order to withdraw such an individual from service. If consent were required, then allocation of the scarce resource would be practically impossible. However, it is recommended that the triage officer consult with the patient or the guardian before taking action so that the reasons for the action can be explained.

---

## Commentary on the Philosophical and Ethical Aspects of the Policy

There are two basic approaches employed within our society to address the problem of allocating scarce resources: the rights-based approach and the consequences-based approach. The committee's approach attempts to include elements of both approaches; therefore, we will give equal consideration to both approaches.

### Consequences and Scarcity

The consequentialist begins the study of distributing scarce medical resources by affirming that the problems associated with allocating expensive medical technology are basically problems of justice. Furthermore, problems of justice are fundamentally moral or ethical problems and are to be treated like any moral dilemma. For consequentialists, since all moral dilemmas are to be solved by developing social rules that produce "the most good for the most people," scarce medical resources are to be allocated the same way.

Although allocating resources at the hospital level (microallocation) is our main focus, one cannot understand micro principles without some reference to principles used to distribute scarce resources within the larger society (macroallocation). Furthermore, the principles used in the micro policy often cannot be justified without reference to macroallocation principles. We thus need to turn to macroallocation philosophy, Once again the philosophical work of John Stuart Mill is of primary importance.

### Laissez-Faire Justice

Mill recommended that whenever we face a problem involving justice, we can do so with very little philosophy. According to Mill, we need only one principle: his principle of utility. The principle tells us that we ought to maximize the good for the greatest number of people. In Mill's view, this ethical rule, in conjunction with relevant factual information, is sufficient to determine how we should justly allocate resources in any given situation. But if one does suppose that the principle of utility is the basic moral rule, how does it generate the supposedly correct rules of distribution?

Mill's answer involves a brilliant piece of analysis. He claims that we know what injustice is. It involves "taking or withholding from any person that to which he has a moral right."[3] According to Mill, a person is unjustly treated when he is made to "obtain a good or made to undergo an evil which he does not deserve."[4] Again, Mill claims that "justice implies something which is not only right to do and wrong not to do but which some individual person can claim from us as his moral right."[5]

For Mill, the basic philosophical problem is to distinguish between the concepts of generosity and justice. He draws that distinction in the following way. When we are generous, we give to someone that which they have no right to or that which they do not deserve. By contrast, when we are just, we give to people what they have a right to or what they deserve. Furthermore, although we are not obligated to be generous, we are obligated to be just. For Mill, just acts are those that someone has an obligation to perform. For example, if I steal your watch, then it is a matter of justice that I return it to you because you have a claim against me. I have an obligation to return the watch. Returning the watch has nothing to do with generosity or charity. More importantly, the state is involved in the watch case. According to Mill, the state has an obligation to coerce me (the thief) to return your watch. On the other hand, if it is your birthday and I wish to give you a watch as a present, then I am acting not on the basis of justice, but on the basis of generosity. The difference between justice and generosity is that, in the latter case, individuals have no obligation to be generous, nor do states have an obligation to coerce me to be generous to you on your birthday.

But how does this help to define what justice is? Mill claims that the principle of utility can adequately specify what rights men and women ought to be given. It is also adequate to determine what obligations men and women have. And, finally, it can determine what are the rights and obligations of government. For Mill, understanding justice amounts to nothing more than understanding two things: the rights and obligations that individuals have, and the rights and obligations that governments have. This is where the principle of utility enters. According to Mill, this principle shows us how to select among competing rules of justice. How?

Mill himself was deeply committed to the *laissez-faire* (literally, this means "allow to do") or the *free enterprise* theory of political economy. Though Mill deviated from the strict free enterprise theory in some limited respects, he did recommend this theory in its broad outlines because he was convinced that obedience to the free enterprise rules of society could produce the most social welfare.[6]

Laissez-faire theorists argue that a strictly free market is the most effective tool for bringing about maximal social welfare. A free market unleashes the power of the individual to produce the highest quality and highest number of goods and services at the lowest possible price. In so doing, free markets, according to Mill, produce the highest possible social welfare. This is very relevant to our discussion because the principle of utility says that we ought to do that which maximizes social welfare. If free markets do produce maximal social welfare, then governments have the obligation to establish these free markets and individual people have the right to interact with one another in accordance with the principles of these free markets. But what is a free market?

One way to understand a free market is to see it as a system in which individuals are permitted to voluntarily exchange or transfer goods or services with one another with minimal government interference. The free market emphasizes competition among all players in a market. According to this theory, it is competition that serves to keep prices of goods and services at their lowest possible levels. The market also serves to maintain a high quality of goods and the highest possible quantity of goods and services. The free market aims to create a context in which goods and services will be provided in a way that maximizes social welfare. If a hospital provides health care services and does not have any competition from other hospitals providing similar services, then the hospital may charge any price it wants for its vital services. Without a competitive market, consumers of hospital services will suffer. If, on the other hand, hospitals are competing for business, they are forced by the free market to charge the lowest possible price and provide the highest possible quality of service.

Laissez-faire theorists argue that government should stay out of the free market. This means that government should not provide services or goods to anyone because it cannot do so efficiently. Government will be inefficient because it will use its power to destroy competition, and without competition maximal social welfare is impossible. For the laissez-faire theorist, the function of the government has nothing to do with producing goods or services. Government secures the common good only when it functions as a mere "night watchman" who guarantees that competing players play according to the rules of free competition or "free enterprise." The government should enforce contracts and prevent fraud and force in the market, but it should not itself engage in market activities.

For Mill this laissez-faire theory was originally formulated with a consequentialist justification. The theory, in other words, should be supported not as a matter of principle, but because it is the best instrument for securing what Adam Smith called the "wealth of nations."

## Laissez-Faire and Rights

Robert Nozick has attempted to give a nonconsequentialist, or what I have called a rights-based, argument for a free enterprise approach to social justice.[7] Nozick argues that justice can be defined in terms of transfer and that there are two principles that determine whether a transfer is just. He says that, first, if the rights to goods or services are *acquired justly* and, second, if these goods or services are *voluntarily transferred,* then whatever results from these voluntary transfers of justly acquired goods is itself just. He argues that such a just transfer often results in unfortunate consequences but that we cannot identify what is unfortunate with what is unjust. For Nozick, it is not that a laissez-faire approach produces maximal welfare that makes the principles of the free market correct. It is unjust to interfere with the voluntary transfer of justly acquired goods and services because this involves *using people for the good of others.* According to Nozick, this is immoral in itself. He argues that the government's attempts to provide education, housing, food, or health care is unjust and maintains that "taxation for earnings from labor is on a par with forced labor."[8] One needs to labor for one's earnings, and if government coercively takes a part of these earnings (even if it then uses the money for good purposes), then government is "forcing labor." If I steal your wallet but use the money to feed the poor, what I have done is wrong because I have "used" you against your will. I have treated you as a means or as a tool. According to Nozick, no one, even the government, has the moral right to transform persons into objects or tools whose voluntary behavior must serve the welfare of others.

Whether one gives a consequentialist or a rights-based analysis of free market principles, it is obvious that these principles are relevant in the context of health care. This relevance is expressed by a modern supporter of this laissez-faire theory, economist Milton Friedman. In his book *Capitalism and Freedom*, Friedman captures the philosophical spirit of Mill's theory when he claims that "if any distribution of things of value is a result of competition in the economic system, then that distribution is just."[9] Because government's role is to be a neutral enforcer of private contracts, the laissez-faire theorist requires that government stay out of the business of providing health care services or products. If a free market is allowed to flourish in health care, then the populace will have the greatest number of services and products that it is possible to efficiently provide at a given time. This laissez-faire approach will justify using "ability to pay" as a procedure for distributing scarce medical resources.

Let us close our account of the laissez-faire theory of justice by emphasizing how important the individual and individual liberty are in this theory. Indeed, it may be described as an individualist theory of justice because it assumes that when the rights of the individual are secured by government, then justice has been accomplished. Securing welfare is a private, not public, matter. The heart of this theory involves the claim that society needs to respect the individual and that this respect is best secured if the state steadfastly avoids interfering with individual choices to secure whatever values the individual decides to secure.

## Egalitarianism

The opposite of this free market or laissez-faire approach is the egalitarian theory of justice.[10] This theory, the heart and soul of Karl Marx's philosophy, emphasizes that individuals are morally equal, an idea that is present in both Mill and Kant. However, for Kant and Mill, moral equality requires only that persons be treated as politically equal. Neither believed that moral equality implied economic equality, as Marx did. Marx rejected the notion that politics and economics could be separated. Marxism argues that the moral equality among persons fatally weakens any attempt to justify differentiations in the distribution of wealth. Like most laissez-faire theorists, including Mill, Marxists believe that the moral equality among persons implies that individuals ought to be politically equal. It would be unjust to give me three votes in the upcoming election and you only one. You and I are morally equal to one another and thus we must be treated as political equals. However, Marx noted that in a laissez-faire society, the rich are able to use their wealth to control elected representatives so that these government officials support the interests of the wealthy classes. In effect, the laissez-faire, liberal ideal of genuine political equality cannot be achieved without achieving economic equality or a classless society.

According to Marx, governments are centers of political power. They have never been neutral with respect to serving interests. Governments have never been mere "night watchmen." Marxists argue that governments have always been prejudiced in favor of the ruling classes and that laissez-faire society simply substitutes owners of industry and commerce for aristocratic landowners. In the laissez-faire state, the government serves the interests of the wealthy by using armed forces to protect their wealth. Free markets, according to Marx, produced new economic classes, and the new wealthy classes have an inordinate or unjust amount of political authority because they can use their economic power to control representative bodies.

Marx's answer to this problem is to create a classless society, thereby ending the economic dominance of the rich. In the classless society, everyone does not receive the exact same amount of goods or services. The Marxist does not require that everyone receive the exact same amount of health care; people who do not need antibiotics need not be given them. Needs and the ability to meet them are the only legitimate bases for just distribution. For Marxists, this means that all means of production within a society should be publicly owned. For Marx, private ownership leads inevitably to political inequality, which, even to the laissez-faire theorist, is unacceptable. Consequently, production facilities such as pharmaceutical facilities must be organized and operated not for the profit of individuals, but for the welfare of the state.

## Marxist Justice

Marx's theory is a collectivist theory of justice because justice is viewed primarily from the perspective of the society as a whole rather than from the viewpoint of the individual. Nationalizing factories that were formerly owned by individuals and controlling services that were formerly controlled by individuals is just, according to the Marxist, because it produces social welfare. If an action leads to the welfare of the state but harms the individual, then this harm is viewed as unfortunate but not unjust.

This state control of production confers enormous power on the state; thus the problem of how the state ought to distribute benefits remains a dominant problem in Marxist or socialist states. Egalitarianism does not mean pure or absolute equality. Rather, Marxists use the slogan "From each according to his ability, to each according to his need" to indicate that goods and services should be distributed to those who need them and provided by those who have the ability to provide them. If a person is able to provide a service, such as health care, that would contribute to the welfare of people (and therefore to the welfare of the state), then the state has the duty to organize health care systems so that these benefits can be secured. Through these health care systems the state controls all transactions or transfers so that maximal social welfare is achieved. For Marxists, the health care system should be fully centralized and placed under government control in order to create a health care delivery system that provides as much health care to individuals as the state can afford. Allocation of scarce medical resources is as inevitable in the Marxist state as it is in the laissez-faire state.

Like the laissez-faire theory, Marxism can be viewed from either a consequentialist perspective or a rights-based perspective. For example, the economist Robert Heilbroner in his book *The Worldly Philosophers* argues that Karl Marx rejected the laissez-faire approach to the economy because, while the free market did work to expand total wealth in the industrialized nations of Europe, it tended to concentrate the overwhelming bulk of the wealth in the hands of a few people.[11] This concentration of wealth left the majority of people in a state of virtual misery. In this reading of Marx, the free market failed to meet the consequentialist ideal of securing maximal social welfare because the majority of people were excluded from the benefits of increased wealth and lived lives that were short, nasty, and brutish.

However one can also give a rights-based interpretation of the Marxist view of justice. In *Capital*, Marx claimed that in the free market the worker must sell himself. "These laborers, who must sell themselves piecemeal, are a commodity, like every other article of commerce."[12] For Marx, the free market requires that men and women be treated as objects that can be sold or bought in much the same way as cloth or iron ore. The marketplace exploits men and women in the sense that it presents them with choices such as "work for wages that only preserve life, or die." Although most workers do "consent" to work rather than starve to death, their choices are not genuine because the context did not allow the worker any genuine alternatives.

## Welfare State Justice

Let us now turn to an alternative to both egalitarianism and the laissez-faire approach to justice. This approach is dominant in the twentieth century because, in the minds of many social and economic theorists, it offers a compromise between the individualism of the laissez-faire theory and the socialism of Marxism. This theory is closely associated with contemporary forms of government in the West. Indeed, all Western governments endorse some programs that provide material services (welfare) to various groups within the larger society. The welfare may involve education, housing, food, or health care. In this contemporary political theory, the government is not a "night watchman" that merely enforce private contracts, nor does it own all the means of production. The government is somewhat involved in providing goods and services to the disadvantaged. In some cases, such as education, it is directly involved, while in other cases it supplies housing or food subsidies. Sometimes the government merely regulates a private industry. We may call such governments "welfare states." The philosopher John Rawls, in his seminal work *The Theory of Justice,* has spelled out one account of the principles that support this welfare state.[13]

Rawls's theory may be understood as an alternative to Mill's purely consequentialist approach to justice. What troubled Rawls was Mill's assumption that the principle of utility was the "only ethical principle" that one needed. In Rawls's view, we need more than the utility rule to manage conflicts involving justice. The principle of utility itself only requires those who distribute scarce resources to use allocation rules that produce as much social welfare as possible. It does not tell us how to divide the good that is produced. For example, suppose a system of distribution X was effective in producing more good than system Y, but suppose X concentrated the good in the hands of ten people and left millions with only minimal amounts of good while system Y produced a little less overall good than system X but divided it so that everyone had enough. System Y might allow some inequities, but not allow people to be so poor that they died from starvation or lack of shelter or basic medical care. This system might fail to produce maximal social welfare but have the advantage of leaving everyone in a better position. People might prefer Y over X even though X produces more total good.

Rawls believes that the contemporary welfare state, in which basic goods and services such as education, housing, and health care are treated as rights, is preferable to the laissez-faire system of justice, in which good things like education and health care are treated as privileges available for purchase in an open market. The contemporary welfare state is preferable, Rawls continues, not because it will produce more goods and services than the laissez-faire state, but because it is derived from principles of justice that are arrived at by agreement. For Rawls, the basis of fairness is the social contract, not the principle of utility. Justice is contractual, not utilitarian.

However, for Rawls, the principles of justice are not derived from a social contract or social agreement among the governed. This would require us to write a new constitution whenever a person turns 18. He says that the principles of justice are the rules that reasonable people who are "ignorant" of their own social and economic position within society would adopt. This "original position" of ignorance is necessary because human beings tend to design rules of justice that favor the class to which they belong. We must design from the position of hypothetical ignorance.

Indeed, laissez-faire rules are often criticized for being "rich man's rules" because they give significant advantages to those who have already acquired wealth. Correcting for self-interest is necessary to construct rules of distribution that are both unbiased and universal. They apply to everyone because they would be agreed to by everyone in the original position.

Rawls's theory unites laissez-faire and egalitarian elements by recognizing the power that self-interest exerts on human beings. Both Rawls and the laissez-faire social theorists stress that men and women are primarily motivated by self-interest. This motivation can be used, according to Rawls, as the basis of a system of distributive justice that tends toward protecting the weak and vulnerable. How? Imagine, Rawls suggests, that you or I were in the original position, i.e., ignorant of our social, economic, and intellectual status, and had to decide whether to accept rules that help the poor or rules that benefit the rich. According to Rawls, if I knew that I was poor, then surely by virtue of my self-interest I would adopt the rules that favor poor people. For example, I would emphasize the ways that people are equal and argue that economic differences are inconsistent with the moral equality of human beings. If I knew that I were rich, then I would favor rich person's rules by emphasizing the differences between people and argue that these differences require that we treat people differently. But what rules, asks Rawls, would rational, self-interested persons agree to if they were really ignorant of their own economic positions?

One might agree to live in a laissez-faire state governed by free enterprise rules that allow individuals to secure their welfare and forbid governments to give direct aid to disadvantaged individuals. But this choice involves a big gamble for those in the original position. One might lose the gamble and be born poor, in which case living according to laissez-faire rules would not be in one's self-interest. But suppose one decided to live according to poor man's rules, which allowed the government to appropriate the wealth of the rich and distribute it equally to everyone. Let us call such a system "Marxist rules of justice." However, this hypothetical choice poses the same problem as the choice to adopt laissez-faire rules. If people in the original position adopt Marxist rules and they are actually rich, then the chosen rules would violate their self-interest. A system of justice that was substantially weighted in favor of the poor might violate one's liberty to secure what one wants.

## Rawls's Compromise

For Rawls, the fundamental question of political theory is "What would a rational person do in the original position, given these bad alternatives?" In typically American fashion, Rawls turns to compromise. He develops two principles that attempt to picture rational women and men in the original position as if they were compromising between the possibility that they are rich and the possibility that they are poor. The first principle, often referred to as the *liberty principle,* states that "Each person is to have the most extensive basic liberty compatible with a similar liberty for others."[14] This principle emphasizes that in the original position, no rational individual would choose to be at the complete mercy of the state. Individuals need to be protected from a government that would enslave them even if this slavery was beneficial to the majority. The principle of liberty is Rawls's basis for defending rights associated with individual property. Rejecting the individual's right to property involves enslaving the individual.

However, the liberty of the individual is not the only value that is important. If the state only cared about protecting individual liberties, then individuals born with special endowments, including both money and talent, might use their endowments to unjustifiably harm others. A second principle must counterbalance the principle of liberty. Rawls calls the second principle the *difference principle.* "Social and economic inequalities should be arranged so that they are both (a) to the greatest benefit to the least advantaged and (b) attached to offices and positions open to all under conditions of fair equality of opportunity."[15] For Rawls, economic inequalities are permitted. However, he also maintains that "inequalities should be arranged." He rejects the completely free market because such arrangements are abhorrent to such a system. What justifies social-aid arrangements is that though they may benefit the least well-off, rational, self-interested persons in the original position would protect themselves against the possibility that they are actually poor. Inequalities are permitted but only when they serve the least advantaged. People in the original position would accept these arrangements, but only if they benefited the least well-off. In the original position men and women take out insurance policies that protect them against the worst contingencies of life.

For Rawls, human beings are fundamentally equal in their moral worth, and this requires that they be guaranteed a social safety net that protects them from being seriously harmed by being born poor, ill, or ignorant. However, Rawls is also trying to support a modern market economy in which one is free to compete with others for scarce goods. The competition, however, is an arranged competition. These arrangements may involve taxing those who win in the marketplace (the rich) at a higher rate and also giving special incentives to disadvantaged individuals. Managing or arranging competition is permissible because those who win in the marketplace, according to Rawls, do not "deserve" all the rewards of winning and those who lose in the market do not deserve all the harms associated with losing. To deserve all the rewards, one would have to deserve the natural endowments that one used to win in the competition, and according to Rawls, one gets one's endowments from the lottery, i.e., by accident.

Rawls believes that "the difference principle explicates the distinction between treating men as means and treating them as ends in themselves."[16] In the welfare state, individuals have a right to health care because health care is treated as a condition for securing equality of opportunity. Access to health care is on the same moral footing as access to education. If one lacks any chance to obtain a decent education, one is unable to compete on a level playing field with those who are educated. Similarly, if one is ill and unable to secure a decent level of health care, then one cannot compete fairly with those who are able to purchase health care by themselves. Just as access to a decent minimum of education guarantees equality of opportunity, so too is access to a decent level of health care needed to support that equality.

## Justice and Microallocation

But these large macroallocation or government policy issues are not the only matters that the hospital ethics committee must face. Suppose Community Hospital is allocated 15 intensive care unit (ICU) beds and further suppose that 25 patients need those 15 beds on a given night. Macroallocation and social policy cannot solve this *local* problem. Consequentialists and rights-based theorists must offer a solution. We will turn first to a consequentialist approach to microallocation, which involves a patient selection theory that emerged after the development of the renal dialysis technology.

The following consequentialist theory of scarcity was developed by the philosopher Nicholas Rescher.[17] He argues that selecting patients amidst scarcity requires a two-stage approach. The first stage involves what he calls *criteria of inclusion*. These initial criteria are used to screen patients and reduce the total number of people who have access to a scarce resource. In this first stage, Rescher excludes people who are not entitled to scarce resources. For example, if a hospital has been created for veterans, then presumably citizens who are not veterans would not have access to the hospital's services. Rescher also argues for a selection procedure that would favor individuals whose treatment would advance medical knowledge. He recommends that "prospect of success" should be a basic screening mechanism for patient selection. He believes that providing services to those who cannot benefit from them is "wasting the service." Such wasting does not maximize social welfare; it violates the consequentialist principle that we ought to act to maximize social welfare.

The second and final stage is the *selection stage*. This stage is necessary because frequently we still have shortages after the first criteria are applied. Need might still exceed ability to provide. In this second stage five factors are relevant to the decision-making process. The first factor is relative judgments regarding likelihood of success. Here we favor individuals who have only a temporary need for a technology over those who will need it permanently. Second, the life expectancy factor is taken to favor those who have a long life expectancy over those who have a short one. Third are family factors. Rescher argues that the mother of children can be given priority over "the middle-aged bachelor," presumably because more people are dependent on the mother than the bachelor. Fourth, the potential future contributions of the patient ought to be factored into the equation since the hospital is "a trustee of social interest." Finally, because the hospital is a trustee of social interest, Rescher maintains that the patient's past contributions must be factored into the entitlement equation.

There is much that is sound in Rescher's consequentialist approach, and a careful reading of Community Hospital's policy on allocation will reveal that his influence on the policy is considerable. However, there are two substantial problems with the approach. The first we have already alluded to: the principle of utility encourages us to maximize welfare, but it does not tell us how to distribute this welfare. The second problem lies at the heart of Rescher's allocation strategy. In the second stage, he requires that we assess candidates for scarce medical resources in terms of their past and likely future contributions to society. Rescher argues that consequentialism requires this. If one had to choose between a great nurse who contributes to social welfare and a drug addict who has spent vast amounts of his life in jail, the consequentialist principle seems to require us to choose the nurse.

But from a practical perspective, how does one grade past and future contributions? In our simplistic example the choice seemed easy and obvious—but suppose the nurse was a child abuser. And suppose the drug addict was a great jazz piano player. Would these factors change the evaluation? How much? How does one weigh the evil effect of the child abuse against the good effects associated with being a great nurse?

However, the practical difficulties associated with comparing the value of jazz piano playing with the value of nursing seem overwhelming. Hence, the consequentialist requirement to get involved in the process of comparing contributions is generally seen as impractical and even absurd, although in some simple and extreme cases it appeals to our preferences.

## A Rights-Based Approach

The second approach to resource distribution is rights-based. One can look to the U.S. Constitution as a illustration of this approach. The Constitution grants to all citizens, irrespective of their past or future contributions, the right to free expression, the right to a free press, and so on. The Bill of Rights commits the government to distributing rights without regard for social contribution. These rights are negative or noninterference rights. For example, the right to freedom of religion is negative in that the government will not build churches for religious communities but it will use its authority to prevent others from interfering with worship. Nearly all rights were traditionally viewed as negative, but during the twentieth century there has been a shift toward viewing rights in a positive sense. Governments now provide a minimum of service to citizens, and citizens are entitled by government to view these minimum services as rights. Many Western societies view education, housing, and health as rights that people are entitled to irrespective of their social contribution.

Many rights-based theorists argue that equal access to a decent minimum of scarce medical resources is a right. For example, one might argue that access to a decent minimum opportunity to receive critical care in an intensive care unit is a right, like the right to a decent minimum of education. The practical task of the rights-based theorist is to spell out these limitations.

In Community Hospital's rationing policy, the right of access to a decent minimum is contained in the "first come, first served" principle. In the intensive care context, everyone only gets *access* to the opportunity to receive intensive care. If the unit is full on a given night, a person may not actually receive the benefit. The right of access does not mean that a patient is guaranteed to receive the services. If one is fortunate enough to need a service when it is available, then one receives the service irrespective of one's contributions or one's ability to pay. The moral value of the chance rule is not that it is guaranteed to always yield the best clinical consequences. Rather, its virtue lies in its affirmation of the moral equality of all citizens.

Thus, the policy treats access to scarce resources as a right, but a restricted right. The equal access of citizens to an intensive care unit, for example, is circumscribed not only by the availability of the service but also by the amount of benefit that the service can provide to the patient. And it is this last element that illustrates the consequentialist element of the policy. The committee accepted the notion that consequences are crucial to any rationing policy when it asserted that medical consequences such as probability of patient survival, patient's quality of life, the probable length of the patient's life, and the cost of providing the service are relevant to patient selection.

## Criticisms of the Policy

In order to appreciate the policy, we need to see how its most energetic social critics would criticize it. The first assault is based on egalitarian considerations, and the second is based on the principles of free enterprise. Egalitarians like Karl Marx would approach the problem of microallocation from a very economic basis and ask how much of society's resources is being spent on ICU services and what benefit are they yielding to the majority. They would compare this to the amount of money being spent on highly technological and very expensive medical strategies and ask whether this expense produces the biggest overall benefit for most men and women. If they found that the financial resources used to secure a particular medical benefit only aided a small minority and inhibited the distribution of decent care to the majority, then they would oppose this use of funds. Countries such as the former Soviet Union, China, and Cuba spent, and continue to spend, very few resources developing intensive care units because these units are very expensive and benefit only a small number of people.

The free enterprise philosopher also criticizes the hospital's policy, maintaining that although it may be unfortunate that some people lack the money to pay for services they desperately need, it is not necessarily unjust to allow these needs to remain unfulfilled. People have all kinds of desperate needs, but this does not entitle them to use other people's money to satisfy these needs. Unsatisfied need is often unfortunate, but it is not necessarily unjust. For the free enterprise philosopher, the fact that someone may need intensive care services and not be able to afford them is surely unfortunate, but need alone does not entitle someone to the service. What this philosopher finds disconcerting in Community Hospital's scarce resources policy is that it treats very expensive technology as if no one had to pay for it.

Intensive care services to the needy are very expensive, and they are paid for by those who pay premiums for medical insurance. Hospitals will charge their insured or paying patients whatever it costs to keep the doors of the hospital open. In effect, the insured pay for many of the services provided to those who cannot pay. This form of transfer of funds from insured patients to the uninsured is not mandated by the legislature, nor have the individuals who pay for the services voluntarily consented to the transfer. And when transfers are accomplished without the consent of the individual and without the explicit consent of the legislature, then injustice occurs.

## Replies to Criticisms

What responses are open to supporters of Community Hospital's policy? Can the hospital answer both the egalitarian critique and the free enterprise critique of the policy? The egalitarian and the free enterprise philosopher both reject the hospital's policy. This is not surprising since Community Hospital exists in a social and economic context that is neither Marxist nor free enterprise.

Let us begin with the egalitarian critique. For modern hospitals the basis of the rationing policy is that equal access to a decent minimum of health care is all that is mandated by the principles of justice. The egalitarians demand complete equality of access, but Western governments have explicitly rejected this egalitarian or Marxist demand. The decent minimum may best be viewed as a compromise between egalitarian considerations and free enterprise considerations. Both egalitarian and free enterprise perspectives are treated as cogent in recent Western debates over just health care. Rather than identifying with either philosophical viewpoint, Western societies have attempted to transcend both philosophies by developing a compromise that incorporates the virtues of both. The decent minimum is not defended for its own internal logic but because of the practical need to develop a workable compromise.

The criticisms of the free enterprise philosopher offer an deeper challenge to the committee. The state mandates that the hospital provide very expensive and scarce resources to the indigent, but it does not provide the revenue necessary to accomplish this. If the hospital did not provide the poor person with access to this expensive care, then the hospital would lose its license. The hospital's only alternative is to "cost shift" and force those who have insurance to pay for the services of those who do not. Cost shifting is morally suspicious because it transfers funds from the "haves" to the "have-nots" without either individual consent or legislative consent. This is important because even if one accepts the welfare state perspective of justice, transfers of income from haves to have-nots must be approved by the legislature. One cannot have automatic transfers using the license as a lever to coerce transfers.

## The Case of Coretta Anderson

Coretta Anderson is a patient in Community Hospital. She is 81 and is a diabetic who is also suffering from end-stage Alzheimer's disease. For eight months she has had nearly no cognitive function and has been profoundly disoriented. She has significant hypertension and coronary heart disease. In addition, she has significant renal failure and is currently being dialyzed. She was admitted to the hospital yesterday after being transferred from an extended care facility because she has contracted pneumonia. Her family insists that everything be done for her. They want the full services of the intensive care unit brought to bear if her breathing becomes difficult.

The physician in charge of the intensive care unit believes that the ICU service is inappropriate for Mrs. Anderson even if her respiration deteriorates. Her attending physician disagrees and wants everything done for her.

The ICU director believes that she would be best served by continuing her care in the general care section of the hospital.

The ICU staff has been overworked due to spending cuts. As a result, significant reductions were made in nursing staff. The patient care quality level has been reduced. The major question facing the committee is whether Mrs. Anderson should be admitted to the ICU since there is a bed open and her breathing is starting to become difficult. The triage officer who is in charge of admissions has refused to admit her.

### Committee Discussion of the Case

| | |
|---|---|
| Dr. Mary Collins: (Chair) | I would like to thank you for attending this emergency meeting of the committee. Dr. Davis asked me to call it, and I appreciate your willingness to assist us with this case. As with all our cases, let's begin by opening the floor to questions. I have asked Dr. Davis to respond to your questions because he has recently been appointed the triage officer for the intensive care unit. |
| Prof. Martin Fisk: | Given the availability of the bed, why hasn't Dr. Davis admitted her? |
| Rev. Richard Marcus: | Can we get a clear prognosis with respect to the four factors mentioned in our policy, namely, probability of survival given the service, length of survival, quality of life, and cost? The reason I want to look at these factors is that she may be a Category 3 patient. We may admit her based on the chance factor and the availability of the bed, but she may be a candidate for exclusion as soon as another person who needs the service appears on the scene. |
| Vivian Harris: | I would like to know more about the family. What kinds of conversations have you had with the family and what kind of decent care can we provide for her on the general floor? |
| Dr. Philip Davis: | Martin, as usual you get to the heart of the matter quite quickly. My reason for not |

admitting her is that my people in that unit are really overworked. There is a bed that is open, but I am not sure that we can maintain a decent level of care to the other patients in the unit if we become responsible for Mrs. Anderson as well. She is going to require a massive amount of care, and I am worried that if I admit her, my staff will become so overextended that they will not be able to provide a decent level of care to the other patients. The current shortage of critical care nurses is a real issue. My staff of nurses are some of the best in the world, but we are stretched to the limits. In the light of this overextension, I feel that Mrs. Anderson's condition does not warrant bringing her into the unit.

With respect to the four issues that Mr. Marcus has raised, I believe that we would have a chance of pulling her out of immediate danger with five or six days of ICU care. But I must emphasize that this is a very rough "guesstimate" based on my experience with patients in this condition. I have seen patients like Mrs. Anderson spend weeks, even months, in the ICU. But I think that if we provided maximal therapeutic care, we could manage the breathing problem to the point where she could be released from the unit to the general floor. The quality of her life is another matter. This aspect of her situation will never, in my clinical judgment, change. She is not going to return from this stage of Alzheimer's disease. I regard her as having a very low quality of life, and it is, therefore, very difficult for me to provide her with services that could be going to other patients. The renal insufficiency is being managed, but her greatest danger is her heart disease. I do not expect this woman to live for much longer, and so I view the ICU as a technology that will not benefit her but only extend her dying process. In my opinion, it will do more harm than good to her. I regard this pneumonia as her friend, not her enemy. Finally, the cost issue is something that I am not an expert on. Indeed, you would be surprised how little health care professionals know about the details regarding cost. But since I am the one being asked the questions, I will give you my guess. I think we are looking at about $2,000 per ICU day.

The family is divided on the matter. One son believes that we can still help Mrs. Anderson and that we should be doing everything. When I spoke to him and gave him the same grim prognosis that I have given you, he responded by asking me whether there is a chance that she can recover from the pneumonia. When I told him that there was such a chance, he immediately fired back that we should do everything we can to cure the pneumonia. He is very emotionally dependent on his mother and he cannot seem to detach himself from her. He seems unwilling to accept that his mother is dying. The daughter has a more realistic picture of what is happening. She is trying to get her brother to appreciate that the treatment will only prolong her biological existence, but until her brother agrees to withhold treatment, she insists that treatment be provided.

Finally, with respect to Vivian's question regarding the alternative to the ICU, I think that we can keep her on the general floor and provide maximal treatment to her. We can also keep her relatively comfortable with analgesics. Her risk of dying, however, will be greatly increased because I am not going to permit ventilators on the floor.

| | |
|---|---|
| Mary Quigley: | Why can't she be ventilated on the floor? |
| Dr. Davis: | No! If we start doing that, we begin to treat the general floor beds as ICU beds. I do not want to get into that because the quality of care that is needed really is different. My clinical recommendation is that we try to do everything we can for her on the general floor and that we also turn toward a "comfort measures only" approach. |
| Atty. John Quinn: | Phil, let me return to a statement that you made about the family being divided. I do not think they are. The sister wants her mother admitted to the ICU. She may side with her brother reluctantly but she sides with him nonetheless. Is this not right? |
| Dr. Davis: | Yes. |
| Atty. Quinn: | My reason for raising this is that, if I were to go to court on this matter, I could not, at least at this time, make a case for division among the family, could I? If a court made the sister a legal guardian, there is no assurance that she would side with you against her brother. |
| Dr. Davis: | You are correct, John. At this time she is not ready to disagree with her brother. |
| Atty. Quinn: | If this is the case, then I think we had better understand that if we decide to support Dr. Davis's view on this case, then we need to invoke principle 6 of our policy, in which we reject the idea that consent of the guardians is a necessary condition for refusing to allocate a scarce resource to a patient. The sister might change her mind and agree with Dr. Davis, but I do not think that we can count on that. |
| Dr. Collins: | John, I would like to know just how risky this is. I have no enthusiasm for throwing the hospital into a potentially dangerous legal situation. |

| Atty. Quinn: | Obviously, the safest thing to do legally is to provide the treatment, but there is plenty of precedent for following Dr. Davis's recommendations. I think that I could convince a court that refusing treatment based on futility and scarcity was justifiable. However, I want to make it clear to you that we are not in a risk-free environment and that juries are sometimes difficult to predict in these cases. The safest thing is to provide the service and then seek a court-appointed guardian to approve the withdrawal. |
| :--- | :--- |
| Prof. Fisk: | Hold on a minute! We seem to be doing to ourselves precisely what we said we would never do. We said that we would not allow legal ambiguity and the desire to maximize our immunity from litigation to determine our ethical judgment. Aren't we doing that? Let's judge this case in the light of our good sense and our policy. Besides, this family has not raised any hints that they would take legal action against us. |
| Atty. Quinn: | Martin makes a sound point, but we might want to inform the family about our intentions and even advise them that they can seek an attorney. If I were their attorney, I would go after a probate injunction against our refusal to admit her. If the court were to refuse to grant the injunction, then we would be in a very solid legal position. |
| Dr. Collins: | Would a court refuse to grant such an injunction, John? |
| Atty. Quinn: | It depends on how well I make my case! |
| Dr. Collins: | In other words, you cannot be sure, can you, John? |
| Atty. Quinn: | I am a terrific attorney but I failed all my courses in crystal ball reading. |

| | |
|---|---|
| Prof. Fisk: | John, you and I have disagreed about a lot of ethical issues. I am very interested to know your ethical views on this case. |
| Atty. Quinn: | Philosophically, I have no problem with Dr. Davis's approach. I think we need to view scarce resources as existing for those who can benefit from them. And I think that Mrs. Anderson is beyond benefit. |
| Marian Rhodes: | The benefit question, however, may not be an objective matter. The President's Commission seems to feel that questions of what is and what is not medically beneficial are ethical and cannot be treated as purely medical. In short, I am not sure that Dr. Davis is entitled to answer this ethical question by himself. He certainly has the right to contribute to the decision and his opinions are ones that I respect, but the family's views on what is beneficial cannot be disregarded. |
| Dr. Davis: | Marian, you know what end-stage Alzheimer's victims are like. Their neocortical tissue is almost completely destroyed. In what sense can they benefit from treatment? |
| Ms. Rhodes: | Your point is well made, Phil, but as a society we have not yet decided to treat Mrs. Anderson as a nonperson. As of now she is still considered a full person who is merely incompetent; therefore, questions about her interest and her wishes need to be decided by her family and her physician. In this case we have division between the physician and the family regarding her interest. However, I do not think that we can simply disregard the family because they are, in Dr. Davis's opinion, not facing the facts properly. |
| Dr. Collins: | Is there any information on what Mrs. Anderson's wishes were? |

| | |
|---|---|
| Dr. Davis: | I asked the daughter whether her mother had a living will or whether she had ever expressed her feelings about what she would want done in circumstances like these. Her response was that "in her family, we never talked too much about these kinds of issues." |
| Dr. Collins: | So we are really ignorant about the wishes of the mother, aren't we? |
| Dr. Davis: | Yes! |
| Prof. Fisk: | Marian, you seem unwilling to allow Dr. Davis to make this decision. Don't you see that your opposition is inconsistent with our policy regarding the duties of the triage officer? Dr. Davis has the responsibility to allocate the beds in the ICU, and in times of crisis we are going to give him authority over the allocation of resources subject to our policy. Principle 6 clearly permits him to do this, even in the absence of guardian consent. |
| Ms. Rhodes: | But, Martin, don't we have a slippery slope issue here? |
| Prof. Fisk: | In what sense? |
| Ms. Rhodes: | Look, Martin, a lot of the services here in the hospital are highly technological and therefore very expensive. The ICU has no corner on expense. From a financial viewpoint, these expensive services could be considered "scarce" and principle 6 could then be extended to cover all them. Aren't we opening the door to allowing unconsented withholding and unconsented withdrawal of these services on the basis of their expense and, therefore, their scarcity? |
| Prof. Fisk: | This is a possibility, Marian, but I think that it is an unrealistic possibility. And I do not think that the hospital will use principle 6 to override the general rule that routine care cannot be withheld without consent. |

Prof. Carla Thomas:    I would like to turn our attention toward another concern that I have with this case. There is one bed left in the ICU and so, strictly speaking, Mrs. Anderson should have access to it since she is first in line. No one else is seeking access to the unit, are they?

Dr. Davis:    Not at this time, but I fully expect that this will change within a very short period of time. I would be very surprised if we did not have an admission request within 24 hours for a patient who has a far better prognosis than Mrs. Anderson. It is also important to note that a great deal of time is spent on a patient when they are admitted to the ICU. It doesn't make sense to admit a patient like Mrs. Anderson if you think that she is going to be excluded in the very near future.

Prof. Thomas:    Your points are well taken, Phil, but allow me to finish making my original point. Mrs. Anderson's survival probabilities are fair. Her length of life, given the service, is short (perhaps months) and her quality of life is, perhaps, low. The cost is about $12,000 based on six days of service at $2,000 per day. My question is how are we to compute these factors in relation to one another? The policy merely tells us that all these factors are relevant but it does not tell us how to weigh one against the others. Two writers[18] recommend that we simply find some way of quantifying these factors and then divide by the cost or the projected cost of the service. This will give us what they call an Entitlement Index. Is this what you are doing, Phil, when you determine that Mrs. Anderson is not entitled to the service?

Dr. Davis:    It is certainly not as quantitative as that. I am making what I call a clinical judgment that includes these four factors, but I am not using any fixed formula. This is part of the art of medicine. I think it might be too early to box us in with the kind of formula that you have suggested.

Prof. Thomas:    In other words, these are the relevant factors, but there is no way to determine how relevant they are or to compare the relevance of one factor with the relevance of another. For example, I think that you are giving a lot of weight to this woman's quality of life factor and underplaying the fact that she will probably survive, thanks to the treatment. These factors definitely do not carry equal weight in your mind.

Dr. Davis:    That is correct, Carla. I do give a lot of weight to the fact that her quality of life, given the success of the ICU, is going to be very low. I can live with that value, and I think that the committee needs to put some confidence in my clinical judgment. I admit that my judgment is not immune to subjective influences, but the hospital did hire me to exercise my clinical judgment.

Prof. Thomas:    Phil, I have a lot of confidence in your clinical judgment decisions. But if you quit tomorrow and a new triage officer comes on board, then I might have a very different level of confidence.

Dr. Davis:    Well, all I can say is that you need to make sure that you hire a good person to replace me because no triage officer is going to be able to do this job without employing a good deal of clinical judgment. This committee better have some confidence in the person or the whole system of allocation will break down, because the key to allocation involves trusting the judgment of the triage officer.

Dr. Collins:    I want to reopen the issue of the one bed still open. Let me quote from the policy:

"The triage officer will allocate scarce resources on a 'first come, first served' basis, but individuals who cannot medically benefit from a resource (Category 3 patients) will have no entitlement to the scarce ICU service, even if they are next in line for it. Judgments of medical futility will be made by the triage officer." I interpret this in a very strict sense to mean that before we can refuse a patient initial access to a scarce resource, we need to demonstrate that the scarce resource—in this case the ICU—is not effective against the disease that we are fighting. Phil interprets this statement more loosely to mean that we can exclude a patient from the ICU if the treatment cannot improve the patient's overall quality of life.

Now I agree that this treatment will not alter Mrs. Anderson's quality of life. We cannot cure the Alzheimer's disease. However, it is damnably effective against pneumonia and isn't this the disease that we are fighting? Now Phil can claim that he has no interest in fighting the pneumonia, but the family does and that is the crucial matter.

Dr. Davis:    Look . . . let me put my cards on the table. Mrs. Anderson is not suffering from pneumonia. Nor is she suffering from Alzheimer's disease. Nor is she suffering from heart disease. I don't think that she is suffering at all. The part of her brain that is needed in order to suffer anything is completely dysfunctional. She is somewhere between being alive and being dead! She is a "neo-mort," and "neo-morts," in my opinion, cannot compete with the value of full human beings that I can help to return to human life with the help of our ICU! The ICU was never intended to be used to save or sustain "neo-morts" in the

|  | nether world between life and death. It was intended as a means for returning people to health. It just doesn't make any clinical sense to use this technology for the purposes that the Anderson family wants us to use it. |
|---|---|
| Prof. Fisk: | Philosophically I agree with you, Phil, but using our positions of authority to institute our private philosophical convictions, which are not shared by the majority of our community, is something that I want to oppose. I want to emphasize, Phil, that, on the theoretical level, I agree with you. But I think that before we can begin to act on the possibility that Mrs. Anderson is not a person, we have the responsibility to convince the society that people with persistent and profound neocortical dysfunction have lost their status as persons. We have not yet convinced people of this. I think that it is wrong to use our positions of authority to enforce our private values on an unwilling public. |
| Atty. Quinn: | Let me emphasize, Dr. Davis, that the law does not admit your concept of the "neomort." As far as I am concerned, Mrs. Anderson is an incompetent person. |
| Rev. Marcus: | I do not think we can dismiss Phil's point so easily. As we all know, the law is not always a guide to what is ethically right. If it were such a guide, then we would never honor a man like Martin Luther King, who became a national hero by breaking the law. More importantly, in our policy we have given the triage officer, Dr. Davis, significant authority. As I read principle 1, we are merely advisory to him on the matter of allocation. In effect, he does not have to abide by this committee's decision. |
| Dr. Collins: | That is what we decided, but, as Phil knows, I am the chief medical officer of this |

hospital and I had better be able to live with his decision. This "neo-mort" discussion does not give me a lot of confidence. I would hate to think that we are making allocation decisions based on these weak considerations.

Dr. Davis:    But the policy does make me responsible for allocation, and in this case I think that we can refuse treatment. Perhaps we need to achieve more consensus around the idea of the "neo-mort," but we cannot help Mrs. Anderson. That seems basic to me.

Dr. Collins:    Phil, philosophy is fine, but we did not agree to use the idea of the "neo-mort" in our policy. So it cannot be the basis of our decision.

Prof. Thomas:    I think that we need to move on to other matters relevant to this case, so I do not think that we can continue with this issue of whether Mrs. Anderson is or is not a person at this time. However, I certainly do not think that Phil's consideration is irrelevant. If we could continue the matter, I would like to hear a more detailed neuro-logical report on Mrs. Anderson's neocorti-cal status. But let me close by reminding Mary that the whole country has been struggling with the abortion issue for 30 years and the major question in that debate is whether first- and second-trimester fetuses have the status of persons. I think that it is perfectly sensible to ask the same question of individuals who have perma-nently lost their capacity to interact. Rather than being irrelevant, I believe that Phil has raised an absolutely critical issue.

Ms. Harris:    Allow me to follow the suggestion that we need to move on. Does Mrs. Anderson have any kind of insurance? Or must the hospital eat the cost of her care?

| Dr. Davis: | The family is not well off and the children work at jobs that do not provide extensive medical coverage. She has Medicare and Medicaid, but that is woefully inadequate in terms of meeting the cost of the care that her family wants her to have. |
|---|---|
| Rev. Marcus: | Our policy does not specify that ability to pay is a relevant factor in the distribution of scarce resources. I thought that we bit the bullet on this matter. |
| Atty. Quinn: | The policy does not introduce the issue of ability to pay directly, but the policy does admit that the cost of care is relevant. Since she has very little to pay, her cost of care will be very high relative to the hospital. |
| Rev. Marcus: | Atty. Quinn has made a fine logical point, but I remember in our discussions of this matter we decided not to consider ability to pay in our deliberations. I think raising the issue breaks the ground rules of our policy. |
| Atty. Quinn: | I too, remember that discussion. The cost elements in the policy were a compromise that all of us agreed to. I agreed to it precisely because cost and ability to pay are not separate matters. If a person does not have the ability to pay, the cost to the hospital is increased. |
| Rev. Marcus: | That was not my understanding. I believed that cost was the same whether the person does or does not have the ability to pay. I suspect that the word "cost" is ambiguous, and so our compromise was merely a verbal one and did not really resolve our conflict. |
| Dr. Collins: | As chair, I think that we can allow these considerations to be raised, but it was my understanding that they were not going to be accepted as an important factor in the deliberations. |

| Ms. Quigley: | Let me enter this discussion of cost. As you all know, I have owned my own business for many years, and I find it absolutely amazing that so many of you consider the ability to pay as "irrelevant" to the issue that we are considering. I have a business that employs over one hundred people and none of them would be working tomorrow if I considered that the ability to pay was irrelevant. In my world, it is one of the most important factors, and it is not an evil consideration. I have to keep my prices as low as possible and my quality as high as possible in order to attract customers. This keeps me and my employees on our toes. Also, my customers have to pay their bills if I am going to keep providing them with the product at a good price. The money keeps me working hard and it ensures that my customers use my product efficiently. Because it is expensive, my customers do not waste what I sell them. Money is something that simply keeps us all efficient. It is not the big monster that so many ministers and a fair number of doctors consider it. So my vote is to put the ability to pay issue on the table and let's talk about it. |
|---|---|
| Prof. Fisk: | Mary, your company sells computer software programs to businesses. You are not in the business of selling intensive care unit beds. There are significant differences. |
| Ms. Quigley: | What are these differences? My customers now tell me that two years ago my programs were a luxury that increased their profitability but that now they are a necessity. Without programs like ours they could not stay in business. The business environment has changed so radically that yesterday's options are today's essentials. For many of my customers my services now count as vital. |

| | |
|---|---|
| Dr. Davis: | But what is necessary for your business is not the same as what is necessary for your life. ICUs keep people alive. As important as your programs are, Mary, I do not think that we can treat them as being on a par with an ICU. |
| Ms. Quigley: | If your life is your business, then there is no difference. I do not want to burst your bubbles here, but life has more in it than medicine, ICUs, and scarce medical treatment. People prefer things other than medical care, and they express their preferences by spending their scarce financial resources one way rather than another. In short, as valuable as medical care is, our citizens may not, if we gave them the chance, consider medical care as important as you do. The situation is similar with teachers. Teachers insist that education is the "sine qua non" for life. But taxpayers do not hold it as that important. Most school boards are operating on a shoestring because they have to live within very tight constraints. Our citizens do not want to spend as much as professionals want them to spend on things like health care and education. |
| Dr. Collins: | Mary, can you make your comments relevant to the case at hand? |
| Ms. Quigley: | If the Anderson family thinks that this treatment is so important, why didn't they pay for it? I am sure that they have a hundred reasons for not doing so, but in the end, they simply made other choices. That is OK in my book because I for one do not think that these ICUs offer a good value. They are very expensive and they do not return much in terms of the good life. However, the Anderson family will demand these services if they are free. But if they really valued life extension, then they |

should have been saving for it for the past ten years. The point is that this kind of care is not free. The nurses who staff that unit want to be paid and the people who sell this technology to us want cash on the barrel head and the physicians who know how to use this technology want decent compensation. Perhaps if we were rational about health care and did not have a de facto system of forced taxation through the insurance companies, then we would not have so much of this technology that is independent of our free choices.

Dr. Davis:

In what sense is it outside of our free choices?

Ms. Quigley:

If real human beings could decide to buy this ICU stuff, i.e., take money out of their own pockets and buy the rights of access to ICU technology or refuse to purchase these rights, then I think that very few would choose to buy such access. We would not buy it because the clinical data indicate that it does not have a very good return on investment. Am I not right, Phil, that most people with multiple system failures above the age of 75, like Mrs. Anderson, who receive ICU treatment never get out of the hospital?

Dr. Davis:

That is correct but . . .

Ms. Quigley:

Pardon me, Phil, but let me finish! Consequently, this kind of ICU technology would not exist in anything like the amounts that it now does in the United States if people could choose. This is because rational people do not buy what doesn't work or doesn't really help them. The desperately poor clinical data on people like Mrs. Anderson prove this. But why then did we create this ICU technology? It seems to me that we bought it because the medical system that operates in this country functions independently of people's actual choices. In technical terms, the medical industry in the United States is not a market-driven system. In fact, it is in some respects worse than the socialist systems of health care because in the socialist countries, at least some of the trash bag politicians get to choose how to spend money, even though the people do not. Here the system operates to buy and purchase technology without anyone asking whether they want to purchase it. I would love to create products that my customers do not have to freely spend their money on. It would make my job a lot easier.

Dr. Collins: May I summarize your remarks as amounting to an argument that ability to pay should be the only basis for distributing scarce beds in the ICU?

Mary Quigley: To quote Gary Cooper, yup!

Rev. Marcus: Mary's views do not reflect my sentiments at all. I agree that construing health care as a right to a decent minimum of health care is filled with ambiguity. But I am still an advocate of this approach. I think that health care is identical to education or food. All women and men have a right to it. A decent minimum of food is not a privilege like a Cadillac; it is a right that minimally decent societies grant to their members. Just as we have the right to free speech by virtue of being persons, so too we have a right to a decent minimum of health care by virtue of being persons.

However, this view does not imply that providing ICU service to Mrs. Anderson is part of the decent minimum. I am not sure that ICU service is a requirement of the decent minimum.

Prof. Thomas: Mary Quigley's remarks deal with macroallocation. She is arguing that the national policy on allocating medical resources is incoherent. I certainly disagree with a number of her basic assumptions, but at this time, her points are irrelevant to the issue that we must address. Our task is a concrete microallocation task, not a matter of global macroallocation. More importantly, these global matters cannot be resolved by our committee. We do not have the authority to set national allocation procedures, and we certainly have no authority to make "ability to pay" the only basis for distribution of scarce or expensive health care resources. I think that if we tried to employ Mary's criterion on the Anderson case, we would be in danger of losing our operating license.

Dr. Collins:

Mary's concerns are widely felt around the country, and perhaps they may someday resurface as national policy. But we would have to create a new policy on allocation if we were to follow Mary's direction, and the committee is not ready to do that. We should be primarily concerned with the application of our present policy.

Ms. Harris:

May I suggest that we address the issues in this case and make some decisions. All of us are more than slightly busy, and I think that each of us needs to call this one in the light of the policy and our own convictions. I would like to propose that we oppose Dr. Davis's recommendation and admit Mrs. Anderson into the ICU. My reasons are threefold. First, she is next in line for the service and she can benefit from the service in the sense that the service will increase her chance of survival. Second, her guardians are requesting the service and the fact that I would not request this treatment for myself, if I were in this position, is not sufficient to override their decisions. Finally, if at a later point another seriously ill patient requires assistance in the ICU, Dr. Davis can exclude her based on our criteria.

Dr. Collins:    The motion on the floor then is admit Mrs. Anderson and then use the criteria to withdraw her from the unit if another patient needs her bed.

Dr. Davis:    My guess is that if we admit her and spend a lot of resources in the admission process, we will then be forced to withdraw her from the service in order to bring in someone who can benefit from the service. In short, why bring her in if you do not reasonably expect to be able to keep her in the unit for long enough to address the pneumonia problem?

Ms. Harris:    I am ready to accept this consequence in order to affirm that she has a right to equal access of care. Furthermore, I think that the question as to whether she is a person is philosophically fine and perhaps the culture should engage in this discussion, but I think that it would be inappropriate to act on Dr. Davis's private convictions about Mrs. Anderson's status as a person. We are a public, not a private, committee.

Prof. Fisk:    Dr. Davis's convictions regarding Mrs. Anderson's status as a person should be treated as irrelevant because they are both private and idiosyncratic. These convictions might be right or wise or insightful or heinous, but they are not yet considered acceptable bases for action. What is an acceptable basis for action is his claim that he cannot in all likelihood benefit her. What justifies his view is that, statistically, she probably will not benefit from the ICU unit. As far as I am concerned, we have no obligation to provide treatment that is in all likelihood futile. In short, I am ready to go along with Dr. Davis, but my reasons are very different from his reasons.

| Prof. Thomas: | But, Martin, who defines "benefit" and who defines "futility"? There are some clear applications of these terms, such as, it is futile to bleed a person as a means of treating their pneumonia. Or, it is of no benefit to dialyze as a treatment for liver dysfunction. But I am not sure whether it is clear to say that ICU treatment for Mrs. Anderson's pneumonia is "futile" or that Mrs. Anderson will not benefit from the treatment. You and Dr. Davis think it is futile, but the family doesn't and some of us have some doubts. |
|---|---|
| Dr. Davis: | I am not used to you speaking in generalities, Carla. Be specific! What are your doubts? |
| Prof. Thomas: | The first doubt is that you are saying that the life of a severely handicapped person like Mrs. Anderson is not valuable enough to give her a fair shot at the scarce resource. My view of Mrs. Anderson is that she is a severely handicapped person. Nothing more and certainly nothing less. To refer to her ailment as a handicap is a way of capturing the idea that she is one of us. A moral equal. She is a member of our moral community. Hence, she is entitled to meaningful access to expensive treatments for her pneumonia. And meaningful access means that admitting her involves a commitment to a period of time that would allow us to manage her pneumonia. Letting someone in for a few moments only to send her out of the unit before it can yield any possible benefits is absurd. |
| Dr. Davis: | What is the point of calling her a handicapped person? |
| Prof. Thomas: | Remember that the President's Commission specifically states that we are not allowed to withdraw or withhold services from an infant merely because she has Down |

|  | syndrome. The commission states very clearly that Down victims are persons. Down victims belong to our moral community, and if they are persons then so are Alzheimer's victims. If we cannot discriminate against the Down victim, then I do not think that we can discriminate on the basis of Alzheimer's. |
|---|---|
| Dr. Davis: | I am very unhappy with the charge that this kind of triage amounts to discrimination. I see myself as merely preventing the waste of valuable resources by not giving them to Mrs. Anderson. |
| Prof. Thomas: | Waste is a vague term, Phil. You can waste expensive cancer treatment by giving it to house flies, and this is because house flies do not count as part of the moral community. You can also waste such treatment by misapplying it, for example, by giving dialysis to victims of hepatic disease. Both of these are wastes. Providing ICU treatment to Mrs. Anderson is not a waste in either of these senses. Is there another sense in which it is a waste? |
| Dr. Davis: | It is a waste in the sense that admission to the ICU will not statistically improve her quality of life nor significantly extend her life. Furthermore, this pneumonia might be secondary to her heart disease, in which case, a simple provision of antibiotics may not break the back of this disease. What appears at the time of admission to be a five- or six-day stay in the ICU may turn into a one- or two-month stay in the ICU that brings about no improvement in the patient's outcome! Carla, you know enough about medicine to understand that we probably cannot help Mrs. Anderson. Why are you defending this line of reasoning? |
| Prof. Thomas: | Because she is part of the moral community and we need to treat her with respect. |

Prof. Fisk:
But treating her as a full member of the moral community and refusing to give her access to the ICU are not incompatible. To provide her with a good level of care on the general care floor demonstrates our respect for her as a person. Consider an analogy from the university. You would never admit a student into an upper-division mathematics class who has not demonstrated that he has sufficient knowledge to benefit from the class. If he lacks the prerequisite knowledge, then it is a waste of our educational resources to let him in. You discriminate against this student because being unable to benefit from the class is legitimate grounds for discrimination. In the moral sense the problem we face is nearly identical. Mrs. Anderson cannot benefit and so it is permissible to discriminate against her.

Dr. Collins:
We have a motion on the floor, and we need to act on it if we are ever to do anything else with our lives.

Dr. Davis:
I oppose this motion! It is bad medicine and it is bad ethics.

Prof. Fisk:
I agree with Phil. What about you, John?

Atty. Quinn:
I am with Phil Davis on this matter. I cannot see giving this ICU service to individuals who can only marginally benefit from it. I think that it is important to say, however, that our policy only permits the triage officers to refuse admission to individuals who cannot benefit from a service. What we say in principle 5D is that only individuals who "cannot medically benefit" from the service will be excluded at the admission stage. The policy is silent on the question of whether we can exclude patients from admission based on the fact they can only marginally benefit. My sense

of this case is that Mrs. Anderson can only marginally benefit from the service, but based on the policy alone, this might not be enough to exclude her from admission to the unit.

In effect, what Phil Davis is doing is extending the notion that we can, under pressure, exclude those who are only marginally benefiting from a service. We did not agree to this in our policy formation stage, but Phil wants to extend his authority and I agree with him. He wants to extend the authority to exclude marginal patients even when we are not under pressure. There is, after all, a bed that is still available.

| | |
|---|---|
| Ms. Rhodes: | Would someone mind telling me what the difference is between saying that someone cannot benefit and someone can only marginally benefit from a scarce resource? |
| Atty. Quinn: | As I see it, Marian, the difference is that in the first case we can agree that there is no benefit and in the second case we cannot reach agreement. |
| Ms. Rhodes: | But if we cannot agree as to whether the service would be beneficial to Mrs. Anderson, don't you think that we need to err on the side of safety and give her a shot at the service? A few days in the ICU will allow us to firm up our clinical picture and then maybe we will decide to withdraw her. I support the motion on the floor. |
| Atty. Quinn: | Let's have a vote and get on with our business. |

The vote is three in support of the motion and six opposed.

| | |
|---|---|
| Dr. Collins: | This motion has failed. Can I ask Atty. Quinn to offer an alternative motion? |

*Committee Recommendations*

| | |
|---|---|
| Atty. Quinn: | Yes! I move that we support Dr. Davis's recommendation to exclude Mrs. Anderson from the ICU service. |
| Dr. Collins: | Any further discussion? (No discussion is offered.) Since there is no further discussion, let's make this judgment. |

The vote is six in support and three opposed.

| | |
|---|---|
| Dr. Collins: | Phil, I think that you need to contact the family as soon as possible and inform them. Perhaps you need to remind them that we will continue to provide Mrs. Anderson with maximal therapeutic care on the general floor of the hospital. |
| Ms. Quigley: | Aren't you going to inform the family that their mother was excluded from treatment on the basis of a triage or rationing decision? |
| Dr. Davis: | I plan to tell them that there was nothing that I could offer their mother that would be more beneficial to her than to continue her care on the general floor. Furthermore, if they bring up the ICU issue, I will tell them that, due to the severity of her illness, she was not a candidate for treatment in the intensive care unit. |
| Ms. Quigley: | But you do not plan to tell them that she was excluded on the basis of triage. |
| Dr. Davis: | I do not see the point. |
| Prof. Thomas: | Phil, avoiding this topic introduces a significant element of dishonesty between you and the family. You are not disclosing relevant information to them. |
| Dr. Davis: | Committees like this function well, but when they interfere in the relationship |

|                |                                                                                                                                                                                                                  |
| -------------- | ---------------------------------------------------------------------------------------------------------------------------------------------------------------------------------------------------------------- |
|                | between a doctor and his patient, I think they overstep their bounds.                                                                                                                                             |
| Dr. Collins:   | Our business is concluded for today. Thanks to all of you for coming on such short notice. I will keep you informed about any further developments in the case of Mrs. Coretta Anderson.                          |

## Questions for Further Discussion

1. Atty. Quinn said that it is the legally safest thing to provide the treatment. How should the committee react to this, assuming of course that he is right?
2. The policy does not explicitly permit the ICU director to refuse admission based on marginal benefit. Dr. Davis seems to extend his authority to do precisely this in the Anderson case. Is this ethical in your opinion? Justify your answer.
3. Carla Thomas is expressing doubts about the role of clinical judgment in the case. What is meant by clinical judgment in Dr. Davis's response? Evaluate whether this is a legitimate response.
4. Can cost questions be separated from "ability to pay" questions?
5. How does one approach the question of defining "decent minimum" of health care?
6. Marian Rhodes wants to "err on the side of safety" and provide service to Mrs. Anderson. Evaluate this response and justify your evaluation.
7. Is denying Mrs. Anderson access to the intensive care unit an instance of discrimination against the handicapped or discrimination against the aged? Justify your answer.
8. Mary Quigley believes that intensive care units do not provide a good return on investment and that, consequently, few individuals would actually sacrifice very much for them if they had the choice. Is she right?
9. The hospital has been cutting back on ICU staff for reasons of economy. Would this justify the ICU staff's decision to reduce the quality of care in the unit, or should the hospital be required to reduce the number of beds in the unit?
10. Should Dr. Davis be required to reveal to the family that his decision was based on triage and that the committee approved his decision to withhold ICU treatment?

# More Cases Involving the Policy

## Suppose the Government Abandoned Dialysis

Last week the federal government informed our fictional hospital that under a new federal health care system it will be necessary to cut its dialysis payments by 75 percent, thus forcing the hospital into the following dilemma. The hospital must bear 75 percent of the costs of running the dialysis unit or the hospital must drastically reduce services to victims of renal failure. The former action would quickly bankrupt the hospital, and the latter decision would require the hospital to decide who shall receive the limited aid. Design a policy that the hospital can follow in order to take the second option.

## The Case of Carl Petersen

Carl Petersen, a 74-year-old widower, previously in good health, has suffered a massive cerebral vascular accident. He was admitted into the local community hospital's medical intensive care unit, which is now operating at full capacity. The patient was mildly alert, confused, and oriented only to person upon admission. He was aphasic with complete left-sided hemiparesis. Within the next couple of days, the nursing staff noted a progressive deterioration in his mental status. The patient had no advance directives.

Five days after admission the patient went into respiratory arrest and was placed on the ventilator. The attending physician noted that there was sharp division among the patient's children regarding the present course of treatment. The two oldest sons wanted to remove their "suffering" father from the ventilator and "allow him to die in peace." On the other hand, the youngest son and daughter believed their father could recover. The patient continued on the ventilator for the next week with no improvement. The physician was working hard to achieve unanimity among the children with respect to the correct course of action. On several occasions, the attending physician had described to the family the poor prognosis, yet the family remained bitterly divided with no signs of coming to an acceptable resolution. At about this time, the hospital's triage officer contacted the attending physician and informed him that the scarce ICU resources required him to take action to remove the patient from the service. The attending physician said "I need more time" to bring the family around to this.

## Futility Scarcity and Blood

J. D. is a 50-year-old who is presented to the emergency room suffering from end-stage hepatic failure. On this admission, he is transferred to the intensive care unit of the hospital. He is losing blood through his naso-gastric tube, his rectal tube, and his Foley catheter. Physicians are unable to stabilize his condition and he continues to bleed. The patient is very confused, although awake, but does not recognize people or respond to simple commands or questions. He is transfused several units of blood every few hours as he continues to bleed. The prognosis is poor, but the family continues to want everything done. The patient continues to bleed despite all efforts. After seven days of treatment the patient dies. Before dying, however, he utilized over one hundred units of a rare blood type. How should an ethics committee manage this problem?

## Further Reading

Aaron, Henry J., and William B. Schwartz, *The Painful Prescription: Rationing Hospital Care* (Washington, D.C.: Brookings Institution, 1984).

Callahan, Daniel, *Setting Limits* (New York: Simon and Schuster, 1987).

Childress, James F., "Rationing of Medical Treatment," in *The Encyclopedia of Bioethics*, ed. Warren T. Reich (New York: Free Press, 1978).

Childress, James F., "Who Shall Live When Not All Can Live?" *Soundings* 53 (1970): 339–55.

Churchill, Larry, *Rationing Health Care in America* (Notre Dame, Ind.: University of Notre Dame Press, 1987).

Daniels, Norman, *Just Health Care* (New York: Cambridge University Press, 1985).

Engelhardt, Jr., H. Tristram, and Michael A. Rie, "Intensive Care Units, Scarce Resources, and Conflicting Principles of Justice," *Journal of the American Medical Association* 255 (9) (March 7, 1986): 1159–64.

Knaus, William, "Rationing, Justice, and the American Physician," in *Journal of the American Medical Association* 255 (9) (March 7, 1986): 1176–77.

MacIntyre, Alasdair, *After Virtue*, 2nd ed. (Notre Dame, Ind.: University of Notre Dame Press, 1984).

MacIntyre, Alasdair, *Whose Justice? Which Rationality?* (Notre Dame, Ind.: University of Notre Dame Press, 1988).

Nozick, Robert, *Anarchy, State, and Utopia* (New York: Basic Books, 1974).

President's Commission for the Study of Ethics Problems in Medicine and Biomedical and Behavioral Research, *Securing Access to Health Care: The Ethical Implications of Differences in the Availability of Health Services, Vol. 1 : Report* (Washington, D.C.: U.S. Government Printing Office, 1983).

―――, *Securing Access to Health Care: The Ethical Implications of Differences in the Availability of Health Services, Vol. 2: Appendices, Sociocultural and Philosophical Studies* (Washington, D.C.: U.S. Government Printing Office, 1983).

Rawls, John, *A Theory of Justice* (Cambridge: Harvard University Press, 1971).

Rescher, Nicholas, *Distributive Justice* (Indianapolis, Ind.: Bobbs-Merrill, 1966).

Sandel, Michael, *Liberalism and the Limits of Justice* (Cambridge: Cambridge University Press, 1982).

Strauss, Michael J., et al., "Rationing of Intensive Care Unit Services," in *Journal of the American Medical Association* 255 (9) (March 7, 1986): 1143–46.

Winslow, Gerald, *Triage and Justice: The Ethics of Rationing Life-Saving Medical Resources* (Berkeley: University of California Press, 1982).

## Notes

1. *Von Stetina* v. *Florida Medical Center*, 2 Fla. Supp 2d 55 (Fla. 17th Cir 1982), 436 So Rptr 2d 1022 (1983), 10 *Florida Law Weekly* 286 (Fla., May 24, 1985).
2. The President's Commission for the Study of Ethical Problems in Medicine and Biomedical and Behavioral Research, *Securing Access to Health Care*, vol. 1 (Washington D.C.: Government Printing Office, 1983), p. 4.
3. John Stuart Mill, *Utilitarianism (with Critical Essays)*, ed. Samuel Gorovitz (Indianapolis, Ind.: Bobbs-Merrill, 1971), p. 44.
4. Ibid., p. 44
5. Ibid., p. 48.
6. John Stuart Mill, *The Principles of Political Economy* (New York: Appleton and Co., 1888).
7. Robert Nozick, *Anarchy, State and Utopia* (New York: Basic Books, 1974).
8. For Nozick such taxation is morally equal to what the Nazis did in the forced labor camps. Many have criticized this analogy since income taxation results from legislative activity while the Nazi forced labor camps were not authorized democratically.
9. Milton Friedman, *Capitalism and Freedom* (Chicago: University of Chicago Press, 1962), p. 161–162.
10. A good source for Marxist thought is *The Marx-Engels Reader*, ed. Robert Tucker (New York: W. W. Norton and Co., 1978).
11. Robert Heilbroner, *The Worldly Philosophers: The Lives, Times, and Ideas of the Great Economic Thinkers*, 6th ed. (New York: Simon and Schuster, 1986).
12. Karl Marx, *Capital*, trans. Samuel Moore and Edward Aveling (New York: Simon and Schuster, 1986), p. 264.
13. John Rawls, *The Theory of Justice* (Cambridge: Harvard University Press, 1971).
14. Ibid., p. 60.

15. Ibid., p. 83.
16. Ibid., p. 180.
17. Nicholas Rescher, "The Allocation of Exotic Medical Lifesaving Therapy," in *Ethics* 79 (3) (April 1969): 173–86.
18. H. Tristram Engelhardt and Michael A. Rie, "Intensive Care Units, Scarce Resources and Conflicting Principles of Justice," *Journal of the American Medical Association* 255 (9) (March 7, 1986).

# 8

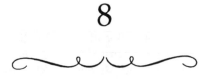

# AIDS

## Introduction to the Problem Area

During the late 1970s AIDS (acquired immune deficiency syndrome) appeared on the medical scene, and since that time it has become a worldwide epidemic. AIDS is caused by the human immunodeficiency virus (HIV), which attacks and destroys the T lymphocyte cells that provide a necessary link within the body's immune system. Without a functioning immune system, the individual becomes subject to a wide variety of illnesses ranging from rare types of pneumonia such as pneumocystis carinii to rare cancers such as Kaposi's sarcoma.

The disease is transmitted primarily through bodily fluids such as blood or semen, and therefore precautions similar to the ones traditionally employed for the hepatitis B virus are employed in the hospital. The disease is not transmitted through casual contact with AIDS victims either in the home or within the health care setting. Patients who exhibit the symptoms of the disease die because at present there is no means available to destroy the virus or protect the T cells from its onslaught. There are only a very limited number of drugs that have been found in clinical tests to extend the life of the AIDS victim. The best known of these is AZT.

What makes the disease doubly difficult for health care providers is that the ethical problems associated with the human immunodeficiency virus are as resistant to resolution as the medical problem of curing or preventing the disease. In this chapter we will examine six categories of AIDS-related ethical problems. A comprehensive hospital AIDS policy therefore presents a number of major obstacles.

### AIDS and Scarcity

Our first ethical dilemma may be the most obvious way in which AIDS touches the hospital. As the number of AIDS victims grows, so does the demand for AIDS-related hospital services. Community Hospital exists within a large American city. It is not surprising that the hospital has a significant AIDS population within its area. Furthermore, although AIDS itself cannot be cured, the secondary diseases associated with AIDS are treatable. This treatment frequently involves a substantial number of therapies that are available within the hospital. Therefore, the total amount of money spent on a particular AIDS victim can be very high. In the United States it is not at all difficult for a typical AIDS victim to consume over $200,000 in hospital services prior to succumbing to the disease.

The question of how many of the medical resources of Community Hospital should be expended on treating the AIDS patient is primarily a microallocation problem. Hospitals throughout the country continue to inform and lobby Congress and their state legislatures concerning national and statewide AIDS policy. However, despite these efforts, hospital boards have little control over these larger political and economic issues. Therefore, we will concentrate on the narrower problems involving microallocation. For example, the reader will note that the triage officer in charge of the ICU is provided with guidelines regarding the allocation of services to AIDS victims.

## AIDS and Informed Consent

The next area of concern to the hospital ethics committee is informed consent. As we have already mentioned in Chapter 3, the concept of informed consent involves four distinct conditions: adequate disclosure, patient understanding, competence, and voluntariness. The AIDS crisis challenges the hospital on all of these fronts. For example, many health care providers are anxious to gain information concerning a patient's HIV status, and they are often tempted to secure this information by performing HIV tests on the patient's blood. This desire may be based on understandable clinical considerations, such as the presence of AIDS-related pneumonia. However, if these tests are performed without the informed consent of the patient, then we face the problem of violating the patient's autonomy.

One may argue that such consent is not necessary because the test is noninvasive and involves no physical harm to the patient. Furthermore, many tests on blood products are routinely carried on at the hospital without securing the informed consent of the patient. If it is not required in these routine areas, it ought not to be required in the context of AIDS.

One difficulty with this response is that AIDS victims frequently do not wish to be tested. Their reasons for refusing to be tested are varied. Many potential AIDS victims are concerned that information on their HIV status will leak out, thereby increasing their risk of being fired from their jobs or losing their insurance coverage. These fears may or may not be well-founded, but it is clear that they are genuine concerns that motivate potential AIDS victims to treat their HIV status as confidential information.

Providers on the other hand are often anxious to determine the HIV status of a patient not only to develop the most coherent health care plan, but also to protect themselves against infection. With this information, the health care providers can increase safety precautions and thereby decrease their risk. But the health care worker could use this information as a basis for refusing to treat the HIV patient. The HIV victim or the person who suspects that he is HIV positive is often frightened to be tested because the results of the test may produce discriminatory reactions on the part of the hospital or the health care provider.

## AIDS and the Patient-Professional Relationship

In addition to challenging the hospital on questions concerning rationing and informed consent, the AIDS crisis has also confronted health care providers within the hospital on issues surrounding the patient-professional relationship. Fear operates among the providers as well as the receivers of health care. In 1987, cardiac surgeon Dr. W. Dudley Johnson publicly declared that he would not operate on individuals infected with the HIV. Physicians like Dr. Johnson argued that the danger to him and his wife was too high, therefore he had no duty to treat HIV victims. Surgeons and surgical nurses are especially concerned because of their proximity to patients' blood. The policy will speak to this issue in very concrete terms, but the reader is asked to note that the philosophical commentary gives special attention to the concept of "virtue." This is because it is difficult to understand the professional response to AIDS without appreciating the peculiar virtues of health care professionals.

## AIDS and Society

The next ethical dimension that needs to be addressed by the hospital ethics committee policy on AIDS is the relation of the individual AIDS patient to the society. A number of social policies that have been suggested for dealing with the AIDS crisis would restrict the rights of individual AIDS victims in order to protect society. Various schemes have been developed to mandate testing of particular social groups. Homosexual men, intravenous (IV) drug users, or prisoners are candidates for mandatory testing. Mandatory testing for jobs or insurance have been proposed.

Although the hospital cannot determine the attitudes of the society as a whole, it must live with those attitudes even when they significantly complicate the operation of a hospital in a modern city. The hospital's ethics committee addresses these issues not because it aims to control social attitudes toward AIDS victims, but in order to educate the hospital staff concerning the duties of medical professionals. Perhaps the most important social attitudes that affect AIDS patients are those associated with "social deviancy." Many AIDS victims are homosexual men or IV drug users. Homosexuality and drug use are "socially deviant behavior" in the sense that they are disapproved of by many individuals in contemporary American society.

However, social deviance may or may not be associated with illegality or immorality. There is a continuum ranging from socially permissible deviance to behaviors that are viewed as immoral and illegal. For example, individuals who sing on crowded elevators may be socially deviant, but they are not violating the law or committing an immoral act. Furthermore, despite the fact that homosexuality is considered immoral by a significant number of individuals in our country, it is for the most part a legally permissible behavior in the United States. IV drug abuse is viewed as socially deviant in a stronger sense. It is viewed by many as immoral. It is also illegal. The borders between these categories of social deviancy, immorality, and illegality are not precise, and frequently the health care provider needs to exercise a good deal of judgment to distinguish where a behavior belongs on the continuum.

The attitudes that health care providers should exhibit toward socially deviant behaviors associated with AIDS is a vital question in bioethics. It is addressed in our policy because typical health care providers meet all three types of deviance in their treatment of AIDS patients.

### AIDS and Confidentiality

The fifth area in which AIDS presents significant ethical conflicts is that of confidentiality or privacy. Keeping medical information private is one of the foundations of patient confidence in general, but it is especially significant to the AIDS victim. AIDS patients frequently need to be assured that they will not be penalized for fully disclosing their symptoms and that full disclosure will not lead to discriminatory behaviors on the part of professionals. Often such patients feel terribly alone and isolated from the community. This sense of alienation often promotes anger and resentment. Patients often act out these feelings toward the health care professional because the professional is viewed as the representative of an uncaring and antagonistic society. Such patients can anger the professional who is unaware that these feelings are operating. It is very easy to personalize these aggressive behaviors and unknowingly abandon patients who are crying out for help and comfort.

But patients are not the only source of difficulties. Professionals with consciously or unconsciously hostile or fearful feelings toward AIDS patients can diminish the quality of care that these patients receive. These negative feelings are a two-way street, originating from both the patient and the health care provider.

AIDS can also be a significant threat to innocent third parties who are having sexual contact with AIDS victims. Health care professionals frequently feel obligated to inform these third parties that they are placing themselves at risk by continuing the sexual contact. This, of course, comes into direct conflict with the patient's right to privacy if the patient refuses to allow the health care provider to reveal this information. In the best scenario, the AIDS victim agrees to inform his or her partner of the victim's HIV status. However, occasionally AIDS patients may refuse to inform their partners, and this places the health care provider in a difficult position. Does she respect the privacy of her patient and thereby increase the risk of spreading the disease to another person, or does she reveal the information to the third party and thus undermine the patient-provider relationship?

---

## Community Hospital's Policy on AIDS

*Purpose*:    The purpose of this document is to spell out the policy of the hospital on the following seven questions related to the AIDS epidemic. This policy does not pretend to be a full and comprehensive AIDS policy. Our goal is merely to address a limited number of problems.

*Questions:*

1. Do patients infected with the HIV virus constitute a threat to health care workers at Community Hospital? Do health care workers infected with HIV constitute a threat to patients at Community Hospital?
2. What is the position of the hospital as it relates to informed consent and the AIDS patient? More specifically, are there any reasons that would justify bypassing the rule of informed consent in the context of AIDS care? Can we secure tests for HIV without first securing the informed consent of the patient?
3. What safety precautions should we initiate to halt the spread of AIDS within the hospital?
4. Should AIDS patients be treated differently from ordinary hospital patients?

5. How should AIDS treatment be allocated?
6. What is the hospital's position on confidentiality as it applies to AIDS patients?
7. Can health care providers refuse to treat AIDS victims?

*Responses:*

1. HIV infection produces fatal disease. The mode of transmission of HIV is comparable to HBV (Hepatitis B virus). Epidemiological studies do not indicate that being a health care worker increases the risk of acquiring the disease. In a study involving 40,000 victims of HIV, with recorded employment data, 2,232 (5.6 percent) were found to be health care workers. Approximately 5.6 percent of the American people work in health-related fields, so if health care employment were actually irrelevant to HIV acquisition, one would expect this percentage of health care workers to be infected. However, some cases of transmission from patients to health care workers have occurred. The hospital requires strict adherence to the guidelines spelled out in "The Centers for Disease Control Recommendations for Prevention of HIV Transmission in Health Care Settings." Special care must be taken with respect to avoiding injuries involving needles and other sharp instruments. No mandatory testing of staff will take place at the hospital.
2. The hospital's policy on informed consent applies fully and completely to all AIDS victims. The attached statement from the hospital's informed consent policy is particularly relevant: "Informed consent for treatment should be secured." Treatment is interpreted by this committee to include diagnostic tests to determine the HIV status of a patient. Mandatory testing that would override the patient's right to consent violates the informed consent policy of the hospital.
3. All patients of the hospital are to be treated as HIV positive. This requires that all patients be treated as risks to the staff. Specific safety recommendations have been issued by the infectious disease department, and the committee has fully endorsed these recommendations.
4. No forms of discrimination against AIDS victims will be tolerated at Community Hospital. The bodily fluids of AIDS patients must be treated as potentially dangerous and precautions should be taken. No other form of isolation is deemed appropriate at this time.
5. At this point the hospital has not set allocations for distributing resources according to disease categories. We have not, for example, set any limits on the allocation of resources for victims of leukemia or Alzheimer's disease. It is, therefore, inappropriate at this time to allocate a specific amount of resources for the treatment of AIDS.

6. All medical communications between a professional health care provider such as a nurse or a physician and the patient should be treated as confidential. This principle is of special importance to the AIDS victim. AIDS victims are often discriminated against if their diagnosis is not treated as private information. Violating this principle is a matter of utmost seriousness and should be considered only as a last resort. If, for example, the only means for avoiding significant harm to others is to violate confidentiality, then the physician is permitted but not obligated to violate the principle.

7. As a general rule physicians should not refuse to treat AIDS patients. If a physician cannot treat an AIDS victim, the physician is obligated to secure competent medical care for the patient.

---

## Commentary on the Philosophical and Ethical Aspects of the Policy

### The Virtue Approach

The rights-based approach to ethics and the consequences-based approach have thus far directed our philosophical inquiry into the problems of bioethics. While these approaches are very useful, we cannot presume that they are the only guides to understanding ethical conflict. Indeed, the problems associated with AIDS open the door to a third perspective. This third perspective, which we may call the "virtue approach," is another philosophical approach to understanding bioethics. It focuses on the idea that bioethical conflicts are best understood as involving competing images of what constitutes the *ideal health care professional*.

Discussion about professional ideals is appropriate because HIV-infected patients present some level of risk to the health care professionals who are exposed to their bodily fluids. According to James Allen there is an "extremely small" probability that a health care professional will contract the disease from those she serves, but there is still some danger.[1] Although several studies document that employment in the health care field is not a risk factor that increases the likelihood of acquiring HIV, needle sticks and other forms of direct exposure to HIV fluids have produced some seroconversions.

The rights-based and consequentialist approaches are vital to understanding the way in which bioethical problems are understood in the United States, but they do not place the individual caregiver at the center of the discussion. The rules of morality take center stage in these perspectives. They do not represent ethical challenges as deeply personal decisions that involve one's own self-understanding. Nor do these traditional approaches attempt to provide us with a picture of the "ideal health care provider." The rights-based approach and the consequences-based approach tend to concentrate on the health care provider's obligations, which are frequently understood as the minimum requirements of the professional. These perspectives emphasize the duties of the physician rather than the ideals of the profession. They represent a modern view of the professional as someone in conflict with society who is trying to find out what she is minimally obligated to do. They tend to see ethics as a tool for resolving conflict between the individual and the society. By contrast, in the eighteenth century the state was viewed as a threat to the individual, and rights were needed to protect the individual against the encroachments of the state. Philosophers pictured ethics as a tool for minimizing the ways in which the state can obligate the individual.

The consequentialist and rights-based approaches tend to treat virtues such as compassion and courage as *extras within the moral life.* One cannot obligate the man on the street to be compassionate toward others; rather, one only minimally obligates him to avoid harming others. Compassion, courage, integrity, wisdom, and such qualities are more than what are necessary because they are not universally required of everyone as part of being a rational person. Enlightenment philosophers pictured human beings as primarily concerned with their own self-interest. Distractions from self-interest, they believed, should only be tolerated if one had an obligation to fulfill. Virtue was an extra—something you might plan to do when you retired. It was, in the jargon of philosophers, *supererogatory.* According to this tempting modern view, virtues are praiseworthy if one has them, but one cannot be blamed for lacking them.

Even the professional is depicted as someone who can get along without virtue. What makes the health care professional unique is not her virtue but, rather, her decision to accept social obligations beyond those of the ordinary citizen. A physician is not someone who is virtuous but merely someone who has made a bargain. He has contracted with society to take on these added duties because society grants something in return. Becoming a physician is not essentially different from buying a car: it is a trade that one makes. Becoming a doctor merely involves new duties, not the requirement to become virtuous.

The approach that we are employing in this chapter takes the Greek philosophical view that ethics necessarily involves an inquiry into virtue. If we understand an obligation as something whose presence we "sense" internally rather than externally, then we may interpret modern ethicists as affirming that we only sense an obligation when we consider the consequences of our actions or the rights of others. The virtue approach denies this assumption and maintains that we sense the presence of an obligation when we consider the ideals of our profession or way of life. If I am a physician, for example, I may say that I am "obligated to care for plague victims," not because of any objective rules to do so, but because of my own sense of what it means to be a doctor. From this perspective, reflection on the virtues of the ideal health care professional is just as essential to determining our moral vision as reflection on individual rights and social consequences. More specifically, virtues are essential to determine the extent of one's obligations. Virtues help the individual determine the extent to which a general obligation applies in a given case. For example, how far would an ideal physician go to protect the privacy of her patient? If the state coerced the ideal physician to reveal information, how should she respond? Virtue cannot be construed as an extra or merely a matter of supererogation because how we determine the extent of our obligation is profoundly affected by our ideals.

## Why Virtue?

But why bother with this virtue approach? What reason do we have for thinking that virtues and personal ideals are essential to the moral life? Put another way, what reason do we have for thinking that theories that emphasize consequences or rights are incomplete? Two very important arguments have recently been offered to establish that a virtue-based ethic is fundamental. The first is offered by Gregory Pence.[2] He argues that the rules that determine the rights and obligations of health care professionals can always be subverted by those professionals who have their own interests as primary. These rules, even if they were objective, would not produce responsible behavior. To disregard virtue is to disregard what it is that motivates people to behave in accordance with supposedly correct rules. Pence uses human subject research as an example. He claims that a devious and uncaring researcher can always get around the requirements of an informed consent document and thereby get the patient to do what the researcher wants. Rules simply do not protect the patient against the professional who lacks virtue or good character. Pence's general philosophical point is that moral character is indispensable for securing what is best for the patient, and that no set of rules can guarantee that the patient will be protected from the uncaring, selfishly motivated physician or nurse. Furthermore, because modern bioethics tends to emphasize public rules rather than virtuous character, contemporary patients are suffering.

Another, more abstract argument is offered by Alasdair MacIntyre in his book *After Virtue*.[3] MacIntyre argues that both the consequentialist and the rights-based theories that we have assumed throughout this text are a part of a larger cultural and philosophical project that has failed. He calls this project *The Enlightenment*. According to MacIntyre, Kant and Mill are both members of the Enlightenment because they both held that reason by itself could supply a minimal ethic that bound all people no matter what tradition they emerged from. This minimal ethic could serve as a basis for revising traditions that were unreasonable. For Mill and Kant reason contains this universal minimal ethic, therefore it takes priority over religious or cultural traditions that are historically conditioned. Because traditions like Judaism or Christianity are historically particular, their moral principles cannot be universally binding. Individual visions of God were so diverse and so historically conditioned that religion could not secure the universality required of the moral life. But unlike religion and tradition, reason could provide a set of rules that were binding on everyone. The principle of utility and Kant's categorical imperative were supposedly derived from reason. The Enlightenment philosophers believed that mind was a storehouse of truth in the sense that it contained the very general principles of method by which the truth could be acquired. The mind was not only the foundation for growth in scientific knowledge but also the means by which one could resolve the fundamental conflicts within any culture.

According to MacIntyre, the main difficulty with the notion that ethics ought to be based on something standing over and above social traditions is that it cannot be done. His argument for this sweeping claim is rather simple, but certainly not simpleminded. He argues somewhat pragmatically that the sign of an adequate philosophy is its ability to resolve practical moral problems that are experienced by ordinary people. For example, should we permit active euthanasia or abortion? According to MacIntyre, we could multiply such examples interminably. The common thread that unites these questions is that our society is unable to answer any of them, and this inability is derived from the Enlightenment assumption that ethical problems can only be solved by pure reason. The Enlightenment claimed to be able to solve these problems, but it cannot. Without substantive ethical traditions, ethical problems are unresolvable. MacIntyre claims that reason is silent on all of the major ethical questions facing our society. If a philosophy's mark of adequacy is its ability to resolve practical ethical problems, then Mill's consequentialist approach and Kant's rights-based approach are failures.

MacIntyre's assault on the concept of pure reason is based on the notion that pure reason is simply not universal. As many anthropologists and sociologists (and, most recently, many feminist thinkers) have pointed out, there is no shared set of intellectual assumptions that all men and women in all cultures share. MacIntyre argues that the empirical absence of such shared ideas indicates that pure reason is another name for Western reason, not reason itself. It cannot be universalized without coming into conflict with the empirical facts of sociology and anthropology. Reason, therefore, suffers from the same historical particularity as any religion.

But does this mean that ethical problems are unresolvable? For MacIntyre, if resolution requires finality and universality, then the answer is "yes!" However, if resolution can admit change over time, if it is tied ultimately to the character of the individual decision maker, then according to MacIntyre, the answer is "no." He argues that moral problems can be addressed within the broader confines of a cultural or religious tradition that contains substantive principles concerning the meaning and purpose of individual and social life. To solve moral problems one needs principles that are richer than pure reason can supply. A tradition is needed to provide someone with a character or set of motivations. Reason cannot supply us with tradition. Traditions are tied to moral communities, and moral communities are often defined in terms of shared religious perspectives on the nature, meaning, and purpose of human life. More importantly, MacIntyre argues that these traditions are somewhat immunized against rational critique since reason itself is and needs to be defined in terms of a broad social context.

### Narratives and Moral Conflict

MacIntyre treats traditions as narratives in which men and women play a part. When a nurse or a doctor is faced with a moral conflict such as whether she should treat HIV victims, the question should be not what the rational moral law dictates in this situation but rather "What stories do I find myself a part of?"[4] For MacIntyre, a story or narrative is not pure history. It involves some myth. It is about our dreams and our ideals as well as the facts. It is a narrative about how, over the years, health care professionals have accepted the responsibility to accept the risks associated with caring for the sick. When those who tell the story of being a nurse or a physician are themselves members of these professions, they see themselves as part of this narrative history.

The story of being a doctor is neither pure history nor pure fiction. As early as the fourteenth century, physicians who ran from the plague were viewed by both physicians and laymen as being negligent.[5] Stories reflect a social ideal. They may present some individuals as models and others—like those who fail to treat the dangerously ill—as not "true" nurses or doctors.

MacIntyre rejects the idea that there exists a minimal ethic, shared by all persons, that is derived from reason. Rather, traditions and stories define the meaning and purpose of a physician's life. They affirm the ideals that he strives to reach. Furthermore, the ethical principles of a tradition spell out *what is a virtuous person* in the light of these traditions, stories, and ideals.

MacIntyre's rejection of the spirit of the Enlightenment leaves us with a fundamental question: to what tradition does he subscribe? His answer is quite straightforward. He is a Christian within the traditions of Augustine and Aquinas. When he faces a moral difficulty, he faces it not as a pure reasoner but as a traditional Christian influenced by the ethics of Jesus as interpreted by the Christian philosophers Aquinas and Augustine. But there are a number of difficulties associated with this approach. First, if tradition is necessary for resolving ethical debate and people in a pluralistic culture do not share the same ethical tradition, then how can these problems be resolved? Must we force everyone into a common tradition in order to make the resolution of bioethical problems possible? MacIntyre's approach suggests that if we are to achieve ethical agreement, then we must diminish the amount of cultural diversity that exists in the modern world. Cultural diversity cannot, for MacIntyre, be something that enriches a society because it necessarily undermines agreement. MacIntyre does little to defend this controversial thesis.

Secondly, our society is a pluralistic one in which there is a deep and binding commitment to individual autonomy or liberty. We aim at tolerating not only nonconforming cultures but nonconforming individuals. The medieval Christian cultures that spawned and nourished these great philosophers had little respect for individual freedom. Within these cultures individuals were, for the most part, forced into social roles that they could do little to alter. The course of their lives was largely determined by the caste into which they were born. If MacIntyre refers to himself as an Augustinian Christian, does this mean that he is recommending that we return to a social order in which serfdom and outright slavery were condoned? Or can one pick and choose, as a modern pluralistic citizen would, among the various elements of a religious tradition?

## Virtue and Greek Philosophy

With these criticisms in mind, let us turn briefly to the ancient roots of this concept of virtue, namely, the writings of Plato and Aristotle. These Greek philosophers did not believe that a good consequence could be easily defined in terms of physical pleasure or mental happiness as the nineteenth-century consequentialists believed. The word "good" applied, they believed, primarily to character traits or virtues. Consequently, ethics was primarily treated as an enquiry into the character of the ideal person. Good character was the end of ethical inquiry, not obedience to abstract principles involving rights and obligations.

Plato and Aristotle did not think that all rational persons ought to have the same character. What it meant to have a good character or to have virtue depended on "one's place within society." Individuals had souls and souls were not all the same. For Plato, some souls were golden, some were silver, and some were bronze. By this he meant that one could only understand the good soul by analogy with the good state. As the state had three parts—leaders, soldiers, and workers—that were functionally differentiated, so too the soul had three parts: a rational part, a spirited part, and an appetitive part. As the virtues of the soldier were not the virtues of the leader (the former requiring courage and the latter requiring reason), so the virtues of the doctor were not the virtues of the businessman. For the Greeks, there was nothing fundamentally missing in the businessman who lacked compassion. For the businessperson, compassion is an extra, an accidental property. One doesn't need it to run a business. Indeed, it might get in the way.

For the Greeks, however, compassion was not accidental to medicine; it was an essential character trait for the physician. As an object cannot be a true triangle if it lacks three angles that equal 180 degrees, so a person cannot be a "true physician" if she lacks compassion. For the Greeks, one's role in society determined who one was, and these social roles defined one's virtues. A virtue was not just a disposition to behave in a given way; it involved an ideal of duty that directed one's actions.

## Virtue as Knowledge

The Greeks, of course, did not think that this approach would make men and women perfect. To emphasize philosophically the "ideal images" of the health care provider does not guarantee that ideally virtuous men and women will result. Oftentimes, the ideal itself and what it demands may be difficult to discern. Most of us believe that merely taking a bioethics course is not going to guarantee that a health care provider will behave in an ideal fashion. However, although the Greeks would not have believed that taking an ethics course would make someone ethical, they were deeply convinced that there was a necessary connection between virtue and knowledge. This intimate connection was most forcefully expressed by one of the most influential Greek philosophers, Plato. Plato argued that the connection between virtue and knowledge was so close that it was impossible to be both a truly knowledgeable physician and an unethical physician. Wisdom and virtue were necessarily linked in that if one understood, in the deepest sense of that word, the virtues of the just person, then one would necessarily act as a virtuous person. For Plato, unfeeling or dishonest physicians are merely men or women who do not really know what it means to be a physician. Plato thus equated knowledge with acting virtuously because he held that unethical behavior is always tied to ignorance at a very deep level. For Plato, true education produced virtue.

This is, of course, a very strong claim on Plato's part, and to many contemporary thinkers it is simply false. There seem to be plenty of instances of health care professionals who *know* it is generally wrong to violate the privacy of their patients but who nevertheless do so. Knowing what is good or right does not mean that one will act rightly. But Plato would respond that such physicians only *apparently know* what is involved in being a physician, that it is possible to know *in a superficial sense* that it is wrong to violate the privacy of a patient and to do it anyway. But the person who is truly knowledgeable about what it is to be a physician cannot avoid acting as a virtuous physician.

The upshot of this argument was that, for Plato, if we want to produce virtuous physicians, then we must truly educate them. A deep and profound education is the best thing that a society can do to ensure virtue in health care professionals.

### Virtue as Habit

In response to this cognitive interpretation of virtue, Aristotle, who was Plato's student, argued that while knowledge was vital to the process of producing virtue in the physician, something more was needed. One had to *habituate* the person or train the person to be virtuous. In *The Nicomachean Ethics* Aristotle said, "It is well said then, that it is by doing just acts that the just man is produced, and by doing temperate acts that the temperate man is produced; without doing these no one would have even a prospect of becoming good."[6] For Aristotle, all the knowledge in the world is ineffective for getting obese persons to regulate their eating habits. Similarly, education alone is not going to produce a just or temperate person. Something else is required: practice. Practicing the art of moderate eating gives one practical knowledge about how to stay fit. For Aristotle practical knowledge is a set of dispositions or powers of the soul to accomplish just acts.

### Virtue and Religion

Religious philosophers and theologians such as Thomas Aquinas were profoundly influenced by the Greeks but argued that, in addition to knowledge and habituation, a theological or transcendent element was needed to produce virtuous behavior. For many Christian theologians, no amount of practice or knowledge could produce a person who was able to act in accord with Christian ideals. God's grace was also necessary. The Christian philosophers of the early Middle Ages created the doctrine of grace in order to account for altruistic behavior, which they construed as unnatural. However, although many Christian philosophers of the Middle Ages rejected the idea that either knowledge or practice was sufficient to produce virtuous persons, something did link these competing Greek and

Christian philosophies: namely the belief that the essential problems of ethics were about the nature of virtue. They agreed about the ends of ethics, i.e., the production of virtuous people. They disagreed about the means.

## AIDS and Virtue

But even if we accept the idea that virtue is essential to the study of ethics, we must still ask whether virtue *requires* the physician or the nurse to treat the HIV patient. If there is a duty, what is it? Daniel Fox's review of the history of medicine suggests that professional societies during many periods have addressed the problem of dangerous epidemics by hiring "plague doctors."[7] The duty to treat was thus recognized by professionals, but they often discharged that duty without fulfilling it themselves. This approach construes the duty to treat plague victims as real but one that could be discharged by hiring someone else to do it. This presumably allows the health care professional to remain "virtuous" without placing himself at risk.

The difficulty with this strategy is that it is unlikely to be practical in the case of AIDS.[8] Thousands of "plague doctors" would have to be hired and thousands of patients would have to be transferred. More importantly, just as police officers or firefighters do not hire others to do their dangerous work, so the doctor does not hire substitutes. These professions are by their very nature dangerous.

Edmund Pellegrino has argued that while doctors have a duty to treat HIV patients, duty cannot be derived from virtue.[9] He says that "as necessary as virtue is to medical ethics it is not sufficient." But rather than pointing us to a consequentialist or rights-based theory of moral duty, Pellegrino offers the ideal of the "good physician." He argues that it may well be in the physician's self-interest to refuse to treat HIV patients, but it is the duty of the "good physician" to treat them anyway. The physician has a duty in some limited sense to "subordinate" his self-interest to the professional or altruistic aims that are embedded in the medical profession. Pellegrino gives three reasons for this position. First, the medical needs of HIV patients are real and constitute a claim on the health care professional. Just as persons in a burning building have a claim on firefighters, AIDS victims have a moral claim on physicians. Need obligates both the firefighter and the health care professional. Second, if the health care professional had acquired her medical knowledge independent of society, then perhaps she could employ her medical skill without reference to social needs. But this knowledge was secured thanks to taxpayer-supported schools and hospitals. The taxpayers invested in medical education, and part of the implicit contract between the society and the profession is that when part of the society is threatened, those whom we educated will protect us. Finally, Pellegrino claims that the contractual language of his second point does not express the deeper, more "true relationship" between the doctor, his patients, and society. To become a doctor, one enters into a mystical relationship modeled on the Old Testament relationship between God, the individual, and the people of Israel. Pellegrino rejects the notion that one can give a "purely secular" account of this relationship.[10]

The major difficulty with Pellegrino's critique of virtue as a basis of the duty to treat HIV victims is that his arguments for that duty are themselves based on his own vision of "what it is to be a good physician."[11] Following MacIntyre, we may say that virtue applies primarily to traditions or professions. One might agree that the medical profession has a duty to treat HIV victims, but the individual physician may be so frightened of contracting HIV himself or so concerned about the welfare of his wife that we excuse him from the duty. Police officers and firefighters are often transferred to desk work when they are unable to face the rigors of "front line" work. That we excuse *some* health care professionals does not mean that we excuse *all*. The duty may apply to the profession as a whole but not to each and every physician.

But how do individuals become ideal or virtuous professionals? For Plato, it is through true education of the student. For Aristotle, the young student must be habituated to caring for those who threaten his own self-interest. For Aquinas, something more is needed: God's grace.

### Virtue and Existentialism

More than any other contemporary thinkers, twentieth-century existentialist philosophers have faced this problem of differentiating between knowing what is right and acting rightly. In particular, Albert Camus wrote extensively on the problem faced by physicians who deal with patients who are infectious and, therefore, dangerous.[12] For Camus, the problem of the virtuous physician is an existential one in that physicians who must decide how to relate to AIDS patients cannot solve it without figuring out their identity.

In Camus's most famous medical novel, *The Plague*, a physician faces a plague that represents a profound threat not only to the welfare of society but also to that of the physician. The novel is in many respects a study of a particular physician's responses to the fact that a plague has assaulted his town. Camus spends little or no time on questions concerning the rights of health care professionals or patients. There is no sustained discussion of the consequences of possible alternatives. Camus had rejected both the rights-based and the consequentialist views concerning what was right and wrong and was therefore completely uninterested in proving that his hero, Dr. Rieux, was obligated to stay with his patients. Nor is there any theological ground offered for saying that Dr. Rieux had to stay with his patients. Theology plays an important role in the novel only in the sense that it is ridiculed for its attempt to offer a theological explanation for the plague. (The plague was said to be God's tool for punishing the sinful people of the town.) Moreover, Camus disregards the Aristotelian notion that Dr. Rieux should stay in the plague-ridden town because he is habituated to do so. For Camus, Dr. Rieux will not be happier in any sense of the word if he stays with the plague victims.

Rather, Camus portrays Dr. Rieux as staying in the plague-ridden town *because he is a physician.* The hero's very identity as an individual is caught up in the identity of being a physician. For him, leaving the plague victims would mean giving up *who he has chosen to be.* It is important to note that other characters in the novel consider leaving the town even after a quarantine has been imposed, but Dr. Rieux does not lash out against them in anger. When he is asked why he chose to stay, he does not attempt to show that more good would be accomplished by staying, or offer any reasons based on respect for persons or the principle of universalizability. In fact, he never condemns people for trying to escape the plague. His reasons for staying in the town where death will find him are, in some respects, very simple. He merely says that he is a physician and that is why he cannot leave.

Camus writes beautifully about how as a young man, Dr. Rieux had entered medicine in order to rise out of his family's lower-working-class status, but it was not very long until the young Dr. Rieux realized that becoming a physician was more than a means for climbing the social ladder. Becoming a physician was going to affect his very identity as a person because being a physician required him to face his own mortality almost every day. Becoming a physician had destroyed many of his illusions regarding life, including the illusion of immortality that the young sustain. The brute fact of dealing with dying patients on a daily basis gave him an awareness that the one fundamental truth of life is that it ends in death and that the joys and pleasures of life are "fleeting and far between." But medicine had given something more valuable than pleasure or more important than physical comfort: it had given him an identity. *He was a physician rather than someone who merely used medical science to make a living.* To leave the plague-ridden town would mean giving up who he was, and for Dr. Rieux that was unthinkable.

This modern and contemporary book places us into the life of a man who is facing death not in terms of any abstract ethical calculus involving social consequences or individual rights, but in terms of his own individual identity. The central question for Camus, as for Plato, is not what is right, what is required, or what produces the best consequences but rather "who am I?"

Camus's concern with what it means to be a health care professional indicates that the questions involving virtues are still at the heart of bioethics. But what are these health care virtues? To address this problem we will focus on five virtues that are associated with medicine. This list is not exhaustive. Many bioethical dilemmas can be recast as conflicts among the virtues. For example, honesty will often be thrown into conflict with compassion. There is no obvious way to resolve these conflicts because the virtues are not presented in any precise hierarchical pattern.

## Five Virtues in Medicine

*Compassion*    The first virtue that we will address is compassion. Compassion can be construed as an ability either to feel for the sufferings of other persons (sympathy) or to have an intellectual awareness of the sufferings of others (empathy). Both sympathy and empathy are associated with a desire to return the person to a state of wholeness. Gallons of ink have been spilled trying to distinguishing these two forms of motivation, but they are both essential virtues of the good health care professional.

Before we move on to a more detailed study of compassion, it is important to ask why compassion is a bioethical virtue. What, for example, distinguishes it from the desire for money or the desire to avoid litigation? Both of these desires can also motivate patient care. What differentiates the desire to relieve the sufferings of others from the desire to earn money? Why is one a bioethical virtue and the other not? Suppose that a nurse provided excellent medical care to his patients merely because he wanted to keep his job. Why is this considered, at best, morally neutral?

The desire for money and the desire to avoid lawsuits are not considered virtues even though they can yield excellent results. They are not virtues because they only achieve medically beneficial results *in normal contexts*. In *The Plague,* Dr. Rieux does not stay in the plague-ridden city of Oran in order to avoid litigation, nor does he stay for the money. Money and litigation have become irrelevant. These motives may be effective replacements most of the time for the virtues of compassion and courage, but not when the "going gets tough." If we place the physician in a dangerous situation where her well-being is at risk, then these motives break down and fail to achieve the goals of medicine. Very few of us would face death to avoid a lawsuit. Dr. Rieux has deeper reasons for staying in the dangerous city. They have to do with his decision to be a physician.

But is Dr. Rieux's motive intellectual or emotional? He is not a very emotional man. He seldom laughs or expresses deep emotions. He seems to understand just that the people of Oran need him and that they suffer. He does not cry when each and every victim falls, but he understands their suffering and acts appropriately. However, he is not a completely cold fish.

He loves his wife and misses her, but he also has a sense of the primary decision in his life, which is to be a physician. In short, he thinks of himself more as a physician than as a husband. Therefore, he decides to stay with his patients rather than go to his wife.

In short, compassion can be understood emotionally and intellectually. The crucial question is not whether the emotional or the intellectual compassion is primary, but how these two different psychological states can interact with each other. Our thesis is that intellectual awareness can initiate coherent responses when emotional involvement might cloud and inhibit them. There is a tendency to dismiss emotive compassion from medicine, but to do so would be a grave error. Our emotions frequently allow us to see things that we would miss without them. Consider the case of the physician who is providing the highest of technological care to a patient who is dying. Sometimes health care providers cannot see that the technology is separating the dying patient from his family. Frequently, the intellectual response to relieving suffering may prevent us from seeing what the patient really needs. The emotional and the intellectual aspects of compassion are both vital in bioethics.

*Courage*    The second virtue that we will address is courage. Courage is not an intellectual virtue. Plato thinks of it as something belonging to the spirit of human beings, not the mind. The brightest of men and women often lack it. We may think of it as an ability to face danger and act in a way that treats fear of death or the fear of pain as important but not decisive. To treat death, injury, or the loss of one's reputation as unimportant is not courageous but foolish. It is vital to note that great courage can be demonstrated in achieving monstrous ends. For example, Hitler's seamen in the U-boat fleet during World War II demonstrated unbelievable courage in fighting the Allied surface fleets. But the cause that they were defending was evil. Because a soldier is courageous is no indication that she is right. Courage is something that we fully admire only when it is directed toward a good end.

It is tempting to describe the courageous person as one who does what is appropriate without being controlled by his fears. This, I think, is an error. Courageous acts are frequently inappropriate. For example, the father who kills his terminally ill son who is suffering and who has begged his father to kill him in order to relieve the incurable pain has committed an act that many would consider inappropriate. At the same time, we may consider it courageous. Dr. Rieux places himself at great risk by caring for the plague victims of Oran. To describe his actions as appropriate suggests that his actions are merely well-suited to achieve an end. But this is not the same as describing his actions as courageous. To admire the courageous act is to assume that the act was not the person's only choice. Rather, it was an act that was imposed on the individual by his own sense of identity. To consider an act courageous is to admire it for emerging out of the individual's deepest personal ideals.

*Tolerance*    The next virtue does not often appear on the list of classic virtues, but it is one that is especially important in the modern pluralistic society. It is tolerance. To be tolerant is to be able to endure beliefs or behaviors that deviate from one's own standards. The tolerant person avoids harming or restricting the rights of those who behave and think in ways that he finds offensive. Tolerance does not require agreement; indeed, it presupposes significant disagreement in values. The tolerant person has her own values but can live with the conflicting preferences of others. Tolerant people have the ability to recognize and perhaps even learn to emotionally or intellectually appreciate human beings who adopt vastly different religious, philosophical, or behavioral lifestyles.

In the seventeenth century, after enduring a seemingly endless series of wars that were fought to suppress one religion or other, governments in the West became increasingly tolerant of deviant religious expression. It was not complete tolerance and there were notable exceptions, but the trend toward religious toleration became embedded in Western culture and enshrined in the U.S. Bill of Rights. What brought us to this tolerance was neither philosophical wit nor poetic sentiment. Europe had to be devastated with two hundred years of religious warfare first. The fierce and brutalizing consequences of war forced nations and individuals to realize that it was in their interest to foster tolerance. The citizens of the modern state are thus required to be tolerant in ways that citizens in earlier epochs would have never accepted.

Westerners tolerate all manner of subjectively offensive behavior in order to secure social harmony amid divergent beliefs and values, and health care providers are at the cutting edge of this tolerance. This is because caring for patients frequently requires an understanding of their private behaviors, and without tolerance one cannot work with the patient to secure his welfare. Many AIDS victims are drug abusers or homosexuals, and these behavioral patterns or lifestyles are construed as deviant by a large portion of society. Intolerance toward these behaviors can inhibit care and, therefore, lead directly to increased illness and death.

But what is involved in tolerance? Is it a matter of feelings or is it simply a matter of action? For example, can the nurse have negative feelings and attitudes toward his AIDS patient because the patient is a drug addict? Can he have these feelings and still be a tolerant health care provider? Can actions and attitudes be separated? Our assumption will be that tolerance primarily applies to actions rather than attitudes or feelings. We prefer this approach because determining the feelings of all health care providers is too difficult. It would require an offensive amount of state interference to disallow negative feelings toward drug addicts or homosexuals. But preventing intolerant action based on these feelings is another matter. Professional organizations such as the American Medical Association (AMA) can oppose intolerant action without requiring that health care providers have the "correct" feelings. One can certainly feel negative toward homosexuals without being intolerant. However, one begins to be intolerant when one believes that one's negative feelings toward the homosexuals or drug abusers justifies discriminatory action or inaction. The heart of intolerance, we suggest, is not negative feelings. It is the belief that one's feelings about a patient's lifestyle permit one to treat that patient as if she did not belong to the moral community that binds us together.

More importantly, intolerance frequently blocks or prevents our feelings of compassion from operating. Intolerance allows us to marginalize and separate the AIDS victim from the moral community. Rather than treating the victim as "one of us," intolerance transforms him into "one of them." Intolerance permits us to behave toward "these patients" in ways that imply that they are less than suffering human beings seeking our help. The victim is isolated from our concern and comfort. This alienation during a terminal illness can augment the suffering of the AIDS patient.

Tolerance in the health care professional, on the other hand, requires that he focus his attention and concern on the individual's suffering rather than on her religion, politics, or sexual lifestyle. When these other factors affect health, then certainly they need to be discussed. Gay lifestyles can increase the risk of acquiring AIDS, so the gay patient and the physician need to discuss these relevant connections frankly. The goal of this discussion is not to instill in the patient guilt concerning his lifestyle but to ensure health and quality medical care. For just as it is improper to attempt to make the Catholic or the Jewish patient feel guilty for his religious choices, it is improper for the physician to use his position to make the homosexual patient feel guilty for his sex life. Discussions between the physician and the homosexual patient need to be informative, and in order to exchange information, tolerance and nonjudgmental behavior are vital.

Tolerance does not, however, require that the health care professional have no personal preferences and values. Nurses or physicians often have political, religious, or ethical convictions that are very strong. Many physicians believe that homosexual acts are wrong and therefore that those who regularly commit homosexual acts are immoral. Such convictions are perfectly compatible with being a tolerant physician. The tolerant medical professional does not give up his values; he merely refuses to make religious or political sentiments a necessary condition for treating a patient. Nor does the tolerant health care professional view her position of medical authority as a tool for pressuring patients to conform. Medical authority is distinct from moral authority.

*Honesty*    Let us now turn to the virtue of honesty. This virtue, we suggest, is the basis of the patient-professional relationship. If the patient cannot trust that the health care professional is being truthful, then the relationship loses its foundation. The same thing holds for the health care professional. If the health care professional cannot trust that the patient is replying truthfully to appropriate questions, then the professional has no basis for coherent patient care. Sound treatment is fundamentally dependent on the assumption that the patient has provided honest responses to all the relevant medical questions. Furthermore, honesty involves not only a commitment to avoid directly deceitful communications with patients but also a more subtle commitment to avoid withholding information that a patient needs.

All these elements are present when dealing with AIDS. Health care professionals need to know whether patients are in "risk groups," so, despite the difficulties associated with being frank about one's sexual activities, patients ought to be honest. If the patient can require honesty on the part of health care professionals, then the health care professional can require the same level of honesty from the patient. The same would hold true for the HIV-infected physician. It would be inconsistent to hold that the patient is obligated by honesty to reveal his HIV status to the physician without holding also that the HIV-infected physician is obligated to reveal his status. However, the virtue of honesty does not by itself legitimize mandated testing for all patients or professionals. To say that the parties should be honest does not necessarily imply that the parties should submit to testing.

*Faithfulness*    The next virtue that will concern us is faithfulness or loyalty. The virtuous health care professional is faithful to his patients. But what does faithfulness entail? Traditionally, fidelity has been interpreted as a commitment to continue caring for a patient even after he becomes difficult to manage, dangerous, or recalcitrant. Faithfulness has generally been separated from issues concerning the initiation of treatment. The implication here is that, if one simply refused to initiate treatment with a class of patients, then one could not be viewed as having any fidelity obligations to them. One did not have fidelity obligations to individuals who were not yet one's patients. Viewed negatively, one is only unfaithful if one abandons a current patient. If faithfulness is a virtue, then its corresponding vice is abandoning patients. Abandonment is usually treated as an activity of refusing to continue treating a specific patient.

But it seems clear that the concept of fidelity extends beyond these limits. It seems to apply even to individuals who are not one's patients. Dr. Rieux does not have a patient-doctor relationship with all the citizens of Oran, and yet he is loyal and faithful within the limits of physical abilities to all the victims of the plague. Emergencies affect fidelity. The physician who happens upon an auto accident victim on the side of the road and who refuses to treat this person without adequate justification may be viewed as abandoning this individual. More specifically, the dentist or nurse or surgeon who refuses to treat AIDS victims who are not already his patients is likewise lacking in fidelity.

Viewed positively, one is faithful to patients when one continues to help them even when the treatment relationship is cost-inefficient, inconvenient, or dangerous. Faithfulness frequently requires courage and is often based on compassion, but it is more than either of these. To be faithful does not merely involve acting on a particular desire. It involves defining oneself as unique. The ordinary person flies from danger and we do not blame him. The health care professional, like the police officer or the firefighter, takes rational precautions in dealing with dangerous medical risks, but like the good police officer or the good firefighter, she does not run.

The assumption that medicine was an inherently dangerous profession was common prior to the dawn of antibiotics. To care for the sick involved fundamental risk to the provider of health care. Like police work and fire protection, health care work was considered a threat to anyone who entered it. But at the end of World War II, antibiotics seemed to transform this state of affairs by making it safe to practice medicine. For the past 40 years our society has not emphasized the danger that was at one time obvious to anyone entering medicine.

The coming of AIDS has brought us back to an earlier period in medical history. Once again health care professionals need to consider their career choices because along with these choices come dangers. Many physicians and nurses need to reexamine what it means for them to be health care professionals. They entered a profession under the assumption that it was safe work, similar to accounting or the law. AIDS has altered this assumption because antibiotics do not cure AIDS. AIDS constitutes a genuine, albeit low-probability, life-threatening danger that health care workers must face. Like Dr. Rieux the health care worker must ask, "Who am I?"

## The Case of Dr. John Doe

Dr. John Doe is an orthopedic surgeon with privileges to operate at Community Hospital. On a number of occasions Dr. Doe has made it known that he requires any patient that he suspects of being at risk of AIDS to submit to an HIV test. If they refuse to submit to the test, he refuses to take them as patients. If they submit to the test and are HIV positive, he refuses to operate on them. He refers them to other orthopedic surgeons who do not have the same degree of concern regarding AIDS.

He justifies this policy by arguing that his risk of acquiring the disease increases with the number of AIDS patients he treats. Without adhering to this policy, he believes that it is likely that he will contract the virus. Orthopedic surgery, he claims, involves a great deal of what he calls "carpentry work." It is not uncommon to puncture gloves during orthopedic surgery and he states that he cannot put himself and his wife at risk. Operating on AIDS victims, he contends, is not a minimal requirement of the profession. It requires being a hero, and, according to Dr. Doe, it is unethical to require any person, even a physician, to be heroic.

What actions, if any, should the hospital ethics committee take in response to Dr. Doe's policy? What action should they take toward his refusal to treat AIDS victims?

## Committee Discussion of the Case

| | |
|---|---|
| Dr. Mary Collins: (Chair) | Once again I wish to express the hospital's gratitude to you for working on this committee. I know that many of you research the cases that come before us and we appreciate all your efforts. I sent this case to you last week and I want to open the discussion by asking for questions. I have asked Dr. Doe to attend the first part of our meeting. When he has answered your questions and made a brief statement, we will discuss the case in private. |
| Dr. Philip Davis: | Dr. Doe, why isn't it your duty to treat AIDS patients? |
| Prof. Carla Thomas: | Dr. Doe, what do you do with emergency surgical cases? |
| Marian Rhodes: | Dr. Doe, how do you select patients for HIV screening? Do you check their arms for needle tracks or do you ask them if they are gay? Also, who pays for the test and the backup tests if the initial tests are positive for HIV? |
| Vivian Harris: | Do you routinely screen all your patients for HIV? |
| Mary Quigley: | Are there other orthopedic surgeons who accept these AIDS patients that you refuse to treat? |

| | |
|---|---|
| Ms. Rhodes: | Do you break relationships that have been already established if the patient has HIV? If so, you seem to be violating your role as a fiduciary. What do you do if there is no other orthopedic surgeon who will take the patient? Also, do you inform the new physician that the patient is HIV positive? |
| Rev. Richard Marcus: | Is it legally permissible for you to screen these patients in this way? |
| Ms. Harris: | What is the reaction of the nursing staff to this screening procedure? How deep is the feeling among the staff that a HIV screening procedure for surgical patients is necessary? |
| Dr. Collins: | If there are no other questions, I will turn the floor over to Dr. Doe. He will respond to your questions. |
| Dr. John Doe: | Let me begin by saying that I have adopted this view after long and hard thought. My wife and I have also talked over this decision at great length. I believe that caring for AIDS victims is heroic work. I have the greatest respect for physicians who provide this service. But I did not consent to become a hero when I agreed to become a physician, and I do not see how society can require me to be heroic. |
| | Second, in my opinion, physicians have contractual relationships with their patients. If I choose not to enter into contractual relations with patients who are HIV positive, then that is my right. If the doctor-patient relationship is based on the mutual freedom and autonomy of both parties, then coercing me to treat AIDS victims is a violation of my freedom and autonomy. I simply do not accept that being a fiduciary requires me to continue treating AIDS patients. Finally, if one is not permitted to refuse to enter into a contract, then how can you describe the relationship between the |

physician and the patient as free? A contractual relationship is characterized by
freedom, and if the freedom of one of the
parties is removed, then the relationship
cannot be construed as contractual and
autonomous.

Third, I believe that none of you would
claim that physicians have the duty to care
for patients who cannot pay their bills. No
one would take away my privileges at the
hospital for demanding payment. The poor
suffer as much as the AIDS victim. The
poor die as slowly as the AIDS victim. In
short, if you cannot obligate a physician to
care for the poor patient, then you cannot
require the physician to care for the AIDS
patient. If a physician chooses to aid the
poor, then that is praiseworthy, but it is not
his duty. We cannot require the physician
to do this.

If physicians treat AIDS victims, then
they are not acting out of duty. If you give
physicians the right to refuse patients who
are impoverished, it seems to me that you
must give physicians the right to refuse
patients who threaten their lives. With
respect to the details of my policy, I screen
patients, if I have any suspicions whatsoever that the patient may belong to a risk
group. If they give any indications of being
gay or being a drug user, I require the test.
At present I do not routinely require the
test for all patients, but I am considering a
change in that direction.

Regarding the issue of transmission, I
think that all of us would agree that there is
some possibility of transmission from the
patient to the surgeon during surgery.
What motivated my decision to require an
HIV test was a deepening sense that
transmission was more than a slight
possibility for the orthopedic surgeon. I
believe that I am at significant risk.

Regarding emergencies, if the person is a patient, then I operate. If I do not know the person, then I will probably not accept the work. The emergency room physicians know my views on this and they do not call me.

Regarding my selection procedure, I simply go on gut reactions. If there is any hint of intravenous drug use, I require the test. If, for any reason, I think that a person has been involved in homosexual behavior, I require the test. This, as you might imagine, offers less than solid protection against transmission, and I believe that in a short time I am simply going to require all my patients to submit to the HIV test prior to surgery. This solves any problems surrounding discrimination, but it really increases the cost of medicine to the vast majority of my patients.

Regarding payment for the test, I assume the patient, or the patient's insurance company, is responsible for all the costs relative to treatment. I have been reluctant to require all my patients to take the test because of the cost factor. My views on this matter, however, are changing. I am now coming to the view that this may be a necessary cost for safe medical care.

If patients show up positive, I advise them to see their general practitioner so that proper medical treatment can begin. I also give them the names of other orthopedic surgeons. I then send a note to the physician whom I have referred the patient to, informing him or her about the positive results of the HIV test.

How that surgeon chooses to deal with this patient is his business. I have not heard of any cases where AIDS patients who needed surgery were not provided with surgery. I believe that providing this information is sufficient to discharge any responsibilities that I might have toward the patient.

If a patient refuses to take the test, I simply refuse to accept him as a patient. Patients clearly have the right to know my HIV status, and if I refuse to either submit to a test or reveal to them the results of the test, then they surely have the right to refuse to accept me as their physician. I simply want an equivalent right.

The nurses I work with have mixed feelings on this issue, as I myself do. They are torn, as I am, over this issue, but while *some* of them feel that my refusal to treat AIDS patients is wrong, nearly *all of them* believe that we have the right to require surgical patients to submit to testing.

I realize that this view is inconsistent with the rule that physician and nurse safety can be secured merely by assuming that everyone is HIV positive. Surgical teams act very differently when they are dealing with an AIDS victim, and the level of security is vastly improved when we are aware of the HIV status.

Ms. Rhodes:

Allow me to interrupt you on this, Dr. Doe. You are correct that the hospital has advised and ordered all personnel to assume that all bodily fluids of all patients are HIV positive. I agree with you that the reality is that this order requires a significant alteration in behavior, and, quite frankly, this change in behavior has not yet occurred throughout the hospital. Old, unsafe habits die slowly, and although we have not as yet had a case in which AIDS was transmitted to a staff member from a patient, I think that given the relaxed attitude around the hospital, it might happen soon.

But you are testing not for the purpose of increasing safety but for the purpose of turning patients away. Screening to increase safety may be permissible but screening to exclude patients is more dubious.

Atty. John Quinn:

If nurses and physicians began to contract the disease, I assure you we would have more than a change in behavior. We would have a large number of staff choosing not to work at the hospital. Furthermore, if medical staff suddenly started coming down with patient-transmitted HIV, then Dr. Doe's screening policy would suddenly seem mild, calm, and full of sweet reason.

But the point I want to stress is that Dr. Doe has made an assumption that he is at "significant risk." This claim needs more than just theoretical possibility to justify it. To my knowledge, no orthopedic surgeon has contracted the disease from a patient. Without this kind of evidence I do not think that we can just accept his claim that he is at high risk. Without evidence that a significant percentage of surgeons have become HIV positive through patient contact, I am not going to accept his claim.

Dr. Collins:

What about the legal issue? Is it legal for Doe to screen out AIDS patients and refuse to care for them?

Atty. Quinn:

At this time I know of no statute in our state that would make this a criminal offense. However, there are liability issues. Is it permissible to require the test of some patients without requiring it of all patients? Secondly, can the physician refuse to treat on the basis of AIDS? Legally speaking, I think that he is placing himself at significant risk on both counts, and I am quite surprised that his behavior has not yet been challenged in the courts.

Dr. Collins:

Since there are no other questions of Dr. Doe, I will ask that he leave us, so that we may continue our deliberations on this matter. Dr. Doe, if you would like to make a final statement, please do so.

Dr. Doe:    Thank you, Dr. Collins, for asking me to attend this meeting and for allowing me to defend my views. Since I feel that screening for AIDS prior to surgery is widely accepted among so many physicians, I will only summarize my reasons for refusing to perform orthopedic surgery on AIDS patients. Such surgery places everyone in the room at significant risk of death. It also places our wives and husbands at considerable risk. I simply do not feel that it is my duty to expose myself and my wife to this risk. Furthermore, since there are surgeons who are willing to treat such patients, I do not feel that my actions have harmed anyone. Thank you for listening to my views on a matter that is vital to all surgeons and surgical teams.

Dr. Doe leaves the meeting.

Dr. Davis:    Let me begin by saying that the issue of Doe's legal liability is not relevant to these proceedings. Quite frankly, I do not care about whether it is legally prudent for him to take this action. Our problem has to do with its ethical legitimacy and I want to lay my cards on the table. I think that his screening policies and his decision to refuse treatment to AIDS patients is ethically bankrupt. He has abandoned an entire class of patients, and I think that we need to respond quickly and aggressively to his behavior. I think we need to offer him the opportunity to change his screening policies, and I think we need to have him reconsider his decision to refuse to treat AIDS victims. If he refuses to change these policies, then I think we need to recommend to the administration that we revoke his privileges to practice any surgery at this hospital. If it gets around that we condone this behavior, then a lot more physicians and perhaps nurses are going to start to refuse treatment to the AIDS victim. We must send a clear signal that the ethics committee considers such behavior unethical.

More importantly, our policy on AIDS speaks to this issue. Response number 6 asserts that physicians "should not refuse to treat AIDS patients" and that is precisely what Dr. Doe is doing. This closes the door on the issue as far as I am concerned.

Dr. Collins:

I am not sure that it closes the door, Phil. Our policy says nothing about screening, and it is silent on penalties. I myself am very sympathetic to the right of the surgeon to know the HIV status of the patient, and I am not at all sure that patients can demand service if they refuse to cooperate with the legitimate safety requests of the physician.

Refusing to treat patients who are HIV infected is, of course, a different matter, and I am more than slightly upset with Doe's position on that issue. But the screening matter is something that I think is very important to address, and so is the issue of penalties. I worry about the ethics committee imposing penalties. This might undermine our effectiveness at the hospital.

Prof. Martin Fisk:

There is also another consideration. Is Dr. Doe able to treat AIDS patients? There seem to be strong psychological factors influencing his decision. He may be psychologically unable to place himself at any risk whatsoever. It may be impossible for him to reach the ideal of treating AIDS patients. We have not examined this issue with him, but the fear of death can sometimes paralyze a human being, and I do not feel that it would be wise to penalize him so severely

| | |
|---|---|
| | if he were psychologically unable to care for these patients. |
| Ms. Quigley: | I find myself feeling a bit awkward defending a physician's freedom, especially against other physicians, but here it goes. What we are talking about in this case is requiring a person to risk his life in order to help other persons. In my mind, this is a very difficult thing to require someone to do. I certainly have never done it in my life and I am reluctant to require others to do it. I think that it would be praiseworthy of Doe to treat HIV patients, and I am thankful that not all orthopedic surgeons feel as he does. But I am not going to require him to do what is praiseworthy. |
| Dr. Davis: | Health care professionals are not ordinary men and women, Mary! We have special duties that transcend the duties of ordinary citizens. Society has created the medical profession, and when we accepted the rights and privileges of being health care professionals, we accepted the responsibility of treating dangerous patients. I am obligated to place myself at risk. |
| Ms. Quigley: | I do not remember reading in the medical oath that physicians must be willing to risk death. Are these statements a part of the medical oath, Phil? If so, I want to see them. They might be implicit in your interpretation of the oath, but I am not sure that they are written into it. More importantly, I might grant that physicians and nurses have some level of obligation to risk harm. But death is another matter!<br><br>There is a continuum of risk with AIDS, and I do not think that our society has defined what precise level of risk a physician is ethically obligated to assume. This becomes a matter for personal decision. Even though I am unhappy with Dr. Doe's decision, I am willing to be tolerant. |

| | |
|---|---|
| Dr. Davis: | It might help everyone to remember that my view, which many of you think is very harsh, is not idiosyncratic. The AMA's Council on Ethical and Judicial Affairs published a policy entitled "Ethical Issues Involved in the Growing AIDS Crisis." The following quote speaks directly to the issue before us: "A physician may not ethically refuse to treat a patient whose condition is within the physician's current realm of competence solely because the patient is seropositive." |
| Prof. Fisk: | This same statement, Phil, is silent on questions of penalties for physicians who refuse to abide by this ruling, isn't it? |
| Dr. Davis: | Yes. |
| Prof. Fisk: | Phil, what if we penalize Doe? What would be the consequences of this? You say that doing nothing constitutes de facto approval of his actions. I am not sure of that. Perhaps we might want to avoid penalizing him and, instead, highlight the AMA's council recommendations at the next grand rounds discussion of AIDS. Perhaps we would be better off praising other surgeons who have a greater willingness to do surgery on AIDS victims than Dr. Doe. In effect, I am suggesting that we might be better off rewarding positive behavior and placing less emphasis on punishing behavior. |
| Dr. Davis: | Martin, you have raised two issues. First, do I believe in positively reinforcing caring behavior? The answer is yes. I fully support any plan that would highlight physicians and nurses who care for AIDS victims. But positive reinforcement isn't enough. To do only that assumes that treating AIDS victims is optional. I do not agree with this. If you are abandoning AIDS patients, it seems to me that we do not need you here at Community Hospital. This is the most |

serious epidemic that we have faced in this century, and the number of AIDS victims that are going to need health care in the next ten years is going to be very high. Condoning abandonment will devastate patients and stain the profession of medicine.

Rev. Marcus: If we permit or condone health care professionals opting out of caring for AIDS victims, aren't we going to concentrate the risk in the hands of a few who are willing to treat AIDS victims? For example, if there is only one orthopedic surgeon, Dr. X, who will operate on AIDS patients, aren't we condemning him to a very high level of exposure?

Ms. Quigley: Dr. Doe isn't coercing Dr. X to treat AIDS patients, is he? In your hypothetical case, if no one is coercing Dr. X to operate on these patients, then no one is "condemning him." Condemning a person implies coercion, and, since there is no coercion, there is no condemning.

Ms. Harris: Mary Quigley, Rev. Marcus, and Dr. Davis seem to be at ethical loggerheads on the issue of punishing Doe. They are arguing about whether such care is obligatory. This debate is an important one, but I would like to turn the discussion away from obligation and in the direction of virtues. This shift is necessary because there is no way to resolve the debate about whether it is a minimum requirement of being a physician to treat AIDS patients or whether it is heroic and, therefore, not obligatory to treat such patients. I think that health care ideals are just as relevant to this case as legal rights and social consequences. Phil's approach is to view Dr. Doe as someone who is violating the rights of patients or as someone who is acting in a way that is inconsistent with social welfare. Mary's view is that he is not violating a minimal requirement. He is simply choosing not to be a hero. It is not unlike the debate over how many angels can fit on the head of a pin. Therefore, I would like to take a new tack. I would like us to consider the idea that Doe may be acting in a way that is inconsistent with the ideals of the profession.

Dr. Davis:

Vivian, I think I understand Mary's view. She holds that providing orthopedic surgical care to the victims of AIDS is heroic and, therefore, it is not a duty. My view is that Doe's behavior is a violation of our duty to avoid abandoning patients. He has, in my opinion, abandoned AIDS victims who need his help. However, I am not yet clear on what you mean by violating the ideals of the profession. Vivian, how is your view different from Mary's? Can we penalize people for violating the ideals of the profession?

Ms. Harris:

I think that it is an alternative view rather than a compromise. At this stage of the AIDS crisis, I am opposed to penalizing people. I am totally opposed to our committee punishing or recommending punishments for anyone. That undermines our role in the hospital. Penalties are administrative matters, not ethics committee matters.

I am far more anxious to discuss how a virtuous physician or a virtuous nurse would respond to the AIDS crisis. I want to establish educational programs that redirect ethics away from matters concerning minimal obligations, social consequences, and individual rights. I want to refocus our attention on what it means to have a set of personal ideals that play an important role in living a meaningful life as a health care professional.

For example, although we run many educational programs on ethics here at the hospital, I have never once heard any conversation about what it means to be a compassionate, honest, or courageous health care professional. I have never once heard anyone speak about what these virtues have to do with the AIDS crisis. We are so tied up with legal minimals that we forget what it means to belong to an ancient profession devoted to fighting human suffering. When we are not concerned with minimal obligations, we focus on social consequences that we can hardly ever determine with any kind of accuracy. This overemphasis on obligations, rights, and consequences has distracted us from talking about what really matters from an ethical perspective: the virtues of compassion or courage or tolerance.

Living virtuously gives our lives meaning in ways that following our obligations does not. Being compassionate, honest, courageous, and tolerant allows us to feel good about being a nurse or a physician. Being virtuous gives us the sense that our work is more than a way to earn a living. Seeing our work as offering opportunities for courage or honesty or integrity gives our lives a dramatic sense that can sustain and comfort us through life's tears.

Prof. Fisk:  But concretely, Vivian, what are the implications of your view for the case at hand?

Ms. Harris:  I am not sure what the practical consequences are. I think that Dr. Doe is violating an ideal of the medical profession. And I think he needs to rethink what it means to be a physician. I think he needs to remember that personal courage and compassion are as important to the meaning of the word "physician" as knowledge of biology or chemistry. Perhaps he needs to be converted into being a physician once again, much as a person might rediscover what it means to be a Jew or a Christian. Medicine might be more like a religion than we previously thought.

Prof. Fisk:

I am not comfortable with this kind of ethical discourse. For me, ethics is basically a search for a tool to resolve conflict. For you, Vivian, it seems to be a search for professional ideals.

Ms. Harris:

Martin, both you and Carla have mistaken the law for ethics. The law is our best tool for resolving conflict. It seems to me that ethics is something else. It is a search for a personal identity that makes being a health care professional meaningful and rewarding. Money and prestige cannot compensate for the oceans of tears that penetrate medicine.

Prof. Fisk:

Vivian, ethics seems far less concerned with ideals and virtues than it does with rights, consequences, and obligations. My sense is that AIDS patients have a claim on society as a whole rather than on specific physicians. That claim against society places an obligation upon society to find health care professionals, including orthopedic surgeons, who freely consent to care for AIDS victims and then provide AIDS victims access to these physicians. If Dr. Doe does not voluntarily consent to care for these patients, then we cannot hold him responsible for their care.

Dr. Collins:

But Martin, yours is a futuristic possibility. It is not the way care is handled at this time.

Prof. Fisk:

Correct! Right now, we have the vague feeling that all physicians have the obligation to care for AIDS victims. This vague, ethical feeling leads to inadequate care of AIDS victims. If we gave up this vague feeling and replaced it with a specific bureaucracy that is responsible for AIDS care, then patients would be cared for. Society has not grappled with the task of creating a comprehensive social approach to the care of AIDS victims. And until we take that step, we are going to be tempted to impose harsh penalties on physicians who are psychologically unable to place themselves at risk.

Patients can demand service from physicians even if they constitute a slight danger to the provider, but I do not think that we can coerce the physician to be courageous. Taking away Dr. Doe's privilege to operate at this hospital puts an end to his professional life in this area. I also think that it would be difficult to replace a surgeon of his caliber and experience. We might want to consider *all* the actual and possible consequences of taking away his privileges. Let us not cut off our noses to spite our faces.

Ms. Harris:    Martin, your last comment suggests that we need to create "plague doctors." This approach demeans the profession by allowing doctors and nurses to abandon their promises and their patients. You say that society has an obligation to provide health care to these victims, but society is an abstraction. *It doesn't do anything!* Only individual doctors and nurses can do anything for AIDS victims.

In the context of death, one needs to talk about existential choice and individual commitment to the AIDS victim rather than developing another bureaucracy to allow people to avoid the meaning of being a doctor.

| | |
|---|---|
| Prof. Thomas: | Vivian, I agree with Martin in the sense that firefighters and police belong to social agencies—bureaucracies, if you will—that address social problems. These men and women face dangers that are probably greater than the dangers faced by physicians and nurses who fight AIDS. Firefighters voluntarily choose a life that is threatening to their well-being. Because of this choice we can explicitly obligate them to take on risky behaviors. Where I disagree with Martin is on the question of developing an entirely new bureaucracy of AIDS physicians and nurses. Health care professionals have already consented to risk danger just like the firefighter and the police officer. |
| Ms. Harris: | Carla, your analogy with the police is only partially correct. Hospitals that employ nurses or physicians can obligate them to care for AIDS patients. They hire on knowing that is a condition of employment. But vast numbers of physicians are private entrepreneurs. They have no superior officer or boss that will fire them for not caring for AIDS patients. Except within contexts like the military, there is no hierarchy that can order physicians to treat AIDS victims. In general, nobody can order the private physician to care for the AIDS victim in the way a fire captain can order a firefighter to enter a burning building. Private physicians are at liberty in ways that firefighters are not. Medicine is not organized along military lines. |
| | But there is a more practical consideration! Community Hospital cannot hire special AIDS doctors and nurses. It would be practically impossible to create a special staff separated from the already existing medical staff. We will not recreate the special class of "plague doctors" and become the laughing stock of this city. All |

of us who are on staff at the hospital have equal obligations to treat AIDS patients.

Dr. Davis:    But, Vivian, how is this last claim different from my view that Dr. Doe is simply violating patients' rights and is obligated to treat them?

Ms. Harris:    There is a big difference. For you, Phil, Dr. Doe is violating social requirements, but I do not think there is an adequate basis for defending the view that one's moral or ethical requirements are equal to one's social or legal requirements. My view is that he needs to reevaluate what it means to be a virtuous physician and he needs to reconsider his original commitments to medicine. He needs to imagine how the ideal physician would behave! Deciding to become a doctor always involves deciding to shoot for an ideal of behavior and Dr. Doe has forsaken the ideal. There is a big difference between saying that something is a violation of a social requirement and saying that the behavior fails to achieve the ideals of the profession.

Dr. Davis:    But look, Vivian, if you call treating an AIDS patient a medically ideal behavior, then something less than ideal behavior must be allowed since we cannot require doctors to be ideals. In your view, we could not penalize his behavior. You are just accepting Mary Quigley's view.

Ms. Harris:    Perhaps legally we cannot require doctors to be ideals, but morally and ethically I think that we need to hold them up to high ideals. The whole point of ethics is to place before health care professionals not the minimum requirements but the ideals or virtues of their profession. I think that we need to find ways to bring Dr. Doe back to the ideal.

| | |
|---|---|
| Rev. Marcus: | Why not simply use the religious language? Dr. Doe needs to be converted with respect to what it means to be a doctor! |
| Atty. Quinn: | Rev. Marcus, that sounds like a great Sunday sermon, but we are faced with a practical task in this committee. We are not involved in purely theological or philosophical debate. Do you have a practical recommendation regarding what we should do with Dr. Doe? |
| Rev. Marcus: | Well, I do not think that we should revoke his privileges nor do I think that we can condone his actions. Perhaps we need to have him spend some time with physicians who see their responsibilities differently. I would propose that we set up some meetings with him and a number of other selected physicians and have some serious conversations about these matters. Maybe we can reorient him to the shared ideals that mean so much to so many physicians who care for AIDS patients. |
| Dr. Collins: | Once again, time is driving us as much as any issue. Can we come to some kind of resolution on this matter? I sense that there is little support for Dr. Davis's call for stiff penalties for Dr. Doe. |
| Ms. Quigley: | Neither punishing staff nor recommending that staff be punished is our role. I for one would want to leave this matter to the administration. |

## Committee Recommendations

| | |
|---|---|
| Prof. Fisk: | I would like to recommend that we draft a letter to Dr. Doe and that it contain a number of ethical recommendations. |
| Ms. Rhodes: | This is a soft reaction, and at this time it seems appropriate to me. Is everyone in agreement on this general reaction? |

There is a consensus on this approach, although Dr. Davis goes on record as opposing it.

| | |
|---|---|
| Prof. Fisk: | I would be willing to draft the letter to Dr. Doe, but I need some consensus as to what it should contain. |
| Ms. Rhodes: | The first thing it should contain is the AMA statement on caring for the AIDS patient. He needs to realize that he is out of step with his professional organization. |
| Prof. Thomas: | I believe that we need to have a formal and regular ethics program on the topic of AIDS and we need to recommend that Dr. Doe attend it. I do not know whether we can require him to attend, but we certainly can recommend that he do so. |
| Ms. Harris: | I think we need to gather together a bibliography of essays on the topic of caring for the AIDS patient, especially essays involving courage and compassion for AIDS victims. |
| Dr. Collins: | Martin, will you prepare this letter and see to it that it contains these recommendations? The committee will approve it at our next meeting. Is there anything else that we need to do regarding this matter? |
| Dr. Davis: | We need to hope that no one finds out just how anemic our response to this issue has been. Dr. Doe avoids his duty and the ethics committee fails to take decisive action. |
| Dr. Collins: | Phil, you did not convince us. Perhaps you need to go home and develop some stronger arguments for your view. Let me close this meeting with some words of thanks. As the medical director I have to meet with Dr. Doe, and the ideas that were expressed here have given me a clearer sense of how I will deal with him. |

## Questions for Further Discussion

1. If you were Dr. Collins, what would you say to Dr. Doe when you met with him?
2. Dr. Davis holds that being a physician requires Dr. Doe to provide surgical care to AIDS victims. What is his argument for this view? Can you make his position more precise?
3. How do you think other physicians and surgeons would respond to withdrawing privileges from Dr. Doe?
4. What are the legal obligations of physicians with respect to AIDS victims in your state?
5. Does Dr. Doe's refusal to operate on AIDS patients demonstrate his lack of courage and/or his lack of compassion?
6. Dr. Doe and Mary Quigley believe that physicians should be at liberty to refuse to care for AIDS victims. What would be the social consequences of adopting this view? In the light of these consequences, how would you evaluate their view?
7. Very little time was spent on viewing the problem from the perspective of patient or provider rights. How would these perspectives affect the evaluation of Dr. Doe's case?
8. How would you respond to Dr. Davis's charge that the committee has given an anemic response to the case?
9. Should the committee spend more time trying to estimate the exact level of risk that orthopedic surgeons face in treating AIDS victims?
10. If you were an orthopedic surgeon, how would you handle the problem of operating on AIDS victims? Should all patients who are in need of surgery be required to submit to an HIV test?

# More Cases Involving the Policy

## Dr. Marriot

Dr. Bill Marriot is a well-known, 51-year-old, married emergency room (ER) physician at Community Hospital. After ten years as an ER physician, he has achieved the respect both of his colleagues and the community. He is a skilled, dedicated, and sensitive physician.

Dr. Marriot is admitted to his hospital with unexplained weight loss and fever. He undergoes multiple diagnostic blood tests. The fevers continue and he remains in the hospital several days. Dr. Sims, who is Marriot's physician, calls in the infectious disease service because she is concerned that Dr. Marriot may be HIV positive. In fact, the HIV Eliza and Western Blot tests prove to be clearly positive. Dr. Sims approaches Dr. Marriot with what she thinks is devastating news. To her surprise, Dr. Marriot reveals that three years ago he tested positive for HIV. Dr. Marriot pleads with Dr. Sims not to disclose his HIV status to the administrators of the hospital.

Dr. Sims comes to you as a member of the ethics committee for your advice on her ethical obligations in this case. What do you tell her? What are your reasons for your advice?[13]

## AIDS and the Family Practitioner

Dr. Smith is a family medicine physician who practices in a small community health clinic. He seroconverted to HIV positive six months ago. His health is still good and he continues to care for patients. He believes that since he is not a surgeon, he does not constitute a genuine threat to his patients. However, he knows that if he revealed his status, many of his patients would seek other medical care. Is Dr. Smith ethically obligated to share this information with his patients? Is he obligated to stop giving medical care to patients? Is he obligated to share this information with his superiors at the health clinic?

## AIDS and the Married Couple

Mr. and Mrs. Jones are patients of Dr. Smith. Dr. Smith informs Mr. Jones that Jones has seroconverted to HIV positive. Jones requests that Smith keep this information private and that he say nothing to Jones's wife. Jones claims that he and his wife are no longer "sexual partners" and that, therefore, he is no threat to her. Mrs. Jones is coming in next week for her yearly physical/pelvic exam. Is Dr. Smith obligated to divulge any information to Mrs. Jones?

## Revealing HIV Status to a Relative

A 68-year-old male presented with significant mental status changes and weight loss. An accurate history could not be obtained from the patient. His sister, however, reported that her brother had been living a homosexual lifestyle and voiced concerns about the possibility of AIDS. An HIV test was performed and the results were positive. The sister repeatedly questioned physicians and nurses about the HIV status of her brother, who was still judged incompetent. The physicians did not want to disclose the HIV status of an incompetent patient to a family member. Do the surrogates who authorized the HIV test have the right to the results of the test?

## Further Reading

AMA Council on Ethical and Judicial Affairs, *Current Opinions, 1986,* Principle VI, 9.11.

Amundsen, D. W., "Medical Deontology and Pestilential Disease in the Middle Ages," *Journal of the History of Medicine and Allied Sciences* 32 (1977): 402–421.

Annas, G., "Not Saints but Healers: A Health Care Professional's Legal Obligation to Treat," *American Journal of Public Health* 78 (July 1988): 844–849.

Arras, J. "The Fragile Web of Responsibility: AIDS and the Duty to Treat," *Hastings Center Report,* Apr.-May 1988, at 10,12 (special Supp.).

Banks, (AIDS and the Right to Health Care, 4 Issues L. & Med. at) 167.

Emmanuel, E. J., "Do Physicians Have an Obligation to Treat Patients with AIDS?," *New England Journal of Medicine* 318 (25) (June 23, 1988): 1686, from the American Medical Association, see "A.M.A. Rules That Doctors Are Obligated to Treat AIDS," *N.Y. Times,* Nov. 13, 1987, at A14, col. 1, and from the Surgeon General, see "Doctors Who Shun AIDS Patients Are Assailed by Surgeon General," *N.Y. Times,* Sept. 10, 1987, at A1, col. 4.

See, e.g., Fox, *The Politics of Physicians' Responsibility in Epidemics: A Note on History, Hastings Center Report* (April 1988): 5.

Gostin, Lawrence O., "The AIDS Litigation Project: A National Review of Court and Human Rights Commission Decisions, Part II: Discrimination," *Journal of the American Medical Association* (April 18, 1990).

Gramelspacher, Gregory P., and Mark Siegler, "Do Physicians Have a Professional Responsibility to Care for Patients With HIV Disease?" *Issues in Law and Medicine* (Winter 1988).

Lo, Bernard, "Obligations to Care for Persons with Immunodeficiency Virus," *Issues in Law and Medicine* (Winter 1988).

Pellegrino, E., "Altruism, Self-Interest and Medical Ethics," *Journal of the American Medical Association* 258 (1988): 1939–1940.

Peterson, L. M., "AIDS: The Ethical Dilemma for Surgeons." *Law, Medicine & Health Care* 17 (1989): 139–144.

Sheldon, Mark, "HIV and the Obligation to Treat," *Theoretical Medicine* 11 (1990).

Turner, C. F., H. G. Miller, and L. E. Moses, eds. *AIDS: Sexual Behavior and Intravenous Drug Use* (Washington, D.C.: National Academy Press, 1989), Chapters 6 and 7.

Walters, L., "Ethical Issues in Prevention and Treatment of HIV Infection and AIDS," *Science* 239 (1988): 597–603.

Winslow, C. E. A., *The Conquest of Epidemic Disease: A Chapter in the History of Ideas* (Madison: University of Wisconsin Press, 1980), p. 118.

Zuger, A., and S. H. Miles, "Physicians, AIDS, and Occupational Risk: Historical Traditions and Ethical Obligations." *Journal of the American Medical Association* 258 (1987): 1924–1928.

**Notes**

1. James R. Allen, "Health Care Workers and the Risk of HIV Transmission," *Hastings Center Report* (April 1988): 2.
2. Gregory Pence, *Ethical Options In Medicine* (Airedale, N.J.: Medical Economics, 1980).
3. Alasdair MacIntyre, *After Virtue*, 2nd ed. (Notre Dame, Ind.: University of Notre Dame Press, 1988).
4. Ibid., p. 201.
5. Darrel W. Amundsen, "Medical Deontology and the Pestilence Disease in the Late Middle Ages," *Journal of the History of Medicine and Allied Sciences* 32 (1977): 403–21.
6. Aristotle, *Nicomachean Ethics*, in *The Basic Works of Aristotle*, ed. Richard McKeon (New York: Random House, 1941), (1105b5–18).
7. Daniel Fox, "The Politics of Physicians' Responsibility in Epidemics: A Note on History," *Hastings Center Report* (April 1988): 5.
8. For a good discussion of the problems associated with hiring plague doctors, see John Arras, "The Frail Web of Responsibility: AIDS and the Duty to Treat," *Hastings Center Report* (April 1988): 11.
9. Edmund Pellegrino, "Altruism, Self-Interest, and Medical Ethics," *Journal of the American Medical Association* 258 (14) (October 9, 1987): 1939.
10. Our discussion of Albert Camus's famous novel *The Plague* is relevant to this claim. The hero of the novel has no religious commitments, but he cares for the sick nevertheless. Camus offers an existentialist account of virtue.
11. Pellegrino, op. cit., p. 1940.
12. Albert Camus, *The Plague*, trans. Stuart Gilbert (New York: Random House, 1948).
13. My thanks to George Kanoti and Sandy Pirwitz for this case. On this case be careful to ask the important questions. You may need to provide additional assumptions.

# 9

## Medical Research Involving Persons

### Introduction to the Problem Area

The modern ethical problems associated with human subject research had their contemporary origins in the tragic events that occurred in the Nazi concentration camps during World War II. Jews, Gypsies, homosexuals, and members of many other groups that the Nazis excluded from the moral community were systematically used as research subjects in medical experiments.

The concentration camp inmates were not voluntary and willing participants in medical research. They were forced by their jailers to submit to heinous experiments. The Nazis rationalized this treatment by attempting to separate Jews, Gypsies, and homosexuals from the human community. The Nuremberg trials that followed the war punished many of the perpetrators of these "crimes against humanity." More important for our purposes, the court issued a code regarding human subject research that ought to be followed by any civilized community. This series of recommendations has been extremely influential in the development of our social and ethical attitudes toward human subject research. The following is a summary of the ten recommendations offered by the Nuremberg Court.

Human subject research should:

1. proceed on the basis of voluntary consent of the subjects.
2. be designed to yield fruitful results for society that cannot be developed using any other means.
3. be preceded by animal experimentation.
4. avoid unnecessary harm to the subjects.
5. avoid the death or disabling of the human subjects.
6. be designed so that the benefits to humanity outweigh the risk to the individual human subject.

7. be based on proper preparations aimed at protecting the human subject.
8. be conducted only by qualified scientists.
9. be designed so as to allow the subject to withdraw at any time.
10. be designed so that the researcher can stop the experiment at any time he or she feels that it will generate unnecessary harm to the patient.

## Two American Cases

The misuse of research subjects is not, however, something that only happened in Nazi Germany. There is an American history of research abuse as well. Perhaps the most famous case of abuse is the Tuskegee studies of untreated syphilis, in which researchers used impoverished and uninformed black men to study the natural course of the disease. The study began in 1932 when the standard of care for syphilis was treatment with drugs containing arsenic and bismuth. Over 200 men infected with the disease constituted a control group. *They received no treatment.* These men were not informed of the availability of curative beneficial medications. They were tricked into submitting to painful spinal taps that were called "special free treatment." This group was followed by the researchers even after the development of penicillin, which cured syphilis. Finally, this research was carried out under the auspices of the U.S. Public Health Service.

The second event was the Willowbrook studies, in which retarded children were deliberately infected with the hepatitis B virus. In the mid-1950s, Dr. Saul Krugman and Dr. Joan Giles led a research team at Willowbrook State Hospital in Willowbrook, New York, and noticed that infectious viral hepatitis was rampant among the retarded children. The hospital was overcrowded with retarded children and newly admitted children would in all likelihood become infected within 12 months. Researchers believed that studying the problem would be very beneficial to future patients. Over 800 mentally retarded children, were intentionally given viral hepatitis and used to study the disease clinically. The parents were informed of the experiment, but admission to the hospital was contingent upon their agreement to participate in the study.

## Protectionism

These cases and a host of others indicated that human subjects, especially children and other vulnerable people, needed to be protected, not from monstrous researchers like the Nazis, but from well-intended but overzealous researchers who were often more concerned with aiding future patients than protecting present subjects. Researchers often see the possible benefits of their research for future generations and occasionally forget their duties to those in front of them. In order to minimize the possible harms to individual subjects, the U.S. government developed several protective strategies.

*The Random Clinical Trial*    The first, and from a scientific viewpoint the most important, tool that government employed was to formally establish a method for establishing both the safety and the effectiveness of research drugs or procedures: *the random clinical trial (RCT)*. This methodology is based on the comparison of two arms or groups, e.g., A and B. Both groups are composed of individuals who are suffering from disease D. The method begins from the point of theoretical equality. Treatment T is being compared with treatment T2, and both treatments are believed to be equal with respect to safety or effectiveness against disease D. T and T2 may be drugs or procedures that are being compared with respect to some medically significant characteristic. T, for example, may be a drug that is hypothesized by researchers to be effective against D; it is given to the individuals in group A and withheld from the members of group B. The members of group B are given T2, which may be either a placebo, if there is no treatment for D, or a treatment that is currently the best weapon against D. The two groups are then studied over a period of time. If the members of group A have clinical results that are superior to those of group B, than treatment T is judged to be clinically superior to the alternative treatments.

The term "random," however, is crucially significant. In the RCT, patients are randomly assigned to groups A and B. This means that neither the patient nor the researcher knows whether the patient is receiving treatment T, a placebo, or an alternative treatment for D. This is called a "double-blind clinical trial" and is the most widely used method for verifying the effectiveness and safety of a treatment. The random factor prevents bias on the part of researchers and patients. For example, if a researcher was convinced that his treatment was effective, he might unconsciously assign to Group A individuals who have an overall better chance of recovering from D than the people he assigns to B. If this happened, the test results would be biased in favor of the researcher's hypothesis.

Finally, clinical trials usually are divided into three different types or phases. In the Phase I clinical trials, questions of safety and effectiveness are not directly addressed. Rather, in this phase a drug is studied with respect to how it is tolerated and how it operates within the body, for instance, how it is metabolized or excreted. The goal of such studies is not to determine safety and/or effectiveness, but they may indicate that a drug is promising. Phase I studies do not involve large numbers of research subjects because there is so little known about the drug that, from an ethical standpoint, we are required to risk as few people as necessary.

In Phase II studies, a larger group is studied. The primary aim of these studies is to determine if a given drug shows real promise of being a useful agent. Phase II studies involve larger groups of patients but usually no more than 200. Determining efficacy against the disease process is the primary aim of Phase II studies, but researchers are also very concerned to determine the side effects and risks of the drug. It should be argued that many Phase II studies wind up failing in that they indicate definitively that a proposed medication is not effective. However, if Phase II studies indicate that a drug might be effective against a disease process, then a Phase III study is initiated. At this stage, a larger group of people (sometimes over a thousand) are studied. In these studies the goal is to determine, with a relatively high degree of exactitude, the level of the drug's effectiveness and its side effects.

*Institutional Review Boards*    The government's second protectionist tool is the institutional review board. This board is composed of researchers, physicians, nurses, institutional administrators, and lay persons who are empowered by federal rules to approve or disapprove research that is carried on within an institution. All research studies must be reviewed by this board. The primary goal of such boards is to guarantee that research neither unnecessarily harm patients nor violate their rights. Whenever a hospital or other research institution initiates a research proposal or joins a team of researchers in a clinical trial, the study must be reviewed by an institutional review board.

A typical dilemma that an institutional review board might face is one involving the use of control groups. Frequently, RCTs are used to determine the effectiveness of a drug against diseases that have no treatment and are universally fatal. In such cases the patients in group B are given placebos— usually sugar pills. Boards frequently disagree about the ethical legitimacy of using living individuals as control groups when historical information regarding patients that have already died might serve as an effective control group. Defenders of the use of living subjects criticize the accuracy and validity of historical control groups. Furthermore, they argue that, although there might be "theoretical" support for the effectiveness of a drug or procedure, there is no solid empirical evidence. Many drugs that look good on paper fail the test of efficacy when tested in the crucible of the randomized clinical trial.

The clinical trial employed in the evaluation of AZT illustrates this dilemma. There were some early suggestions based on admittedly insufficient statistical data that AZT (azidothymidine) was an effective treatment for AIDS. These insufficient data were drawn from a Phase I trial. A random clinical trial employing a placebo control group was initiated to compare using AZT with doing nothing. Critics of the trial argued that all the victims of the disease should have been given the AZT because the disease is universally fatal. In this case the conflict between the researcher and the physician becomes primary. The researcher's goal is to determine the effectiveness of a given treatment, and doing so requires a control group that sometimes receives an ineffective treatment. Providing this ineffective treatment is compatible with the values of the researcher, but it seems to conflict with the values of the physician.

The physician uses and depends on scientific research but is directly committed not to securing the medical welfare of future patients but to securing the welfare of the present individual patient. A physician who recommends that a patient enter a random clinical trial thus faces a challenge. Should she recommend that the patient enter a treatment program in which it is possible that the patient may receive a treatment that is known to be ineffective?

*Informed Consent Documents*    The third mechanism employed by the government is the informed consent document. We have already discussed informed consent in a previous chapter, but we need to emphasize some aspects of informed consent that are particularly relevant to research. The three most critical aspects of informed consent for human subject research are disclosure of relevant information, patient understanding of this information, and the patient's voluntary consent to participate in the research.

To meet the challenges associated with research, institutional review boards rely heavily on the informed consent documents that *must* be signed by patients who are research subjects. These forms normally include vast amounts of information describing the disease and the treatment program involved in the research. Committees screen these documents with the following eight questions in mind.

1. Is the purpose of the experiment clearly expressed?
2. Is the procedure to be followed defined?
3. Are the side effects explained?
4. Are the "hoped for" benefits presented?
5. Are alternatives presented?
6. Are confidentiality and privacy guaranteed?
7. Are questions of cost addressed?
8. Is the right to withdraw at any time presented?

*Research and Children*    The final area of governmental concern focuses on the role of children or legally incompetent persons. Because of their competence, adults may enter a Phase I nontherapeutic clinical trial. This trial is not intended to benefit the patient. Adults, for example, may freely enter a study in which there is no hope for personal benefit but that may contribute to the care of future patients. We permit adults to place themselves at risk for the benefit of others. Children and incompetent adults, however, are another matter. Therapeutic research aimed at benefiting children is not nearly as troublesome, but nontherapeutic research is very challenging because children are very easily mistreated. The Food and Drug Administration (FDA) does not completely forbid such nontherapeutic research but it does require that it involve *no more than minimal risk to the child.* This restriction, which significantly complicates pediatric research, does not apply to competent adults. However, we must approach the legally incompetent, especially the mentally impaired adult, with the same restriction in mind.

At most hospitals, the institutional review board (IRB) is distinct from the ethics committee. There is no legal requirement for this distinction. Rather, it is based on convention. There are usually two committees in order to distribute the workload. However, for the sake of continuity, Community Hospital's ethics committee will do the work of the IRB.

---

### Community Hospital's Policy on Human Subject Research

*Purpose:*    The purpose of this policy is to set out the guidelines on the use of human subjects in medical research.

*Background:*    Human subject research involves five distinct issues that require sensitivity to conflicting ethical values. First, the hospital follows the principle of the great French physiologist Claude Bernard, who stated in 1865 that "physicians already make too many dangerous experiments on man before carefully studying them in animals." The hospital accepts and, indeed, requires animal research before testing in human subjects. However, the hospital requires that all researchers follow the NIH's *Guide for the Care and Use of Laboratory Animals.*[1] Second, human subject research is often motivated by a desire to help human subjects, but it is also directed at helping future patients. Such research thus has a dual purpose, and this mixed purpose is a primary source of ethical tension. Third, the research itself involves either autonomous individuals or individuals who are represented by guardians. The wishes of these patients and their guardians need to be respected. Fourth, because autonomy plays such a crucial role in human subject research, the issues of informed consent and confidentiality are central to such research. Finally, because access to research protocols is viewed by many individuals as a "scarce resource," questions of access to this resource need to be addressed.

*Principles:*

1. The institutional review board of Community Hospital must approve all clinical, psychological, or social research that involves human subjects and is conducted at the hospital. The responsibilities of the IRB include determining that a proposed research project is aimed at securing beneficial knowledge, that the knowledge could not be secured in ways that do not involve human subjects, and that there is a favorable balance of benefits over harms to both future patients and the human subjects.

2. The committee will adopt the double-blind random clinical trial as the preferred mode of clinical inquiry and will bypass this method only when it is impossible to follow this methodology. Surgical research, for example, obviously need not follow this method.

3. Every effort will be made to secure a fair and just access to experimental protocols when they are in short supply. Discrimination based on race, religion, national origin, or sex will not be tolerated at Community Hospital.

4. The goal of research will be to secure the medical welfare of present and future patients within the limits of respect for the autonomy of the individual research subjects.

5. In order to secure the goal of respect for the autonomy of human subjects, the institutional review board of Community Hospital adheres to the following list of rights:

   a. Participants in human subject research will give their informed consent prior to being entered into a protocol. Subjects are to be informed of all relevant side effects of a treatment. They are to be given an opportunity to ask any and all questions that they have regarding the protocol. This information should be presented to the subject in a written informed consent document. The IRB should take as one of its primary tasks the review and reconstruction of such documents.

   b. Research subjects are to be given alternatives to entering into the protocol, including the alternative of no treatment or palliative treatment.

   c. Research subjects are to be informed of their right to refuse or withdraw from the treatment. No penalties should be imposed because a patient withdraws from a protocol.

   d. Research subjects should be informed of all the costs for which they will be responsible.

    e.  The consent of the subject is to be secured in writing and it should be witnessed.

6. The committee accepts the idea that protocol treatments should be at least as beneficial as any alternative treatment. It is thus unethical to provide a protocol treatment that we know to be inferior to an alternative treatment. Finally, the arms of a clinical trial should be roughly equal with respect to their therapeutic utility.

7. Since placebos are often essential in the random clinical trial, especially in cases where there is no alternative treatment for a disease, the committee accepts their use as long as the patient is informed that he may be placed on the placebo arm of the clinical trial and that he, in fact, may receive a treatment that is known to be ineffective. Such trials should be watched with special care and should be closed as soon as possible. At this point, all persons in the study should be provided the treatment.

8. Legally incompetent individuals such as children and the mentally ill may be admitted to therapeutic research. However, special attention should be paid to nontherapeutic research involving children or other incompetent persons. Indeed, everything within reason should be done to avoid employing legally incompetent persons in nontherapeutic research, i.e., studies that are not intended to benefit the individual but that secure valuable scientific information. The only exceptions to this general rule are research protocols that involve minimal risk or discomfort. A minimal risk is one that is no greater than what the person would encounter in his or her daily life. Because adults may consent to being "used" in nontherapeutic research, participation in Phase I random clinical trials should be restricted (where possible) to consenting adults.

9. No inducements will be offered to research subjects as an incentive to participate in the research. Because inducement is difficult to avoid when employing prisoners in medical research, the committee is very skeptical of such research.

10. Prisoners and inhabitants of mental institutions have been unethically employed as research subjects in the past. Therefore, it is understandable that we should wish to protect them against being used in scientific experiments. In the recent past, such protectionist concerns have led to the exclusion of such individuals from research protocols. The committee considers such protectionist concerns noble but only if they do not entail excluding such persons from the benefits of human subject research.

# Commentary on the Philosophical and Ethical Aspects of the Policy

## Research Involving Competent Adults

Since most human subject research involves competent adults, we open our discussion with the ethical issues that are present when researchers use competent adults as research subjects. In consequentialist terms, the fundamental philosophical problem associated with doing research on adult humans involves the potential, and sometimes actual, benefits and harms. Such research has two possibly conflicting goals. Human subject research is based on the consequentialist imperative to secure the good of present and future patients. The consequentialist also requires that researchers obey another imperative: to respect the wishes and interests of the individual patients who serve as subjects. Since society can benefit from research that may harm the individual subject or violate his wishes, it follows that we must find some way to balance or weigh the harm to the individual against the benefits to society.

However, from a rights-based perspective, the "balancing" or "weighing" metaphor of consequentialism is fundamentally suspicious because it suggests that we may, if the benefits to future patients are high enough, use a human subject against her will. The rights-based theorist suggests that the fundamental ethical problem has nothing to do with "balancing." Rather it is to develop a policy that will protect the rights of human subjects. For the-rights based theorist, no balancing is necessary since the rights of the individual are always primary. If an individual is used as an object, then the research is unethical no matter what the results. The end cannot justify the means.

Many attempts have been made to form a compromise between the rights of the individual subject and the welfare of patients who are served by continuing research. For many philosophers, the linchpin of any such compromise is the principle of informed consent.

## The Informed Consent Compromise

This conflict between the rights of the individual and the needs of society was resolved in the West by drawing a compromise between individual autonomy and social utility. According to this compromise, competent patients could enter into socially beneficial research if they did so autonomously and if there were sufficient protections built into the research process that would protect vulnerable patients. Society's need for research could be satisfied, but only if society respected the right of the patient to refuse to participate. Society could have the benefits of research but only if significant restrictions or obligations were imposed on the researcher.

Furthermore, the potential conflict of interest between the researcher's role as physician and his role as researcher could be resolved by rigorous attention to securing the free and informed consent of human subjects. We may call this the *informed consent compromise*. According to this compromise, the researcher is obligated to provide to the subject accurate information concerning all aspects of the research experiment or protocol and to guarantee to the subject that every reasonable effort will be made to protect him from harm. These obligations are imposed on the researcher by the society as a means of protecting the autonomy and the welfare of the human subject. This informed consent approach to human subject research has had a profound influence on the development of the hospital's policy. The emphasis on informed consent and the requirement to respect the individual's privacy and confidentiality are largely motivated by the belief that the ethical conflicts surrounding human research can be settled by respecting the autonomy of the research subjects. Furthermore, one can only respect the autonomy of the patient and secure the welfare of future patients by pursuing research based on the informed consent of the subjects.

## A Case Involving the Informed Consent Compromise

But the compromise still leaves a number of ethical questions unanswered, especially for research involving double-blind clinical trials. Indeed, we may say that this new clinical method is challenging the adequacy of the compromise. The following case is a good illustration of the problems associated with research and informed consent. We will appeal to it throughout this commentary.

In the late 1960s, oncological researchers began running clinical trials on osteosarcoma, a cancer that begins in the long bones of the body. Standard treatment at the time involved surgery. Evidence existed that treatment with chemotherapy (Adriamycin and methotrexate) offered some theoretical protection to the patient with undetected metastases (cells that spread cancer). If there were detectable metastases following surgery, then nothing except palliative treatment was offered. The patient died. Genuine controversy existed about whether the chemotherapy offered any protection beyond the benefits associated with surgery alone.

Patients whose cancer had not obviously metastasized (spread) were surgically treated for osteosarcoma. After surgery they were divided into two groups. Group A was given surgery with chemotherapy and group B was given surgical amputation alone. Random clinical trials were initiated comparing the two groups. These trials seemed to yield decisive results.

Members of group A had substantially superior results to those in group B. Consequently, by the early seventies, surgery in conjunction with chemotherapy became the standard of care for patients without metastases.

However, following the first clinical trials, a new diagnostic procedure, the CT scan, was developed that was far superior at detecting metastases following surgery. The improved diagnostic procedure immediately made many researchers skeptical of the original clinical trials, which were done with inferior X-ray methods. Critics argued that the results of the earlier clinical trials were potentially defective because they were based on an inferior diagnostic tool. Perhaps the chemotherapy was irrelevant to the improved results of those who received it. Perhaps those who died early in the first trial did so because the X-ray machines did not discover the metastases. These critics argued that if the more accurate CT scan were employed, then perhaps patients who had surgical amputation alone would have had better comparative results. Given the negative side effects of the chemotherapy, it was argued that amputation alone was a preferable treatment if the chemotherapy did not offer a significant advantage in terms of survival.

A new trial was therefore initiated using the CT scan to identify patients without metastases. This test would rule out the possibility that the chemotherapy was only apparently effective in extending the lives of those with osteosarcoma. Early in the clinical trial, interim results became available to the researchers. Only three patients receiving the chemotherapy had extension of the cancer. However, 22 out of 31 of those receiving amputation alone experienced spread of the disease. These interim results seemed to indicate that there was a clinical advantage to the chemotherapy.

### Three Problems with the Informed Consent Compromise

This case illustrates at least three different problems with the idea that informed consent can resolve the major ethical conflicts surrounding clinical research. First, such trials often proceed by attempting to show that there is a very low probability that the observed effects of the study are the result of something other than the treatment that is being studied. But what is this probability? And what kind of sample of the population constitutes an adequate basis for establishing this probability? How low does the probability have to be in order to be convincing? It is common among researchers to maintain that a probability of .05 is adequate to establish the effectiveness of a treatment. This means that there is a one-in-twenty chance that the results of the trial could be explained by another, as yet unconsidered, factor. But this decision to treat .05 as the indicator of effectiveness is somewhat arbitrary or conventional. It is easy to imagine a patient in the control group (perhaps receiving a placebo) of a clinical trial who is aware of interim results. If, at a certain point in the research, it becomes evident that there is a lower probability that the treatment is effective or preferable to the alternative, then some patients may wish to withdraw from a treatment early. They may also wish to be given the other treatment because *for them* a lower probability of effectiveness is good enough to warrant that they would be better off with the alternative treatment. The principle of informed consent is not usually interpreted as requiring the researcher to disclose his research conventions, so the informed consent compromise may not resolve the conflicts surrounding double-blind research. The decision to treat .05 probability as the indicator of effectiveness is a convention of science. Such conventions can themselves induce ethical conflict.

Our case illustrates a second inadequacy with the informed consent solution. It is easy to imagine that the individuals who were in the "surgery alone" arm of the second osteosarcoma clinical trial might well have wanted to know the interim results. With that information, they might well have decided to withdraw from the "surgery alone" arm of the clinical trial and request that they be given the chemotherapy. But if the actual practice specified in current informed consent documents is our guide, this interim information is not provided to these patients. Indeed, providing such information would undermine the double-blind validity of the study and undermine the scientific validity of the protocol. If it is to be a double-blind study, everyone must be ignorant of interim results. Revealing this information, according to many researchers, is unwise because early results may be invalidated by subsequent data; in effect, early results can be misleading. There are many possible reasons for thinking that the early results were skewed in favor of the chemotherapy, and most importantly, the sample results were not yet numerically adequate.

Third, the case illustrates the *problem of the null hypothesis*. Ethically legitimate trials involving human beings must satisfy the "null hypothesis" condition. A protocol satisfies the null hypothesis only if all arms of the protocol are therapeutically equal with respect to their treatment efficacy. This hypothesis is vital for the physician, who would be duty bound to advise a patient against entering a random clinical trial if one of the arms was known to be more effective than another. In order to recommend a clinical trial to a patient, the physician must have an argument that establishes the initial clinical equality of all arms of the research. Indeed, one can argue that the purpose of all clinical trials is the same: to show that the null hypothesis is false, that in fact one of the arms actually has better or worse results than its alternatives.

The difficulty with the null hypothesis is that there is some ambiguity about how to prove that the null hypothesis is initially satisfied. More importantly, the principle of informed consent does not require that the researcher establish for the patient that both treatments are equal. In other words, in the absence of clinical experimental information that the experiment is supposed to provide, how does the researcher prove that all arms are equal? Our osteosarcoma case illustrates this problem. It was clearly possible that the old X-ray machines used to detect the presence of metastases were inadequate. One might explain away the apparent benefits that accrued to patients who received both surgery and chemotherapy, as opposed to surgery alone, by saying the X-ray machines did not pick up hidden metastases. This is a possibility. But does this theoretical possibility satisfy the null hypothesis? Mere theoretical possibility is weak ground for establishing that two arms are equal. It is logically possible that cancer is caused by the relative position of the moon but that would not justify clinical trials to disprove the assumption. Surely it was logically possible that the CT scan would show that the early results were incorrect, but does the fact that an idea is logically possible or makes sense indicate that surgery alone was therapeutically equal to surgery plus chemotherapy even after the initial trials with the X-ray machine indicated that the chemotherapy arm was preferable?

Such problems indicate that there are some conflicts between the "autonomy-driven" rule of informed consent and the random clinical trial. One ordinarily does not withhold information from competent autonomous patients, nor does one ask such patients for permission to withhold relevant medical information from them. The principle of informed consent seems to require that physicians share important information with the patient, and the RCT seems to significantly limit the amount of information that one can give to a patient. Few researchers would maintain that persons in the clinical trial are entitled to be informed of interim results, because judgments of "clinical effectiveness" are professional or scientific judgments and not matters that patients are competent to determine. Researchers, who are reluctant to share this information, assume that these matters are scientific, rather than ethical, questions, and therefore they do not need to be shared with the human subject. Furthermore, such interim information may not be scientifically valid, given that it has not been developed from a completed scientific research. Interim results on a trial might indicate that a treatment has a high probability of being therapeutically preferable to its alternative, yet, in order that the trial be completed and the clinical evidence established, most professional researchers would not reveal this information to the human subjects. Early information can be invalidated by later test results.

Reluctance on the part of researchers to reveal interim results, however, seems to be inconsistent with the notion that informed consent on all relevant medical matters is required if the patient's autonomy is to be respected. The rule of informed consent, by itself, does not prove that patients have no right to this information, and yet this information is regularly omitted from informed consent documents.

## Clinical Trials as Waivers

The informed consent approach fails to address many of the problems with the random clinical trial because the rules of the "RCT game" prevent patients from obtaining information that is relevant for decision making. The random clinical trial itself seems to be based on the notion that, at the beginning of a trial, human subjects must waive their right to information. The patient must accept that the research committee will represent her interests against the interests of the future patients who may benefit from a completed trial. The research team is thus empowered to act for both the human subject and the community at large. Such empowerment is inconsistent with the notion that the individual should have the right to determine the ongoing course of her life. The research team continues to face a conflict of interest.

## Research Involving Children

The committee confronted the serious problems associated with research involving legally incompetent persons such as children. The ethicist and theologian Paul Ramsey expressed grave misgivings concerning nontherapeutic research involving children.[2] Nontherapeutic research is aimed at securing knowledge that may prove helpful to future patients. Its purpose is not to help the human subject. Ramsey argued that while research that has the possibility of benefiting a child (therapeutic research) is permitted, given the informed consent of the child's guardian, nontherapeutic research that is aimed at benefiting others is unethical because it involves using children as tools for securing the welfare of others. The general prohibition against using people without their consent argues against the use of children in nontherapeutic research. But no matter how well-intentioned the researcher may be, Ramsey contends that nontherapeutic research should only be open to adults since only the adult is competent to "become a joint adventurer in the common cause of medical research." To use children who cannot consent bypasses the requirement that we can expose children to risk only if the exposure is potentially *beneficial to them*. From Ramsey's viewpoint, it is fine for the physician-researcher to say to the adult, "I can no longer help you, but I would like you to help advance the course of science and assist future patients by participating in an experiment." The patient may voluntarily identify with the researcher's goals and consent to participate in this nontherapeutic research, but children cannot consent. Therefore, the physician should not even offer to enroll the child in such research. Finally, parents or surrogates may only consent for their children to participate in medical research that is aimed at securing some benefit for the child.

Ramsey illustrates this position by reference to the Willowbrook studies. Mentally retarded children were intentionally exposed to viral hepatitis so as to evaluate the effectiveness of gamma globulin in the treatment of the disease. The goal of these studies was to test, confirm, and improve the amount of gamma globulin that was necessary to secure temporary immunization against viral hepatitis. Because the infection was rampant in hospitals for the mentally handicapped, it was argued that no additional harm was done to the children because they would in all likelihood have contracted the disease merely by being a resident of the hospital.

Gamma globulin was known to be a somewhat effective agent against the disease, but in order to improve immunizations for future potential victims of this disease, researchers designed a study to discover how effective it was and at what doses. This research required control groups, which meant that gamma globulin was withheld from specific children even though researchers knew of its value. By inducing the virus into children who had been given the gamma globulin, researchers hoped to test and improve the inoculum. Ramsey admits that the parents of these children had consented to the treatment and that many of the children at Willowbrook were exposed to and contracted the disease simply because they were exposed to other children who were infected. He also admits that the results of the tests were scientifically useful because they verified that higher doses of gamma globulin induced a higher degree of immunity against the disease. The tests improved the vaccine and thereby contributed to the welfare of future children. But incompetent human subjects were intentionally harmed by the research. He also maintains that some of the information uncovered by the Willowbrook study could have been secured by using adults who were exposed to the disease. Adults are preferable because, unlike children, they can give or withhold their consent. If adults had been employed, then the information gleaned from the research could have been applied to the cases of children. But the major issue in the case is that, for Ramsey, no amount of consent on the part of parents justified the intentional exposure of children to the hepatitis virus. This is a disease that threatens the welfare of children. Although the authority of parents over their children is extensive, it does not extend to authorizing acts that harm the children or place them at significant risk of harm.

This position has its origins in the Nuremberg trials following World War II. The trials revealed that thousands of involuntary human subjects, including children and legally incompetent people, had died at the hands of Nazi researchers. *The Nuremberg Code* affirmed that the voluntary consent of the subject in medical research was "absolutely essential" and that the legal ability to give consent was therefore necessary. However, this view that consent was absolutely necessary was described by Franz Ingelfinger, former editor of *The New England Journal of Medicine,* as "extremist." He argued that if one accepted Ramsey's view, then one must condemn vast amounts of nontherapeutic pediatric research that involved only minimal risk. Are skin pricks with needles or venipuncture done in the course of nontherapeutic research immoral? If so, then many advances made in pediatric medicine must be viewed as having as immoral a basis as Nazi research. Ingelfinger argued for a compromise position that was largely adopted by the United States Food and Drug Administration (FDA). This compromise position asserts that where the risks to children are minimal and the potential benefit to children, as a class, is substantial, then the FDA will permit guardians to consent for their children to participate in nontherapeutic research involving minimal risk. A minimal risk is defined as involving the kinds of risks that ordinary daily activities involve. Government regulations seldom contain philosophical justifications for their principles, but we can turn to the work of the philosopher-theologian Richard McCormick as a possible basis for understanding the federal rules on children and nontherapeutic research.

According to McCormick, proxy consent is legitimate in some nontherapeutic research but only where the harm resulting from the research is minimal. His reasoning is tied to a view of justice. He claims that in a situation when a child's life could only be saved if he were given a blood donation from another child, then it would be permissible to transfuse the child donor. The benefits would be enormous for the recipient and the harm to the donor would be minimal. He thinks that, in this situation, refusing to transfuse the blood would require us to assume that the donating child would actually refuse to give the blood if he were of legal age, an assumption that cannot be proven. Parents can decide that the child would wish to donate his blood in order to save a dying person. But in addition to the presumed consent argument, McCormick also argues that there is a moral tradition, called the *natural law tradition,* that affirms that the child "ought to" choose to support the natural good of another's life. This natural law tradition assumes that men and women have moral duties to aid and support one another, and because participating in research involves aiding and supporting others, it follows that all people have the duty to participate in research. Therefore, with the parent's consent, we may submit children to minimal-risk, nontherapeutic research based on this presumed duty that all people have to come to the aid of others.

One difficulty with this last view is that McCormick does not spell out the extent of one's moral duty to others. Nor does he spell out why adults can exercise their voluntary control to refuse to aid others. One would think that if adults, like children, have a duty to aid others, then the rule of autonomy should not extend to them the right to say "no" if a researcher asks them to participate in a research program. If it is a moral duty, then presumably one does not have the moral right to refuse to do it. Yet, for McCormick, apparently adults do have such a right. In effect, by granting the right to refuse to participate in research that aids others, it seems as if our society is refusing to recognize a general duty to aid others by participating in human subject research.

## Research Involving Animals

Community Hospital's policy opens with a quote supporting the necessity for animal research. However, since vast amounts of important medical research subjects animals to treatments that cause suffering and death, animals have claims against us to avoid unnecessary suffering. In Western culture, it is common to assume that human beings occupy not only the center stage in ethics but also the entire stage in bioethics. This means that there are no other beings that are *intrinsically* valuable except humans. The roots of this belief are deep in Western thought and especially the Judeo-Christian heritage. The Bible views animals as "given to humans by God." In Western religion, animals were instruments that humans were free to use. Animals were only extrinsically valuable. This view is compatible with traditional consequentialists, who maintained that only human beings needed to be taken into consideration when one assesses the moral worth of an action or an object. Actions were right or wrong if they maximized good for the greatest number of *people*.

Rights-based theorists held a similar view toward animals. It is men and women that have rights, not animals, insects, plants, or the natural world. Persons could not be used without their consent, but this principle was certainly irrelevant to animals since securing the consent of animals was impossible. Rights emerged from being a person. Nonhumans were not persons; therefore, they had no rights. Because nonhumans had no rights, others had no obligations toward them.

## The Rights of Animals

A number of contemporary philosophers have challenged these Western assumptions about animals. Perhaps the best-known philosophical critic among them is the philosopher Tom Regan. Regan argues that animals can be treated as having no intrinsic value only if we can show that there is an *ethically relevant difference between the animals and humans*. This rule requires us to justify differences in the way we treat individuals by proving that there is an ethically relevant difference between them. For example, you can throw away a piece of paper but you cannot throw away a human being; the human has consciousness, can reason and experience pain, but paper has none of these ethically relevant properties. If we can run experiments on chimpanzees that harm and kill them, but we cannot do this to humans, then there must be an ethically relevant difference between the chimpanzees and the humans. But Regan argues that all of the supposed differences between chimps and humans are "arbitrary," and hence not ethically relevant. For example, one could argue that it is legal to harm and kill animals for research purposes but illegal to harm and kill humans. However, that illegality must be regarded as an irrelevant difference since slavery was legal in 1860 in the United States and equating legal differences with ethical differences would have ethically justified slavery. For Regan, legal differences may correlate with ethical differences, but they do not have to.

One might then turn to the intellectual differences between chimpanzees and humans. Chimps are simply intellectually inferior to humans, and this intellectual inferiority is the ethically relevant difference that justifies the use of animals in research. This was, for example, Immanuel Kant's position. Animals lacked rationality and thus they were not moral agents who demanded respect. Regan's response is that permanently incompetent humans—for example, those in a persistent vegetative state—are intellectually inferior not only to humans, but also to chimpanzees, and yet we do not allow the use of incompetent humans in nontherapeutic harmful research. In short, if we accepted the idea that intellectual inferiority was a difference that justified the use of animals in research, then we would have to permit using incompetent or profoundly retarded humans in research.

Furthermore, if one accepted the principle that superiority of intelligence justified using individuals in nontherapeutic and harmful research, then we would have to say that it would be morally and ethically permitted for intellectually superior aliens from another planet to use us. But even if these aliens were far superior to us, this would not lead any of us to assume that they had the right to use us for their medical research. The conclusion of this argument is that, for Regan, there are no nonarbitrary differences between animals and humans that justify our use of animals in medical research.

Regan's positive view of animals is that animals are the subjects of a life. That is, they are able to experience their lives as faring well or ill. This ability to experience is what unites animals with human beings and it is why most of us think that human beings are inherently valuable. According to Regan, this trait is also something that ethically differentiates plant life from animal life. While it is unethical to experiment using animals, it is morally permissible to experiment on plants.

## The Traditional Arguments

Regan's arguments challenge the fundamental views of the hospital and the research community as a whole. Although a full and complete defense of the committee's decision to allow animal research under government-controlled supervision is impractical, some defense is necessary. The basic argument supporting the animal rights position is that animals have consciousness and, therefore, deserve respect. However, this argument brings in a slippery slope consideration. If we are obligated to respect chimpanzees, then the same arguments require us to respect dogs, cats, mice, rats, and fish. Perhaps even plants, bacteria, and viruses have consciousness. Consciousness is a vague property, and although Regan thinks that it is "arbitrary" to respect only humans, he maintains that we need not show respect to certain other living things such as plants or fish. Regan himself does not offer a precise criterion for where we should cut off our respect. He admits that where we draw the line "is certain to be controversial." The ethics committee held that as long as the animal rights position involved arbitrary commitments, their claim that "the traditional position was arbitrary" lacked sufficient reason. If both positions contain arbitrary aspects, then neither position can be criticized for being arbitrary since what counts against all participants in a debate counts against none of them. In summary, because consciousness is a very vague property, it seems that opening the door to the higher primates would push our culture down a slippery slope that would require us to respect beings such as bacteria or viruses.

# The Case of Herpes Simplex Encephalitis

This case is a famous nonfictional one that took place in 1977 and precipitated much debate during the 1980s. It continues to trouble many members of institutional review boards and hospital ethics committees. We will assume that the trial is being run at Community Hospital and that the members of our fictional committee must address the issues in the case.

Herpes simplex encephalitis is a disease that leads to brain and nerve damage and death. A new drug called ara-A has been developed that appears to be effective in the treatment of the disease. A clinical trial is being run at Community Hospital and two of the members of the research team have brought a number of ethical concerns to the hospital ethics committee. The critics of the research, Dr. Penner and Nurse Dorn, are both participating in the research in that their patients are part of the trial. Dr. Harding represents the majority of researchers at the hospital who support the continuation of the trial. The trial was originally approved by the ethics committee in a somewhat perfunctory fashion.

The major concern of the critics of the clinical trial is that, since there is no cure for this form of encephalitis and since death or significant impairment will likely result, then it is wrong to place some individuals on the placebo arm of the experiment. This is the group that will not receive ara-A. The progress of those on this control arm will be compared to those who receive ara-A. Despite this consideration, the trial was initiated and is continuing at the hospital. Preliminary data indicate that ara-A is effective, but this is unconvincing to many of the statisticians who are in charge of the protocol. Dr. Penner and Nurse Dorn want the study immediately closed so that everyone in the control group can be switched over to ara-A.

## Committee Discussion of the Case

| Dr. Mary Collins: (Chair) | Let me open this meeting by indicating that this is not the first time this committee has addressed this clinical trial.  Twelve weeks ago this protocol came before this committee, and it was one of 11 protocols that were approved during that one-and-a-half-hour committee meeting. We reviewed the informed consent document, and, on the surface, it appeared similar to hundreds of other protocols that we somewhat mechanically review and approve. Dr. Harding, who is a member of our medical staff, made the presentation at that time, and he is also present with us today. He is ready to answer any questions that you might have regarding this protocol. |
| --- | --- |
| | At the meeting six weeks ago, there was little or no substantive discussion of the critical issues in the case. We approved the protocol. However, Dr. Penner, who is a member of Dr. Harding's research team, called me last Sunday and raised a number of substantial and very disturbing aspects of this clinical trial. I want to note that this committee has ponderous responsibilities and that, despite the fact that we are all pressed for time, we cannot avoid our |

responsibilities to patients and researchers who depend on us to provide a careful and rigorous ethical review of the clinical experiments that take place here at Community Hospital. We may have "rubber-stamped" this one!

Prof. Carla Thomas:

Dr. Collins, are you saying that we screwed up in the initial approval of the protocol?

Dr. Collins:

I am not saying that. I voted to approve the trial last time and I may well vote in a similar way at the end of today's meeting. However, it seems clear to me that we approved this trial without addressing some of the important ethical issues in the case, and that very much disturbs me. The agenda for that meeting was enormous. We reviewed 11 protocols and my fear is that we were rubber-stamping these experiments and not giving them a careful reading. There were relevant issues that were simply not even raised at the first meeting. In that sense, I want to say that we may have been unresponsive to our duties.

Atty. John Quinn:

I, for one, am happy that these proceedings are not being recorded, and I would definitely recommend that we avoid inserting any of Dr. Collins's personal judgments into the minutes of the meeting. I certainly do not feel that we were derelict in our duty with respect to this case. If we have more information in our hands today, then perhaps we want to revise our judgment. There is nothing wrong with reviewing and revising our judgment in the light of new information. What I am concerned about is the possibility that the hospital may be liable if this committee openly admits, without careful reflection, that we were derelict in our duty.

Prof. Thomas:

Once again, Atty. Quinn is anxious to protect the hospital against any and all possible threats of litigation. And we respect that quality in John, but if this committee is rubber-stamping and thereby avoiding its responsibility to protect the rights of patients, then perhaps we are being derelict. I remember that meeting. I too felt that we had to cover a great deal of territory in a very limited amount of time. Now it seems as if some critical issues were overlooked. I think we need to look long and hard at our very limited ability to carefully review these protocols. Maybe we cannot do a responsible job and still cover 11 protocols in a span of a one-and-a-half-hour meeting.

Vivian Harris:

I felt very rushed at that meeting too. There were technical issues that came up that I needed to be informed about and the shortage of time made that impossible. I felt that if I asked another question, I would be shot by those of you who had to move on to your other duties and by researchers who were anxious to get approval for their protocols so that they could begin their research. I simply did not understand some of the medical and statistical information. However, if I am going to vote responsibly on these protocols, I think that the members of the committee with the technical know-how are going to have to spend more time educating those of us who need it. If the government and the society want us to review these experiments, and if we agreed to do this work, then perhaps we simply have to make a bigger commitment of time to this review process. Finally, we have to avoid covering such a large number of protocols in one meeting.

Dr. Collins:

I am glad that many of you feel as I do that we need to spend more time on each protocol. Rather than meeting every six weeks, perhaps we need to meet monthly.

| | |
|---|---|
| Prof. Martin Fisk: | Perhaps we can postpone this decision. I know that all of us are swamped with duties and that our schedules are already packed. I might suggest that we respond not by increasing our meetings, but by decreasing the protocols that are employed at the hospital. |
| Dr. Philip Davis: | But, Martin, that will decrease the quality of care at the hospital. |
| Dr. Collins: | We do not need to solve this problem right now. Allow me to turn the meeting over to Dr. Penner and Nurse Dorn so that they can express their concerns regarding the ara-A protocol that we approved at our last meeting. |
| Dr. Penner: | Thank you, Dr. Collins. Let me begin by telling you what I told Dr. Collins last Sunday. Right now, there is little other than palliative treatment that we can offer to victims of herpes simplex encephalitis. Nearly 70 percent of those who contract the disease will die, and nearly all of those who survive will be severely impaired for life.

At your last meeting, the head of our research team, Dr. Harding, made the presentation in favor of ara-A. Even at that time, we were in substantial disagreement over this issue. Dr. Harding feels that without a clinical trial that empirically proves the effectiveness of ara-A, we cannot assume that ara-A is in any way effective against herpes simplex viral encephalitis. He argues that there are hundreds of cases of drugs that looked promising at the beginning of a study that turned out to be useless. Six weeks ago I thought that there was some evidence in support of ara-A and that I would have trouble recommending to my patients any course of action other than ara-A. I expressed my views to him but did not choose to engage the committee with my concerns. |

| Dr. Harding: | Dr. Penner, how can you recommend to a patient a course of treatment that has not been empirically proven to be useful? Medicine is not an occult skill that you pick up in medical school. You have no mystical skill that can detect the medical utility of a drug. The random clinical trial is not a secret method but a mere statistically driven mechanism that is currently the best tool that we have for determining clinical effectiveness. At this time the trial is incomplete, so we cannot determine that the consequences of ara-A are beneficial. |
|---|---|
| Dr. Penner: | There was some evidence for its effectiveness. The drug is one of the most exciting drugs in medicine at this time precisely because it has been shown to be effective against other forms of herpes infections. At this point, I made a clinical judgment. I believed that there was sufficient similarity between herpes simplex encephalitis and these other viruses. Based on this similarity, I judged that ara-A was our best approach to treating patients who are afflicted with this terrible disease. |
| Dr. Collins: | Dr. Penner, you say that you formed a clinical judgment in this case. I thought that you were doing research and that what we wanted you to do was develop research judgments. Do you see a conflict between your role as researcher and your role as a clinician? |
| Dr. Penner: | Yes, there is an eternal conflict between these roles. More important, there is no obviously rational way to resolve this conflict. The two professions have different goals, and when researchers are also clinicians, then there is deep and profound conflict. Researchers take the welfare of future patients as primary, while clinicians take the welfare of present patients as primary. All of us have to decide which is |

more important to us, present patients or future patients. I promised myself when I started doing research that I would never let future patients override my commitment to the patient who is sitting in front of me. The physician can never let the researcher's imperative override his commitment to the patient. For me this would involve bad faith.

Dr. Collins:

I see your point. But what do you mean by a clinical judgment? I thought clinical judgments were ones that were based on solid empirical evidence. It seems that in this case your judgment that we should offer ara-A was not grounded on such solid empirical evidence.

Dr. Penner:

I admit that I did not have clinical evidence for my view. Six weeks ago, I decided to participate in the study only if I could get my patients into the ara-A arm. But since this would obviously destroy the double-blind character of the research, I could not participate.

Dr. Davis:

As a consequence, none of your patients have any access to the clinical trial. Do you think that it is in their best interest to be locked out of access to this potentially beneficial drug because you cannot violate your promises to yourself?

Dr. Penner:

That is something that I have had to grapple with in my own mind, but I cannot compromise on this issue.

Dr. Davis:

Why couldn't you offer your patients the opportunity to decide for themselves?

Dr. Penner:

Look, as a physician, except in rare cases, I do not offer my patients choices among treatments. I usually make the treatment decision that is in the best interest of my patient. If the patient has a problem with my recommendations, then we negotiate. I do my best to listen, and we usually come up with a resolution that both of us can live with. But if I think that ara-A is my drug of choice, then it would be wrong to recommend anything but ara-A as my first choice. Offering them the possibility of a placebo, which I know does not work, seemed wrong when I believed that ara-A was best.

Dr. Davis:

But why couldn't you let your patients make the critical decision?

Dr. Penner:

Because this is not a matter that can be solved merely by respecting the autonomy of the patients. The issue at debate between Dr. Harding and myself is not a debate over patient rights. It is a debate over whether it is ethically permissible to run a random clinical trial on ara-A. My answer is no! Such a random clinical trial involves withholding a treatment from a group of living people who could, in my clinical opinion, benefit from the treatment. We are, in effect, using these people in order to help others, and that seems wrong to me. It violates my commitment to aid those who are ill and provide for them the best treatment.

Furthermore, the trial itself seems wrong because there are other control groups available to us.

Dr. Davis:

You are referring to the use of historical control groups—people who have already died of herpes simplex encephalitis.

Dr. Penner:

Yes! There are hundreds of well-documented cases of herpes simplex encephalitis in historical records of the disease. The course of untreated herpes simplex encephalitis is well known. These historical control groups are minimally adequate as a basis of comparison, especially in the case of diseases that have death or significant impairment as the end point of the disease process. I agree that there are many methodological shortcomings associated with historical control groups, not the least of which is that we might not be sure that some members of these historical groups actually had the disease in question. We may need to limit these groups to individuals who had well-documented cases of the disease.

Dr. Harding: I do not need to remind you that there are over one hundred years of medical research that are inconsistent with this suggestion.

Mary Quigley: Are you saying that we do not need to use living people in order to discover the efficacy of a drug?

Dr. Penner: In cases where death is the end point of the disease, we could use these historical control groups as a basis of determining the utility of ara-A.

Dr. Harding: There are a hundred years of clinical research that warn against the use of historical control groups. The quality of the research is definitely decreased by the use of this approach.

Marian Rhodes: But, Dr. Harding, aren't you potentially sacrificing people's lives in order to secure high-quality research? Isn't it permissible to trade off a little research quality for the sake of avoiding unnecessary loss of life?

Dr. Harding: This is a very large issue. To explain fully, I would need to give you a defense of clinical trials in general and a justification for why they are superior in comparison with historical groups. This is something that we just cannot do in this limited context.

Dr. Penner: Please don't misunderstand my view. Harding is right! Clinical trials in which drug treatments are compared with living control groups are intellectually preferable to comparison with historical groups. I would never dispute this. My view is merely that, although historical control groups are intellectually inferior to clinical trials, they are still "good enough," especially in cases where death or significant impairment is the expected end point of the disease process.

Ms. Rhodes:

It seems to me that, if we had only one arm in the test and gave everyone ara-A and found that we had better results than we had in the past, then we would know that we had the better treatment.

Rev. Richard Marcus:

We are breaking one of the unwritten rules of this committee by jumping immediately into the discussion of the case. Shouldn't we allow for the members of the committee to ask their informational questions before we get into substantive discussion?

Dr. Collins:

Yes! Thank you, Rev. Marcus, for reminding me. I am afraid that I have entered into the discussion prior to entertaining questions. If any of you have questions, please ask them.

Prof. Martin Fisk:

What is it that is making the statisticians reluctant to close the study? Are there any negative side effects associated with taking ara-A and is there any way of taking these side effects into consideration in evaluating the treatment's effectiveness? My concern here is that American medicine is famous for extending the length of life and in the process extending the dying process. In short, do the random clinical trial evaluators take quality of life into consideration in evaluating the results of a trial?

Prof. Carla Thomas:

I know that the scientific literature contains a number of criticisms of the random clinical trial. Are there any systematic alternatives to this kind of trial that are

|  | being considered by the scientific community that do not have the ethical shortcomings of the random clinical trial? |
|---|---|
| Dr. Davis: | I spend my life as a practitioner of medicine. I am not a researcher, though I have participated in a number of research protocols. Research seems very precise, and taking care of sick people has always seemed very imprecise. It is "messy," if you will. How can we be confident, given the differences between messy practice and precise clinical trials, that the results provided by the precise research tools are going to be good predictors of what will happen in the messy imprecise world of clinical management? The RCT may not simulate the management of patients in the real world of medical practice. |
| Dr. Collins: | Are there any other questions? If there are none, I am going to ask Drs. Penner and Harding to respond to the questions. Dr. Harding, will you start? |
| Dr. Harding: | Let me open up by responding to Dr. Davis. I agree with you that the management of patients is a far more complicated affair than running clinical trials. There is an artistic side to patient care that involves appreciation of the individual. Clinical trials do not provide information about the individual patient. They provide information only about classes of individuals. For that reason I also agree with you that clinical trials are not exact replicas of the problems faced by clinicians in the field. However, the patients in any good RCT are *randomly selected*. If they are not, then the quality of the study decreases. This randomness provides a lot of variation or what Dr. Davis calls "messiness." This variation or "messiness" in the subjects is precisely what bestows validity on the study. I agree |

that the variation provided by the clinical trial is not as great as that found in a busy clinician's office, but it is adequate to warrant saying that a treatment is effective. Finally, Dr. Davis knows that patients on protocols exhibit a high degree of variation and complications. It is because of this that we can have some degree of confidence that the drug that is being studied will be effective in the clinical setting.

Dr. Collins:

Can we take the questions in order? What about Prof. Fisk's questions regarding the statisticians' problems?

Dr. Penner:

Let me try to explain the statistical problem. We have entered 28 patients on the protocol. Ten have received the placebo, which is equivalent to doing nothing—which is what we now do. Eighteen have received ara-A. So far we have had seven deaths on the placebo and five on the ara-A. We have had six people on ara-A suffer some severe damage and one person on the placebo has suffered severe damage. Seven of the 18 on the ara-A have returned to reasonably normal health and only two on the placebo have returned to normal health. I am recommending that we immediately close the protocol and give everyone ara-A.

But the statisticians do not agree. They argue that we simply do not have a large enough sample to justify a judgment that ara-A is effective. They argue that we need to look at more people. For example, one additional recovery among those receiving the placebo would make the results profoundly indeterminate. This suggests to them that we do not yet have enough evidence to indicate that ara-A is actually effective.

Prof. Fisk:

How do you respond, Dr. Penner, to the claim that the research is not complete?

| | |
|---|---|
| Dr. Penner: | I think that there is enough evidence *for me*. I am a clinician, not a statistician, and as such, my standards for being convinced are lower than the statistician's. There is enough evidence for me. |
| Prof. Fisk: | You mean that standards of what counts as "sufficient or adequate evidence" are relative to what profession a person belongs to? This seems counterintuitive to me. Are there different standards of evidence for every profession? What is the standard for hairdressers? |
| Dr. Penner: | I knew that this idea would scandalize a philosopher but, nevertheless, that is what I mean. Professions are, in my opinion, a bit like cultures. They differ in their standards of moral correctness. Statisticians hate being wrong and so they set up high standards before they put their reputations on the line. They want to ape mathematical exactitude. The self-image of the physician is not, however, determined by mathematics. The physician is more willing to risk being wrong in order to save a human life. Society permits and, I think, encourages this kind of risk taking on the part of physicians. |
| Ms. Quigley: | What about revealing this information to the patients and letting them decide? |
| Dr. Harding: | That would destroy the double-blind character of the test and, in the process, destroy the scientific validity of the clinical trial. |
| Ms. Quigley: | Would this completely annihilate any validity or would it merely decrease validity? |
| Dr. Harding: | My response is that the experiment would have no validity if the patients were informed prior to closure. It would lose its double-blind character. With respect to Dr. |

Penner's claim that he is convinced that ara-A is effective, I simply do not understand how one can be so loose with one's convictions. He is adopting a very weak standard of proof and that is inconsistent with the scientific approach. What happened to the skeptical attitude that your research education tried to instill in you, Dr. Penner? I know that you want to believe that ara-A is effective. I also want to believe this. I, too, would like to think that we have a solution to a horrible affliction, but I will not yet concede that ara-A is any better than snake oil. Until the completion of the protocol, I regard ara-A as being clinically equal to doing nothing. I hope that the test will undermine the hypothesis of clinical equality, but it seems to me that the data are as yet insufficient to establish this claim. It could be a matter of luck that seven patients on ara-A have recovered.

Let me now turn to the question raised by Rev. Marcus regarding side effects. As you can see, the side effects of ara-A at this point are significant. If we continue the study, we may get more information about these effects. We may even learn something about managing them. We may even come to the position that the clinical side effects are so profound that, even if life is preserved with ara-A, it may be in such a compromised form that many patients and clinicians may choose not to use the drug. I think that determining the kind of side effects and the severity of these side effects is an essential aim of human subject research, and that we cannot determine these effects without completing the study.

Regarding alternatives to the random clinical trial, I am not the one to speak to that issue because I am so convinced that where it is feasible, the double-blind random clinical trial is the best mechanism available for clinical research. It corrects for bias in ways that are, to my mind, excellent. But perhaps Dr. Penner can give you an alternative that is receiving some hearing in the research literature.

Dr. Penner:
Well, to begin with, there are lots of single-blind and no-blind studies that go on in the Western world. Furthermore, historical controls may be an alternative to using living persons as control groups.

Nurse Dorn:
This last alternative is the one that we recommend in this ara-A case, since death or significant harm is the end result of this disease. We dissenters on the research team believe that we already know what the result of doing nothing will be for those suffering from herpes simplex encephalitis. Doing nothing will be worthless. On the basis of the literature, we can apply ara-A and compare it with doing nothing and then decide whether ara-A represents a better alternative. We do not need a face-to-face confrontation.

Ms. Quigley:
I would like to make a comment about Dr. Harding's refusal to inform the patients about interim information. I think there are some real problems with this. At the beginning of the experiment, you tell the patient that he has every right to withdraw at any time and then you withhold from the patient the information that he might use as a basis for withdrawal.

Don't you see any conflict in this approach?

Dr. Harding:
I see your point. But I think that as long as the subject is informed that no interim information will be shared with him, then I do not think that any violation of patient's rights is committed.

Nurse Dorn:
You require then that patients who are entering protocols waive their right to

information that may positively affect the course of their lives and may even prevent their deaths. They have to give up quite a bit in order to get your experimental drugs, don't they?

Dr. Penner:    Allow me to say something more about alternatives to the random clinical trial. There is another statistical approach that attempts to avoid some of the negative consequences of the random clinical trial. We can call it the "play the winner" strategy. It was developed by Zelen. This strategy is not fit for all protocols but is appropriate in research contexts where the outcome is known soon after randomization and application of a treatment. It involves assigning the first member of a study group randomly to one or more arms of a study. That single patient is then followed. If he does well, then that arm is called "the winner" and there is an increased probability that the next patient will be assigned to the winning arm. The opposite also holds true. If the patient does poorly on a given arm, then the next patient has an increased chance of being assigned to the alternative arm of the study. Researches determine likelihood of assignment. This technique is illustrated in a study of respiratory failure in newborns.[7]

Dr. Harding:    Regarding Dr. Davis's question that the random clinical trial does not simulate clinical practice because the former is so precise and the latter so imprecise—so human, if you will. I agree that the clinical trial is mathematically precise and that there is little in clinical practice that simulates this kind of precision. But the randomization is exactly aimed at modeling some of what you call the "messy" aspects of clinical care. For example, by randomizing patients you may wind up inserting into control groups individuals who have characteristics that make the placebo seem effective. Randomizing messes things up, and that is why it is so essential within clinical trials. In short, I do not think that the trial is completely different from messy clinical practice.

I understand what Dr. Penner has said about the difference between statistics and clinical medicine. I agree with him totally that we clinicians do not need to be controlled by statisticians *in every case*. But this case is one that is not, in my opinion, a close call. We do need to enter more people onto this protocol before we can justifiably judge that the medication is effective. We simply do not have a large enough sample to make an efficacy judgment.

Dr. Collins:

I realize that we could discuss these questions forever, but we need to get directly to our case. Are there any motions regarding the case?

Prof. Fisk:

Well, it seems as if there is more than one question facing this committee, and so more than one motion may have to be offered. We are being asked whether the initial approval of the protocol was right, given that there is no alternative to ara-A and that the likelihood of death without ara-A is so high. Second, we are being asked whether it is permissible to close this study given the interim information, which Dr. Harding and Dr. Penner interpret differently. Finally, we are also being asked whether it is permissible to reveal interim information to patients who are on the placebo arm of the protocol, so that they may exercise their right to withdraw.

I think that there are probably other issues in the case that may emerge, but if we could address these three matters, then we would be doing a decent job.

| | |
|---|---|
| Rev. Marcus: | I am ready to offer a motion on the first question. The initial approval of the case was based on the assumption that there was no alternative to the clinical trial to establish clinical effectiveness. We now have a number of possible alternatives, most importantly the "historical controls" model. In future protocols involving experiments that have death or severe harm as a consequence, I think that we need to look at the historical control approach. I think that we need to communicate our ethical interest in the historical control model to national research centers and advise them that we want them to seriously consider this model as well as other alternatives to the random clinical trial. But we are not yet prepared to enter into this novel form of testing, and we need to have this alternative explored. I support it, but I support it because it avoids placing individuals on placebos when we think that the ara-A may be effective. But I think that the historical control group approach needs to be studied. We cannot endorse it without further inquiry. I move that we approve the ara-A random clinical trial and inform the research agency that submitted it to us that we think a historical control group approach is worth considering. |
| Dr. Collins: | Is there any discussion of Rev. Marcus's motion? |
| Ms. Harris: | I do not know whether I can support Marcus's motion because we at this table are not competent to evaluate the technical issues that separate Drs. Penner and Harding. What separates them is whether there is clinical equality between the placebo and the ara-A arms. Harding says there is clinical equality and Penner says no! I am not competent to settle this technical debate. I must say I lean toward Penner, |

|  | but I am not confident in this opinion at all and I am not sure that I am properly educated to make this judgment. |
| Prof. Thomas: | Vivian, think about it! Who bears the burden of proof? If Harding were coming before us for the first time, would we require him to establish that there is a clinical equality between the proposed arms of the trial? We must do this since in the absence of clinical equality we could not randomly insert people into the various arms. We would have to insert them into the one that we thought was best. If you cannot tell whether there is clinical equality, then you cannot approve the trial since clinical equality must be proven before you can approve any trial. Harding bears the burden of proof and he has not established the clinical equality to you; hence, you cannot approve it. |
| Ms. Harris: | Carla, your point is well made but you missed my drift. The lay persons and, indeed, some of the clinicians at this table, by their own admission, are not able to judge the question of clinical equality. My question is whether we should be responsible for adjudicating matters about which we are not competent. |
| Dr. Collins: | Wait a minute now! The federal Food and Drug Administration created institutional review boards (IRBs) to review human subject research protocols in order to protect the rights and the welfare of human subjects. The feds want us to judge whether any individual rights are being violated in this protocol, and they also want us to judge whether the welfare of patients is undermined by this protocol. The FDA wants you to call it the way you see it just as you would if you were on a trial where technical issues came up. I am saying that |

you should do your best to understand the issues and then call it the way you see it.

Prof. Fisk:  I think that, due to the pressure of time and our very busy schedules, we failed to have a thorough discussion of the important ethical issues in the ara-A protocol six weeks ago. Despite the fact that the "historical controls alternative" is possible, the research community is not yet ready to adopt it. This might be a better alternative, but we cannot withhold approval from the ara-A protocol merely because the research community is not giving sufficient attention to the historical approach. I think that we need to continue the fight for using historical controls in cases where death or significant harm is the end point of the disease, but we cannot withhold approval from the ara-A protocol as a means of protest. The more difficult question for me is this business about the interim information. There is some indication that ara-A is effective. The problem for me is whether I can agree to sacrifice the statistical standards of proof out of compassion for these human subjects.

Dr. Harding:  You of all people, Martin, should not need to be reminded of the philosopher Descartes. I know that he is one of your philosophical heroes. He was not only one of the fathers of modern philosophy but also one of the fathers of modern science precisely because he taught us the importance of being skeptical about what we observe. Skepticism is not just at the roots of philosophy but also at the roots of good clinical science. Scientists know better than any of us how easily humans are deceived by initial appearances. I admit that ara-A looks good at this point, but there are hundreds of other drugs that looked good at the initial stages of a trial but turned out to be useless by the time the trial was completed. We know from past experience that initial appearances can be deceptive. These ara-A appearances are initial appearances and so we need to be skeptical of them. Descartes would recommend that if we might be wrong about a result, we need to be skeptical of it until we are more certain. The best thing that we can do for people is to follow Descartes's advice and retain our skepticism about these results.

Prof. Thomas: It is one thing to be skeptical about theoretical matters but quite another to be skeptical about matters pertaining to an individual's life and welfare. I can easily imagine that a physician would believe that we have not statistically established that ara-A is effective but that there is enough anecdotal evidence to convince the physician or the patient that ara-A represents his patient's best option among relatively poor options. The fact that the patient has few, if any, acceptable options changes the clinical context.

Where death is the only alternative to using an unproven drug, perhaps we need to avoid establishing objective standards of clinical efficacy and allow the patient and his physician to make an autonomous decision as to what constitutes enough evidence.

Ms. Rhodes: Professor Thomas's point about letting the patient and the physician jointly decide intrigues me. But does that mean that you would vote against closing the study and giving everyone in the control group ara-A?

Prof. Thomas: Yes! I think we must end the study as a double-blind study, but I think that we simply need to get used to the idea of sacrificing some clinical certainty for the sake of an ethical value. Many people may

decide to stay with the placebo, and I think
that is fine as long as they are given the
facts and the options. Indeed, I would
recommend the following motion.

## Committee Recommendations

| | |
|---|---|
| Prof. Thomas: | I move that we inform all participants in the ara-A study of the interim information and allow them to decide if they wish to continue in the study. |
| Dr. Collins: | I take it that Carla's motion allows us to continue the study on the condition that the subjects be informed about the interim data and that they be given the opportunity to withdraw and receive the ara-A. We have not usually followed Robert's rules in these meetings, but I would like to see if there is any initial support for this idea by asking for a second to the motion. |
| Ms. Quigley: | I second the motion. |
| Dr. Collins: | Can we have some discussion of this motion? |
| Dr. Harding: | But the data become invalid if the double-blind aspect is lost. |
| Prof. Thomas: | That is our decision to read the data as invalid if the double-blind aspect is lost. We can change our decision. |
| Dr. Harding: | That is a scientific question, Carla. The institutional review board considers ethical issues, not scientific issues. You are crossing the boundary between science and ethics and that bothers me. You are not authorized to determine whether the data are valid or invalid. You are not a scientist. |
| Dr. Davis: | What are the possible implications of going this route? Let's not do something before we consider the consequences. |

Dr. Harding:    I cannot be sure, but if you do this without the support of the national group that originated this study, they may well choose to reconsider their decision to use this hospital as a research site. How can they continue to use the hospital for research if we are going to violate their disclosure rules, which they consider essential for doing good science? Clinical research is a bit like a game in the sense that a group of people cooperate with one another, according to a set of predetermined rules. Research agencies send us promising new drugs if we consent to cooperate with their ground rules. Revealing this interim information to patients violates their ground rules. Would you continue to play with someone who violated the rules?

Ms. Quigley:    I am a businesswoman, Dr. Harding, and I am pretty good at recognizing a threat when it is made. Are you threatening this committee with a "shut off" of research protocols if we follow the recommendation that is before the committee? Please tell me that I am misreading you.

Dr. Harding:    No, what I am saying is not a threat, but it is a possible consequence of passing this motion. I think that agencies that may be worried about securing solid data may choose to bypass Community Hospital if you folks are not going to abide by the rules. This motion would destroy a lot of important data, and research groups take such action very seriously. After all, by accepting the ara-A from the research agency, didn't you agree to play by the rules of the providing agency? If they cannot trust Community Hospital to uphold its end of the research bargain, then they are going to have a problem with Community Hospital in the future. I do not

think that it is as much a threat as it is a
fact.

Dr. Collins:    I think that we need to take Dr. Harding's
words seriously. These protocols provide to
our patients the most up-to-date medicine
available in the world, and it's free, for the
most part. I would hate to jeopardize our
patients' access to this benefit. Furthermore,
I think that physicians of good faith could
reach different decisions on the effectiveness of ara-A. I know that, based on the
limited amount of evidence presented so
far, I am not convinced of its effectiveness. I
would want more clinical agreement before
I would require the protocol to be closed.
Dr. Davis, what do you think?

Dr. Davis:    I think that, at this point, we still are not
sure that there is enough evidence to make
ara-A the gold standard of care for herpes
simplex encephalitis. I admit that it looks
promising, but there is not adequate
evidence to warrant invalidating all the
data.
    By the way, Dr. Penner, how did you
get access to this interim information? Isn't
such information supposed to be hidden
from you as well as from the patient?

Dr. Penner:    I promised the person who revealed this
information that I would not reveal his or
her name. But I assure you that it is accurate.

Dr. Davis:    So you got this information from the center
that is controlling the study?

Dr. Penner:    I cannot say. But I assure you that it is a
very reliable information source.
    This issue of withholding the interim
information from caregivers is not without
ethical import. We need to talk about this
matter as well. Can a physician who takes

|  | his patient as primary enter into a relationship with a research agency knowing that it will withhold potentially vital information regarding the welfare of the patients? |
|---|---|
| Dr. Collins: | I do not believe we can address every relevant issue in human subject research! We need to reach some closure on this matter. Carla Thomas has offered a motion to inform the subjects currently enrolled in the protocol and I think we need to vote on it. Can we have a vote on Carla's motion? |

The vote is five in support of the motion, four opposed.

| Ms. Rhodes: | It troubles me that we cannot verify Dr. Penner's interim information. Therefore, if we did inform the subjects, we would be giving them information that we cannot verify! I think we are on weak ground here. Can we obtain a verification of these data? |
|---|---|
| Dr. Penner: | Probably not, but you might try. |
| Dr. Collins: | Dr. Penner, I am going to recommend that, based on the committee's evaluation, we contact the people on the protocol and inform them that there is some information that indicates that ara-A is effective. They should then be given the opportunity to withdraw from the protocol or stay on it as they see fit. |
| Dr. Harding: | Can we have this decision put in writing so that we can use it to establish that it was the institutional review board's decision to take this action and that it was done against my recommendation? |
| Prof. Fisk: | That seems perfectly legitimate. |
| Atty. Quinn: | Dr. Harding, if this research agency does start closing you out of important research protocols and if you believe that their decision is based on this IRB decision, then I hope that you let me know about it. I would be more than happy to inform them |

that such action is tantamount to penalizing us for having a responsible IRB. I am not sure that the federal Food and Drug Administration would be very supportive of this discrimination merely because we have a gutsy IRB that makes hard and difficult judgments.

Dr. Collins:    If there are no other matters before us, I think that we are adjourned.

## Questions for Further Discussion

1. The committee has chosen not to require verification of Dr. Penner's information. Is this a mistake? Does the committee need to verify the information before it acts on it?
2. The committee did not choose to view the original protocol as being unethical on the grounds that the end point of the disease was death. Was this a mistake, since the protocol knowingly provides useless treatments to patients who might be saved with ara-A?
3. Evaluate the statistics in the case and determine whether they provide enough evidence to support the decision to inform the placebo control group.
4. In human subject research how would you define "enough evidence"?
5. Dr. Harding is defending the need to obey the rules of the research protocol. By doing so, is he using people to secure the welfare of others (future patients)? Is this unethical?
6. Do patients need interim information regarding the status of a drug in order to properly exercise their right to withdraw from a research protocol at any time?
7. IRBs are supposed to defend both the rights and the welfare of human subjects. Is disclosing the interim evidence a defense of rights, a defense of patient welfare, both, or neither?
8. There are technical questions that some committee members feel ignorant about. Dr. Collins tells them to make the decision despite this perceived ignorance. Is this a proper response? If not, what alternative would you offer?
9. If you were a human subject in this protocol and if you were receiving the placebo, would you feel wronged if they did not inform you of the interim information?
10. If these subjects were told at the beginning that no interim information would be presented to them and if they agreed to participate in the protocol, would that relieve us of any obligation to inform them about interim information?

# More Cases Involving the Policy

## The Use of Animals in Research

Dr. Robert Jones, a surgeon on the staff of Community Hospital, is anxious to begin a research protocol involving the transplantation of baboon livers into humans whose livers are failing. He is working with a team of researchers who believe that they have developed a new drug that will decrease the rejection problem. He is very optimistic about the research and argues that there are simply not enough human livers available for transplantation. Furthermore, although he admits that animals have some intrinsic value, he believes that the lives of humans are more valuable than the lives of baboons. He also argues that if it is permissible to sacrifice animals for food, it must be permissible to sacrifice them to save the life of another person.

## Competency and Research

Cancerous brain tumors remain a difficult problem for oncologists. John Peters has a brain tumor for which his oncologist has no treatment that is likely to be very effective. The doctor recommends that John enter a new chemotherapy protocol and John has consented. However, the oncologist is concerned because John's cancer has already affected his reasoning ability. He has a great deal of trouble with memory and cannot determine how many quarters are in five dollars. He does, however, know his doctor, and he says that he understands the information contained in the informed consent document. However, when he is questioned about the information contained in the document, he gives very confused responses. He does insist that he wants the drug. John's wife thinks that he is better off with a palliative approach to his disease and is unwilling to consent to the research.

## A Desperate Volunteer

John suffers from a fatal disease for which there is no effective treatment. His life expectancy is less than one year. Palliative measures are available and there is a standard treatment that is likely to extend his life an additional two or three months. But John wants more. He wants to try something: his preference is a promising experimental drug. If he can't get that, he will seek vitamin treatment, miracle waters, or whatever he can get. He is desperate for a cure; even more, he desperately desires to fight his disease rather than passively await his death.

John's physician knows of a drug protocol that has some chance of extending the lives of those suffering from John's disease; there is even a chance — though a very small one — that the drug might cure the disease in a few patients. Of course, there is also the possibility that the drug will have no effect or that it might even shorten John's life because of toxic reactions. John understands and he wants to try the drug. "If I die sooner, at least I'll die trying," he says. So the call is made to the researcher running the test and John is scheduled for an appointment.

The experimenter is scrupulous in explaining the situation to John. She explains that in order to measure accurately the subtle effects of the drug — whether beneficial or harmful — the study requires a control group. Some people in this experiment will get the new experimental drug; others — the control group — will receive what is currently regarded as the best standard treatment procedure. The control group will not receive the experimental drug. To preserve objectivity, this is a double-blind experiment. Thus even the researcher will not know whether John receives the experimental drug or the standard treatment. "The drug may not help," she says, "and may actually hasten death. You are being offered the opportunity to participate in a double-blind experiment. This means that you may or may not receive the experimental drug. You may receive the drug that we currently use to treat your disease. You won't know which drug you are getting and I will not either. Our purpose in proceeding this way is to gain knowledge concerning the drug, and without this 'blindness' it is difficult to do so. Once again, this procedure may or may not benefit you, but it is the only way that we can offer you this new experimental drug."

John did not expect anything like this. "Look," he said, "I want the experimental drug. I know what the standard treatment is and I know that I would die on it. I also know I'll probably die on the experimental drug, and maybe sooner, but I'll take that chance. I want at least the hope that I'm taking an experimental drug that *might work*. I don't expect a guarantee that the experimental drug will work; I don't even expect a guarantee that it will not do more harm than good; but I do want a guarantee that at least I'll be taking the experimental drug."

The researcher can offer no such guarantee. If John agrees to participate, then he'll either get the experimental drug or receive conscientious treatment with the standard optimum treatment methods. Participation in the experiment is entirely up to him. He is given very thorough information concerning the experimental drug, the research procedure, and the risks. No one pressures him to be part of the experiment. If he chooses not to be part of the experiment, there are others eager to participate. "I understand, it's my choice," he said. "I can be part of the experiment and take my chances on getting the drug I want, or I can decline and stick with the standard—

ultimately ineffectual—treatment; or throw my money away on faith healers and apricot pits. OK, I'll be a volunteer. Sign me up."

The researcher/physician is concerned that John is being mistreated in this situation. The researcher side of her says that nothing is wrong or coercive in making this offer to John. The physician side says that John ought to be given what he wants. Who is correct?

## Using Prisoners

In a large prison located in the same county as Community Hospital, there are over 300 inmates who have tested positive for the HIV virus. A large pharmaceutical company has recently developed a new antiviral drug that they believe may be helpful in suppressing the virus. A cancer specialist, Dr. Martha Walker, who is attached to the Cancer Care Center of Community Hospital, is anxious to coordinate drug testing, and she believes that the prison is an ideal place to run the study.

Though the prison authorities have not allowed drug testing at the prison for over a decade, they are changing their position because of the large number of prisoners who have seroconverted. Officials have decided to permit the research on the grounds that the prisoners will likely die from the disease and also that, because of cuts in the prison's medical budgets, these prisoners will not be able to receive expensive medical treatment when they become sick.

The research involves a double-blind study in which the drug, X, will be compared with a placebo for effectiveness in postponing the onset of AIDS. One group of HIV-infected prisoners will receive X and another will receive a placebo. There are side effects associated with X, including possible liver, kidney, and heart damage. In addition, many of the prisoners report that they are participating not only because they think the study is their best chance of getting decent medical care, but because the Parole Review Board will regard participation in a research protocol as evidence that they should be released.

Since the research will be coordinated at the hospital, the hospital's institutional review board must affirm that the research is ethically permissible. If you were on this committee, would you support this research project? Would you add any special requirements to the research protocol?

## Further Reading

*The Belmont Report: Ethical Principles and Guidelines for the Human Subjects of Reseach,* DHEW Publication (OS) 78-0012,0013,0014. (Washington, D.C.: U.S. Government Printing Office, 1978).

Freid, Charles, *Medical Experimentation: Personnel Integrity and Social Policy* (New York: American Elsevier, 1974).

Katz, Jay, *Experimentation with Human Beings* (New York:  Russell Sage, 1972).

Levine, Robert, *Ethics and the Regulation of Clinical Research* (Baltimore: Urban and Schwarzenberg, 1981).

*Trials of War Criminals before the Nuremberg Military Tribunals under the Control Council Law No. 10, Vol. II,* Nuremberg, October 1946 – April 1949.

Veatch, Robert, *The Patient as Partner: A Theory of Human Experimentation Ethics* (Bloomington: Indiana University Press, 1987).

## Notes

1. U.S. Department of Health and Human Services Public Health Service, *Guide for the Care and Use of Laboratory Animals,* NIH Publication no. 85-23, rev. 1985.

2. Paul Ramsey, *The Patient as Person* (New Haven, Conn.: Yale University Press, 1970), pp. 1–58.

3. Ibid., p. 12.

4. Richard McCormick, *Perspectives in Biology and Medicine* 18 (1) (Autumn 1974): 2.

5. Tom Regan, "Ill Gotten Gains," in *Health Care Ethics: An Introduction,* ed. Donald van DeVeer and Tom Regan (Philadelphia: Temple University Press, 1987).

6. For a consequentialist approach to the defense of animal rights see Peter Singer, *A New Ethic for Treatment of Animals* (New York: Random House, 1975).

7. For a good discussion of this see Robert Levine, *Ethics and the Regulation of Clinical Research* (Baltimore: Urban and Schwarzenberg, 1981), p. 210.

# 10

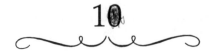

# Pediatric Ethics

## Introduction to the Problem Area

Many of the most difficult ethical problems faced by the modern hospital ethics committee emerge from the hospital's pediatric floors, especially from the hospital's neonatal intensive care unit. The severity of these dilemmas often motivate hospitals to form special *pediatric ethics committees* that deal exclusively with the ethical problems faced by pediatric health care professionals. For the sake of continuity, our committee will remain constant, but nurse and physician specialists from pediatrics will be represented in our dialogue.

There is, of course, a great deal of similarity between medically caring for children and medically caring for adults. The goals of the two enterprises are largely the same: preventing disease, curing disease, minimizing the effects of disease, and relieving discomfort. But there are several factors that increase our ethical perplexity within pediatrics. We can begin our study by examining competence, limited autonomy, and the best interest criterion.

### A Competency Continuum

While all pediatric patients are incompetent from a legal perspective, only some of them are incompetent from an ethical perspective. Infants are completely incompetent, but the same cannot be said of older children and young teens. Teenagers are not only very different from adults, they are also very different from infants. In terms of competency, they are "between the dawn and the daylight." The existence of this gray area indicates that there is no hard and fast line between competency and incompetency. Rather, there is a competency continuum along which there are significant differences in reasoning power and autonomy among pediatric patients.

It must be emphasized that the law is somewhat skeptical of such a continuum. There are understandable reasons for this skepticism. However, physicians and nurses realize the reality of this continuum and must adjust their practice accordingly. Similarly, in bioethics we recognize that we must divide pediatric patients into those who have some autonomous reasoning power (young teens) from those who have none.

Infants lack all autonomous reasoning ability; thus, we cannot appeal in any way to their autonomy to settle critical health care questions. But it is not just the absence of autonomous reasoning ability that makes infant care so perplexing. A presently incompetent patient who was formerly competent may have an advance directive and thus retain autonomous control over his life even when he lapses into incompetence. What makes infant care so ethically challenging is not only the absence of competence but also the absence of former competence.

### Autonomy and Best Interests

The complete absence of patient autonomy in the context of infant care is particularly troubling because we rely so heavily on the autonomy of persons in order to determine what is in their best interests. Our society is marked by a deep and profound skepticism about how to define objectively the best interests of individuals. As a result, our society prefers to appeal to the free choices of individuals to determine what is best for them. But in infant pediatric cases, we cannot do this. We must look to the parents and the physicians. Physicians and surrogates thus play a more extended role in pediatrics and are responsible for defining what is the best for severely ill children.

But while our society grants to these parents this responsibility or role function, it gives them few guidelines as to how one should define the best interest of a child. The extent of the parents' authority to determine the best interests of infants is ambiguous, and this ambiguity creates many of the deepest and most baffling moral challenges for parents, physicians, and society. For example, because our society cannot define the extent of the parents' and the physician's authority, these persons face profound and tragic dilemmas in managing severely handicapped newborns. In a number of celebrated cases involving infants who were born with severe, permanent, and nontreatable diseases, parents have chosen to forgo life-sustaining treatment. Parents withheld such treatment on the grounds that dying was in the "best interest" of the child. But such decisions have often troubled legislative and judicial leaders as well as the general public.

The President's Commission for the Study of Ethical Problems in Medicine and Biomedical and Behavioral Research report entitled *Deciding to Forego Life Sustaining Treatment* discusses a case in which the parents of a newborn Down syndrome baby refused to give permission to surgically correct a blocked intestinal tract; the baby died as a result.[1] The parents based their decision on the claim that a life lived with Down syndrome was not in the best interest of the child. The President's Commission rejected this specific exercise of authority, but it did not reject the general principle that parents have the right to make "net benefit" decisions. This nonfictional example illustrates that society can grant to parents authority to decide the best interest of their children without defining the limits of this authority. Parents are thus given a *general* right to determine the best interest of their children, but when they do make a *particular* choice about what is in the best interest of a severely handicapped child, society may opt to withdraw this supposed right or rebuke them for acting against what it considers the "real" interest of the child.

The source of this conflict between the law and the individual guardian is traceable to society's very understandable and perhaps reasonable desire to avoid writing law that covers every bioethics case. Neither legislators nor judges want the responsibility to resolve all bioethical problems. They are not gods who can anticipate the complexity and the uniqueness of every dilemma. This is precisely what makes the formulation of general laws very difficult. Election to a legislative office or appointment to the bench does not give a person any special insight into how these issues should be addressed ethically. Judges and legislatures clearly have the power to restrict the legal rights of parents, but this power does not ethically validate their decisions.

### The Health Care Provider and Best Interest

Another factor that adds to the complexity of pediatric ethics is that parents or guardians are not the only ones who determine the best interest of pediatric patients. Physicians are also involved in defining what is best for the impaired child.[2] Indeed, many commentators describe such judgments as ones that are "jointly made" by the guardian and the physician. Furthermore, the physician is often pictured as needing input from a health care team, including nurses. However, the problem with these joint decisions concerns the nature and extent of both physician and parent participation. One view suggests that physicians should contribute only medical information and not participate in ethical decision making.

This problem regarding the physician's role in best-interest judgments emerges within a particular historical context. During the past 40 years of bioethical inquiry, the most frequent criticism leveled against clinicians has been that they "medicalized" ethical judgments. *Medicalizing* is defined as attempting to transform ethical questions into medical questions with the aim of excluding patients or guardians from the decision-making process.

In the past some physicians transformed their medical authority into ethical authority by making ethical decisions that should properly have been made by patients or guardians. When physicians medicalize, they mask their ethical values as medical decisions. This not only excludes patients from serious involvement in ethical decision making but also undermines the doctor-patient relationship by introducing an element of dishonesty into it.

The tendency to medicalize continues to be a danger facing physicians, but the criticism itself may have had the unfortunate effect of pressuring some physicians to withdraw completely from the arena of bioethical decision making. This withdrawal is unfortunate for patient care because not only do patients and families want sound medical advice from their physician, but they also frequently need sound ethical advice, especially during times of medical crisis. The problem, therefore, is not *whether* physicians should offer advice on ethical questions that arise in the nursery or the neonatal intensive care unit, but *how* both guardians and physicians should jointly address bioethical questions and manage ethical conflicts.

### Conflict of Interest

Another factor that augments ethical dilemmas in pediatrics is *the family*. Parents who must make critical health care decisions are frequently responsible for other children as well as the pediatric patient. The patient's siblings need the time, energy, and, frequently, the scarce resources of the family. As a result, families are often torn by the demands that chronically ill infants place on their psychological and financial resources.

But if the needs of other family members frequently conflict with those of the impaired child, then parents, as best-interest decision makers, face a herculean challenge. For how can they take into consideration the needs of other family members and still follow the axiom that best-interest decisions must be made in the interest of the patient alone? How can they actually screen out all other considerations? Mothers and fathers who have other children to care for frequently find this principle difficult, if not impossible to follow. Furthermore, even if parents accept this principle, it is difficult to determine when they have successfully disregarded or screened out the interests of their other children and focused exclusively on the interests of their sick child.

### Justice in Pediatrics

A final factor that increases the complexity of pediatric ethics involves a more global consideration. Pediatric patients are young. The life expectancy of chronically ill pediatric patients is, in general, longer than the life expectancy of chronically ill aged patients. In general, therefore, the cost of caring for chronically ill pediatric patients is correspondingly far greater. The cost of being chronically ill for 70 years is much higher than the cost of being chronically ill for 3 years. The question then is how should considerations relevant to anticipated life expectancy affect decisions about the allocation of scarce resources. Many studies seem to indicate, for example, that long-term survival rates for patients over 60 with multiple system failures is quite low. But this is not the case with children who are treated in the neonatal intensive care unit (NICU). Those who survive NICU treatment have long life expectancies. It seems clear that allocation problems are intensified in the pediatric context.

---

## Community Hospital's Policy on Pediatric Withdrawal

*Preamble:*   The policy of the hospital continues to be that, because infants possess an intrinsic dignity and worth, those who are receiving artificial life support will continue to receive this support unless it is medically and ethically contraindicated.

*Purpose:*   The aim of these guidelines is to determine when discontinuation of artificial life support for critically ill infants is ethically indicated.

1. *Application*   This policy will apply to
   a. infants who have irreversible circulatory or respiratory failure; or
   b. infants who have irreversible cessation of all functions of the entire brain; or
   c. infants who suffer from maladies that permanently and completely prevent them from participating in human interaction; or
   d. infants for whom continued treatment serves only to prolong the dying process; or
   e. infants for whom continued treatment does not provide, in the words of the President's Commission for the Study of Ethical Problems in Medicine and Biomedical and Behavioral Research, a "net benefit" to the infant.

*Principles:*

1. The primary individuals who are responsible for the decision to forgo treatment are the child's parents and the attending physician. Every effort will be made to maximize the information given to the parents so that they can make an informed decision. Included in this information should be the following:
   A. as accurate an appraisal of prognosis as possible.

    B.  a report on any significant uncertainties.

    C.  information on the availability of additional medical, religious, or counseling consultants.

2.  In the event that the parents disagree on the issue of withdrawal, every effort should be made to resolve the disagreement, and no forgoing of treatment should take place during this period of conflict. If this conflict cannot be settled in a reasonable amount of time, or in the event that the parents are not available or are not acting competently, a legal guardian should be appointed by the courts as soon as possible.

3.  The best interest of the infant should be the only factor that affects the decision of the family and the physician. The influence of other factors, such as the interests of either the family or the medical caregivers, is discouraged. The question of what is in the interest of the child is often affected by both medical and ethical considerations, and the following three principles are recommended as guides for dealing with these factors:

    A.  If parents make treatment withdrawal decisions that are clearly inconsistent with what is medically beneficial to the infant, then the treatment should be continued and the institution should seek to have a guardian appointed by the court.

    B.  If the treatment is of medically uncertain value and if the parents decide to forgo treatment, then the parents' wishes should be respected. If the parents choose to continue such treatment, then this decision should also be honored.

    C.  If the treatment is medically futile and if the parents wish to forgo treatment, then this wish should be honored. If the parents wish to continue with the medically futile therapy, then the pediatric ethics committee should be called upon to mediate this conflict between the parents and the health care providers. Community Hospital is not committed to providing medically futile treatment. The competent patient's right to refuse treatment does not imply that the patient or his guardian has a right to require the hospital to provide medically useless treatment.

4.  Decisions to forgo infant treatment are justified when the consequences for the infant of continued treatment are so severe as not to provide a net benefit to the infant. However, the existence of handicaps such as Down syndrome alone is not in itself sufficient to warrant a decision to withdraw care.

5.  Physicians and parents are encouraged to use the services of the hospital's Ethics Committee to assist them in developing sound decisions regarding these difficult choices.

6.  To ensure the dignity of infants from whom services are withdrawn, services such as social comforting and analgesics should be provided.

7. Decisions to withdraw treatment should be clearly written in the infant's medical record. All such decisions should be reviewed by the director of the neonatal unit prior to any withdrawal action. Furthermore, health care providers, including nurses and house staff, who are uncomfortable with a withdrawal decision should have an opportunity to submit their views to the chief of service, and every effort should be made to address these concerns.

## Commentary on the Philosophical and Ethical Aspects of the Policy

The relatively new subspecialty of pediatrics known as *neonatology* has precipitated not only a major technological revolution but also a vast set of challenging philosophical and ethical problems. It is appropriate, therefore, to begin our philosophical commentary on the policy by focusing on the following four concepts: "best interest," "medical uncertainty," "medical futility," and "the capacity for human interaction." We will offer a number of alternative philosophical interpretations of these concepts so that the reader can appreciate why imperiled newborns are so disturbing for our culture.

### Best Interest

Our first philosophical difficulty involves the meaning of *best interest*. The expression "net benefit" appears in the application section of Community Hospital's policy and the expression "best interest" of the child appears in principle 3. The two ideas are closely related. Frequently, treatment produces both effects that are in the interest of the patient and harmful side effects as well. To find the net benefit, one must somehow weigh the harmful effects of treatment against the beneficial effects and either continue or discontinue it in the light of this process. Best-interest judgments are to be understood as the results of net benefit judgments, derived from a weighing of the negative and positive effects of treatment.

According to philosopher Allan Buchanan, to make a "best interest" judgment for a child means that the guardian must take two factors into consideration.[3] First, some interests of the child may be more important than others. Second, a decision regarding best interests may advance some interests and undermine others. For Buchanan, these two considerations pose four philosophical questions.

The first question is whether clinical best-interest judgments are objective. Buchanan notes that the problem of determining best interests is the problem of separating one's preferences from what is actually in one's best interest. Since one could make a mistake and prefer what is actually harmful, it follows that preferences and actual best interests need not be identical. Furthermore, it is impossible to identify the best interests of imperiled newborns with their expressed preferences, since they have no expressed preferences. Therefore, some attempt must be made to discover the objective or actual best interest of the child.

The second philosophical question that Buchanan considers vital is how one weighs future benefits against the present and future harms related to treatment. Should neonates be required to suffer long-term discomfort and pain for a chance to become adults? How should the likelihood of severe retardation and severe handicaps affect the process of weighing future interests against present sufferings? Can surrogates take future quality of life as a basis for withdrawing treatment? Buchanan suggests that these problems are all but intractable, especially in situations where medical uncertainty dominates. Often, even skilled professionals cannot determine with certainty what the outcome of an extended course of treatment will be, and this profoundly complicates the defining of best interests.

Buchanan's third question involves a distinction. If interests can be separated into *self-regarding* interests and *other-regarding* interests, how do we take other-regarding interests into consideration? If a child loves its parents, then the interests of the parents are other-regarding interests of the child. In some limited sense, it is the interest of the child to secure the interests of the parents. This comes into play, for example, when we are making decisions about transplanting organs from incompetent children to their parents or siblings. To assist the parent seems to be the other-regarding interest of the child. However, it is easy to see that donating a kidney is not in the *self*-regarding interest of the child, since the child loses half of its reserve renal capacity. If guardians are to make best-interest judgments, how are they to balance the child's other-regarding interests against its self-regarding interests? More important, the notion of other-regarding interests poses a real threat to the child. The concept can be employed as a basis for "using children" and undermining their most vital self-regarding interests. Buchanan responds to this danger by suggesting that guardians should never judge that the child's other-regarding interests overrule its basic self-regarding interests, and that whenever the concept of other-regarding interests are employed, there should be a higher standard of proof applied to establish that the other-regarding interest actually outweighs the self-regarding interest.

Finally, Buchanan believes that the best-interest criterion provides special problems for individuals who are diagnosed as being in a persistent vegetative state. If we assume that some level of cognitive capacity is necessary for having interests, then, since persons in persistent vegetative states have no cognitive capacity, they may have no interests. We will now address Buchanan's first two questions regarding self-interest and postpone responding to these last two questions until we have addressed the philosophical problems involved in managing infants who have permanently lost the capacity to interact as persons.

Although his first two questions direct our attention to some of the critical issues faced by ethics committees within the neonatal context, Buchanan fails to draw our attention to the concept of *objective self-interest*. He seems to think that subjective self-interest based on preference is all that we have to go on, and since neonates cannot express preference, the problems of weighing best interest are "intractable." However, we can turn our attention to the idea of objective self-interest and suggest that there are various philosophical meanings associated with the word "objective."

There are at least two different meanings associated with the idea of objectivity. A judgment may be said to be objective if it is verifiably correct. For example, the claim that "Amoxicillin is an effective antibacterial medication" is "objective" in the sense that the judgment is verifiably correct. Clinical trials have established that this medication is effective against many bacterial infections. The clinical trial is thus taken as the mark or the criterion of objectivity.

The second meaning of "objective" is "impartial." For example, if a jury reaches a judgment without coercive or other unfair influence, then we may call the judgment "objective." A jury's judgment may be objective in this sense without implying that it is objective in the first sense of "verifiably correct." A jury can render an impartial verdict without employing an experimental procedure to do so. However, if the jury finds a defendant innocent and we later discover that each juror had received $5,000 from the defendant, then we begin to doubt the jury's objectivity. Further, a jury may impartially determine that a defendant is guilty without being able to prove it experimentally. The standards of evidence in the courtroom are thus different from the standards of evidence used in the experimental setting.

One might be tempted to require that best-interest judgments be "objective" in both senses of the word. Community Hospital's policy avoids this temptation. The policy requires only that such judgments be objective in the sense of impartial. The primary reason for this is that to require that best-interest judgments be verifiably correct sets a standard that is so high that it will be far too difficult, perhaps even impossible, to satisfy. Best-interest judgments are surely "intractable" in that they cannot be verifiably correct, but they may not be intractable if we view objectivity as impartiality. Consider the case of the anencephalic baby born without an upper brain. We can verifiably ascertain that such children will die within a short period of time, but we cannot verifiably ascertain that such children ought to be withdrawn from intensive treatment. However, this does not mean that parents and physicians cannot make impartial decisions regarding the best interests of the child.

*The Absolutist Criticism*    Critics of the best-interest criterion are primarily concerned with its subjective nature. This subjectivity, they argue, will harm future patients. For example, some parents may judge that it is in the best interest of a child born with Down syndrome to continue living. Other parents may not think so. If we allow subjective choice to operate in this context, what will prevent us from allowing it to operate when a baby is born with a birthmark? The problem at the bottom of this debate is *how does one define the best interest of a Down syndrome baby?* More generally, if the subjective choice of the parents and the physician is allowed in cases of severe deformity such as anencephalia, how can we disallow it in cases such as Down syndrome or birthmarks?

Such critics are often said to hold an *absolutist view of best interest*. This view asserts that life *in any form* is in the best interest of an individual and that everything should be done to sustain life under all circumstances. The absolutist avoids all the problems of best interests and requires that medical professionals do everything they can, under all medical circumstances, to preserve the life of any infant. This view argues that if we fail to follow this absolutist rule, we will eventually slide down a slippery slope that will destroy the moral fabric of society. Furthermore, accepting the best-interest criterion will eventually lead to the termination of children born with the "wrong" sex or color.

*Subjectivism*    The physician-philosopher H. Tristram Engelhardt has offered what may be called a *subjective* response to this criticism, which suggests that we cannot avoid defining best interests in a subjective fashion. This view asserts that because best-interest decisions are indeterminate, no absolute rules can be drafted that will determine how every imperiled-newborn case should be handled. As a result, we must leave such questions to parents and physicians alone. Engelhardt also argues that the slippery slope concern that infanticide will destroy the moral fabric of a culture is undermined by historical examples. Many non-Western societies permit infanticide, and so did many Western societies that preceded our own. The Greeks and the Romans authorized infanticide when a child was born deformed. In Politics, Aristotle states, "Let there be a law that no deformed child shall live."[4] Plato approves of the practice, and according to Engelhardt, infanticide was not only widely practiced in Rome, it was also approved in the very legal system that forms the foundation of Western law. For Engelhardt, Greece and Rome were the foundations of our own society and their moral fabric was not destroyed by infanticide.

In addition to this historical argument, Engelhardt offers us two more philosophical arguments for the legitimacy of infanticide. In the first argument, he tries to prove that saving an infant so that it can live a low quality of life may be an injury against that child. In the second, he argues that infants may not be persons in the "strict sense."

Engelhardt admits that a low birth weight baby who has permanently lost its lung functioning and who has suffered significant upper brain damage can be kept alive with the services available in neonatal units. But he believes that keeping the child alive may involve the imposition of a "wrongful life" on the child. It is easy to imagine that many individuals would not want to be kept alive if living meant permanent respirator dependency. Indeed, keeping such a child alive may involve violating the rule to "do no harm." For Engelhardt, this can ethically justify the decision to withdraw or withhold life-sustaining treatment in the nursery.

This wrongful life argument does not require us to make any judgments about the intrinsic worth of the infant, but Engelhardt's second argument forces us to address this issue. For Engelhardt, fetuses and infants should be viewed as *human nonpersons* because they lack the necessary and sufficient conditions for being persons. Following Kant, he claims that persons can be defined in terms of three factors: self-consciousness, rationality, and the possession of a minimal moral sense.[5] The fictional movie character ET is not a human, but because of his self-consciousness, his rationality, and his moral sensitivity, most of us would grant ET the status of a person. Furthermore, because of this moral status, ET deserves the moral respect due to persons. His nonhumanness is irrelevant to his being or not being a person.

According to Engelhardt, the fetus and the infant may be humans in the sense that they belong to the species *homo sapiens,* but belonging to a certain biological species by itself does not confer on them the status of being persons. Just as the extraterrestrial can be a person without being human, some individuals may be human without being persons. For Engelhardt, infants illustrate this point. Infants do not have the intrinsic value of persons because they lack the rationality, self-consciousness, and minimal moral sense required for being a person. However, while they lack *intrinsic* value, they have what Engelhardt calls *extrinsic* or social value. They are or can be important to other persons. They have their value because of their relation to persons, not because they are themselves persons.

This libertarian view of persons would have profound impact on decision making within the pediatric setting. For example, if a physician and the parents of a Down syndrome baby decided that it was not in the best interest of the baby to continue living, then they could withhold or withdraw life-sustaining treatment, even for treatable diseases or maladies. Because infants are not persons, parents in their role as guardians should have extensive moral authority to determine the "best interest" of the imperiled newborn, including the authority to allow them to die.

### The Procedural Compromise

But there is a position that combines the absolutist and the libertarian views. This view, which has been adopted by Community Hospital, may be called *the procedural approach*. In this view, it is ethically permissible to grant to parents and physicians the right to make withholding or withdrawal decisions jointly, but only in limited contexts and under limited circumstances. The view is neither absolutist nor purely subjective. It involves aspects of both positions.

According to this procedural view, best-interest judgments are not objective in the sense of verifiably correct. However, they can be impartially objective. The philosopher Robert Veatch has described such a proceduralist or contractarian view in his book *A Theory of Medical Ethics*.[6] For Veatch, the basic principles or foundations of ethics are derived from mutual agreement. For the proceduralist, these mutually agreed-upon principles provide a common moral framework within a pluralistic society. However, the nature of this agreement and the substantive principles that are agreed to are hotly contested. What is central to this approach is that both consequences and rights are taken seriously without either one being construed as the fundamental moral point of view.

This "ethics by agreement" approach may be applied to the problem of weighing the harms and benefits associated with neonatal care. In order to impartially define "best interest," we must specify a set of procedures or rules that ought to be followed when making best-interest judgments. The proceduralist thus recognizes the need to appeal to recognized authorities to make best-interest judgments. The proceduralist then establishes rules that balance rights and consequences. These rules determine what restrictions or limitations can be placed on the parent's right to forgo life-sustaining treatment. Procedures define when parents can and cannot exercise authority. For example, one might grant extensive rights to parents but restrict them from making decisions that are aimed at securing their own best interest.

*The Policy as Procedure*    Community Hospital's policy illustrates this procedural view. The application section of the policy specifies to whom this policy will be applied. The policy cannot be applied to children on the basis of sex, hair or skin color, or other such trivial factors. But it will apply to infants who have irreversible circulatory or respiratory failure; infants who have irreversible cessation of all functions of the entire brain; infants who suffer from maladies that permanently and completely prevent them from participating in human interaction; infants for whom continued treatment serves only to prolong the dying process; or infants for whom continued treatment does not provide a net benefit.

One might argue that the list is too libertarian or too conservative, but every effort was made by the committee to construct a list of possible disease categories that would avoid the dangers both of the conservative position and of the libertarian. The policy emphasizes that sound decision making in this area requires that both the parents and the physician consent to the withdrawal and that clinical considerations such as whether the treatment serves only to prolong the dying process ought to play an important role in the decision-making process. Furthermore, the policy is very explicit about the relevance of family interests to the decision-making process. The policy emphasizes that although the family's interests often make withdrawal decisions more difficult, perhaps even tragically so, they are *irrelevant* to the process.

## Uncertainty and Futility

Although the procedures followed by Community Hospital reduce ethical ambiguity, they do not exclude tragic choice as a necessary element within medicine. Tragic choices are those that cannot be made by following rules. It would be wonderful if our procedures could eliminate the necessity to make such choices, but borderline cases are present within pediatrics and, therefore, tragic choice remains an indispensable aspect of infant care. Tragedy enters with the appearance of uncertainty and futility. At first glance, these concepts seem very different but they are closely tied together in the President's Commission report *Deciding to Forego Life Sustaining Treatment*.

In this report, many of the possible conflicts that emerge between physician and family are approached using the "the parental priority model of decision making." This approach recommends that physicians override decisions of parents only when the wishes of the parents are clearly inconsistent with the medical interests of the infant. But parents take priority in two other possible contexts: when treatment is of uncertain value and when treatment is futile. Presumably, when there is significant medical uncertainty that continuing treatment is actually in the best interests of the child, this model would give the parents' wishes priority over those of the physician. For example, consider a situation in which a physician neonatologist is uncertain that maintaining the child in intensive care is going to produce a recovery. If he wishes to continue care because he *hopes* that the child will recover, then the family's decision has priority in questions concerning forgoing treatment. Hoping that a child will recover is different from having a clinically justified belief that a child will recover. If the family wishes to exercise the withdrawal option against the physician's preference for continuing treatment, then the family's preference overrides the physician's wishes. There is parental priority in cases of medical uncertainty. However, within this procedural model, the physician has the right to interfere with a parental choice, but only when the physician is medically certain that forgoing treatment is inconsistent with the infant's welfare.

From the viewpoint of the proceduralist, this parental priority model is generally sound. However, the President's Commission also applied the parental priority model to cases in which continued treatment was known to be *medically futile*. According to this model, if continued life-sustaining treatment is known to be futile, then the parents can decide whether to continue it. *The President's Commission assumed that the ethical principles that ought to govern cases involving medical uncertainty also should govern cases of medical futility.* The commission seems to identify medical uncertainty with medical futility.

However, there are some significant problems with this assumption. It seems clear that when physicians are genuinely uncertain whether continued treatment will benefit an impaired child, then the technological skills of the physician become somewhat irrelevant to the decision to withdraw or continue treatment. Parents should have priority over physicians because the decision to take one course of action over the other cannot be based on clinical science, since uncertainty about clinical outcome is present. But in cases of futility, uncertainty is not present. In these cases, clinical science *is relevant* to the decision.

Why? The answer seems to be that when clinical science can reveal the likely outcome, then the technological information *should* influence what is the most reasonable choice. In such cases the relevance of the technological information is established. Perhaps the most obvious area in which futility judgments based on technological information override the wishes of guardians is the determination of death. When a ventilator-dependent patient is judged to be clinically dead, the physician may remove the patient from ventilator support even if the family does not consent. A patient's guardians do not have to consent to a declaration of death and the withdrawal of ventilator support, even if the patient's heart and lungs are still circulating blood and air. When a physician properly declares that a ventilator-dependent person is dead, then the physician is actually declaring that *further effort is futile and therefore the consent to withdraw is not legally required.* Here, the intimate relation between futility and uncertainty is clear. *Futility judgments are delivered once uncertainty of prediction is eliminated.*

When a judgment of medical futility is justified, is relevant in determining what ought to be done with the patient. But we need to distinguish the *complete* futility associated with declaration of death from *partial* futility. Partial futility is established when nothing more can be done to return a person's organ or limb to full functioning but the person can be saved with removal or amputation. For example, a gangrenous leg may be treated at first but then amputated when continued treatment is judged to be not only worthless for saving the leg but dangerous for the rest of the body. Nothing more can be done to save the leg and the surgeon recommends that further attempts are futile. Further treatment *of the leg* is judged to be medically futile, and saving the person becomes the primary goal of treatment. This judgment involves only partial futility because it does not imply that all further treatment is futile. Other treatments aimed at saving the person, including amputation, may be necessary.

It is important to note that there is a criterion that separates partial from complete futility. In the case of complete futility, no further treatment can be provided that will aid the person. The brain-dead person cannot be helped. The victim of gangrene, on the other hand, can be. With rehabilitative care, he can return to interact with the rest of the human community as a person. As we will see, this distinction between full and partial futility can be applied to more difficult cases but not without attending to the fifth concept that permeates our policy.

### The Capacity to Interact as a Person

In the application part of the hospital's policy (section c), it is asserted that the policy will apply to "infants who suffer from maladies that permanently and completely prevent them from participating in human interaction." This statement affirms that withdrawal of treatment is appropriate when the child has lost its capacity to interact as a person. Community Hospital's policy on withdrawal thus speaks directly to the last two philosophical questions raised by Allan Buchanan concerning other-regarding interests and persistent vegetative state. The policy recommends that the child's best interest be the sole criterion for making judgments regarding withdrawal. It does not recognize the concept of other-regarding interests. In effect, the policy affirms the traditional view that the patient, rather than the patient's family, should be the physician's sole object of concern and that to do otherwise brings the physician dangerously close to conflict of interest.

Buchanan's concerns about persistent vegetative state are taken very seriously by the committee. The policy maintains that withdrawal of treatment is a possible response for patients who have lost their capacity to interact as persons. Practically speaking, this means that the committee rejects the view that whole brain death is a necessary requirement for withdrawal of treatment. Another way of putting this claim is that complete futility can be reached prior to the point of whole brain death. The child with a completely and permanently dysfunctional neocortex, whose brain stem is still functioning, has not satisfied the whole brain definition of death. Such an infant has only partial brain death; one part of the brain still functions. However, although the patient is still legally alive, the destruction of its neocortical tissue produces a significant ethical problem because this tissue is biologically necessary for any and all cognitive activity. This patient has no hope of acting as a person or interacting as a person with others. If one has lost the power to act as a person, it seems plausible to suggest that one has lost the status of being a person.

The reader will recall that significant objections were raised against Engelhardt's view that no infant was a person in the strict sense. It seemed to suggest that color, sex, or other irrelevant factors could be used as a basis for withholding or withdrawing treatment from children. These objections still stand, but the complete loss of neocortical tissue seems substantially different from color or sex, which are irrelevant to the cognitive and experiential qualities associated with being a person. Neocortical tissue is not irrelevant—it is necessary. In short, if persons are defined by cognitive or affective behavior and if an infant has lost or never had these capacities, then it seems that it has lost its status as an *obvious person*.

But once again the committee does not jump from the fact that an infant is not an obvious person to the claim that it is not a person. Rather, it employs the procedural approach to resolve the issue. The consent of the parents as well as the consent of the attending physician is required prior to the withdrawal of treatment, and no judgment is made that the infant can be withdrawn because it lacks the status of a person. Health care providers are reluctant to argue with parents that their neocortically dysfunctional infants are not really persons in the strict sense. It is enough to indicate that such children have permanently lost the power to function as persons. Providers need not bear the additional burden of establishing the philosophical doctrine that these infants are not members of the moral community. A more pressing problem with the Community Hospital's ethics policy is the notion of futility. One can argue that clinical futility has been reached once it is determined that a child's neocortical tissue has been completely and permanently destroyed. This is not a situation in which partial futility exists, as in the case of the gangrenous leg. A person whose leg has been amputated is a handicapped person, not a nonperson! But legs and neocortical tissue are very different. The neocortex makes human behavior possible, and thus the complete loss of this tissue suggests that the person will never recover and therefore that further treatment is completely futile.

But it is vital to point out that the kind of futility that is reached in this neocortical case is not biological futility. Pulmonary functioning, heart functioning, and circulation can be maintained in such cases. The cells can be fed and hydrated. Most important, the whole brain is not dead since the stem of the brain is still functioning. However, despite the presence of these biological functions, one can argue that we have reached the stage of complete futility because nothing more can be done to restore the capacity to interact as a person. No further personal interaction with this patient is possible.

It is essential to emphasize that *interaction with* persons is not the same as *action toward* persons. Health care providers and family members can continue to act toward the infant with complete neocortical destruction. Their actions can be filled with caring and tenderness. But action from this kind of patient toward other persons has ended because the capacity for personal communication has ended. The feelings of pain, pleasure, joy, sorrow, envy, greed, and generosity have ended. Cognition has ended. Consciousness has ended. All of these functions have ended because the seat of these capacities, the neocortex, has been permanently and completely destroyed. Complete and partial futility can, therefore, be adequately distinguished only if we rely on the criterion of incapacity to interact as a person. The presence of this criterion is clearly operating in the determination of brain death. Why else do we declare that a person is legally dead when total brain death is reached? It is because the patient has permanently lost capacity to interact as a person, and it is by virtue of this fact that we construe further care as being futile.

But even if we accept this view of brain death, we are faced with a further question: can complete futility be reached prior to total brain death or, more generally, can complete futility be reached before a declaration of death can be made? The answer seems to be a guarded "yes." Treating patients who have permanently lost complete neocortical function may be considered completely futile because these patients have lost all hope of interacting as persons. Yet they are not wholly brain dead and, therefore, cannot be declared to be *legally dead*. These patients are on the borderline between dead and alive.

The traditional approach to managing these patients is to consult the patient's guardian. We must look to the best-interest criterion as the sole basis for decision making, and the next of kin or other surrogate must make this determination.

Community Hospital's policy emphasizes the role that guardians or next of kin play in withdrawing care from infants who have permanently lost the capacity to interact as persons. While recognizing that continued treatment of such patients is futile, the committee was unwilling to grant to physicians the authority to unilaterally forgo treatment of such patients without the consent of the guardian. At the same time the committee also refused to obligate physicians to do what they consider to be completely futile.

The policy thus contains two principles that are at odds with one another. The principle that requires guardian consent for withdrawal is clearly at odds with the principle that grants to the physician a right to avoid doing what is completely futile. It is easy to imagine cases in which these principles conflict. The committee simply does not have a "cookbook solution" or a set of principles that will resolve every such conflict.

The critic might charge that the hospital's policy is vague or perhaps even inconsistent. Because these principles can push us in opposite directions in specific cases, the critic argues that the committee must reformulate the policy. What response can be offered to this criticism?

One response is to simply admit that in each case the physician has the right to judge that a treatment is futile, not the obligation to do so. Merely having a right does not imply any duty to exercise that right. The conflict between these two principles is genuine. At this time it is unresolved within both our committee and our society. It is something that health care professionals and patients are going to live with for the foreseeable future. The virtue of this response is its humility. It affirms that the hospital ethics committee does not have all the answers. Sitting on such a committee does not by itself give one an intuitive insight into how all the problems of bioethics should be managed. Furthermore, this admission of ignorance allows the artistic side of medicine to take center stage.

Pediatrics, like every medical specialty, is both an art and a science. Since the ethics committee has affirmed both principles and refused to grant priority to either one, the individual pediatrician, confronted with a case in which the principles are in conflict, must address the case wearing her artistic cap. How does the pediatrician as artist address the problem? One approach is to avoid confrontation that pits the family against the physician in a struggle that may be counterproductive. Parents who cannot accept the death of their infant frequently express their love for the infant or their inability to accept the death by resisting the physician who confronts them with a futility judgment. Forceful and strident confrontation between the physician and the parents in which the physician affirms his right to avoid providing futile care and the parents affirm their right to withhold consent to the withdrawal of treatment does not produce effective patient management. Rights talk is a convenient way of operating in the legislature but not in the pediatric nursery. How might the artistic physician manage these conflicts?

First, it is important to note that even if it is the physician's *right* to refuse to administer futile treatment, it is not thereby his *obligation* to do so. At this point in medical history, neither the committee nor the society at large has transformed the right to avoid futile treatment into an obligation. Of course, one can imagine that as medical resources in the United States become more scarce, society may transform what is now a right into an obligation. At present, however, the pediatrician is not obligated to avoid futile treatment in every case.

Second, if a physician decides to continue what she considers to be a futile treatment, it is recommended that she set goals for it. The pressure of specific goals and specific time frames is not unhealthy for the physician who is playing the "futile therapy game." Accepting the futility of continued treatment is often a process that requires time, information, and sensitive artistic communication. A joint search for what is best for the patient is clearly preferable, but without goals and time frames the opportunity for dialogue can be transformed into a nightmare in which families and health care institutions are permanently caring for "the dead."

## The Case of Baby John Fitzer

Baby John Fitzer was born ten weeks ago. His weight at birth was very low due to his short gestation period (27 weeks). He was immediately placed on a respirator and transferred to the hospital's neonatal intensive care unit (NICU). His progress in the NICU since then has not been good. He has suffered at least two quite severe (grade IV) intercranial hemorrhages, and there is a strong indication, based on CT scan review, that significant brain damage has occurred. The neurologist has predicted that if baby John survives, he would probably suffer from severe mental retardation.

Baby John is also suffering from bronchopulmonary dysplasia (BPD), a chronic lung disease that will make him dependent on the ventilator for the remainder of his life. In addition, he is unable to ingest food orally. He requires extensive skilled nursing care to manage not only his ventilator, but also his feeding tube. It is very unlikely that he could be released from the hospital in the near future since his need for professional nursing care is so profound. Even if a nursing home offering the necessary care were to accept him, it is likely that he would require numerous returns to the NICU.

It is not clear at this point whether John is terminally ill. The neonatologist in charge of the case, Paula Reid, feels that at this time John cannot be diagnosed as suffering from a terminal, irreversible disease that will imminently cause death. According to Reid, high-intensity neonatal care can indefinitely prolong baby John's life.

John's parents are upper-middle-class professionals who have two other young children and lead very busy lives maintaining a family life as well as their demanding careers. The Fitzers divide the responsibility of visiting John. One of them comes every third night. They regularly meet with Dr. Reid, and during the first six weeks they have been very cooperative.

But in the last few weeks the strains of having a severely handicapped child have made them extremely upset. They see their careers and their relationship with their other children suffering from the pressures associated with John's birth. Their doubts about his future quality of life and the pressures placed on their family and professional lives have been deepening. Neither one of them has been able to work with the usual intensity, and both have started taking stress-reducing medication. Two weeks ago, both of them told Dr. Reid that "our lives are falling apart as a result of the pressures associated with John's birth." According to Dr. Reid they are at their wit's end and are emotionally distraught.

Last week the parents came to a decision. They want John removed from the respirator and they want him to be allowed to die. Dr. Reid told them that she was concerned that their distraught emotional states may be leading them to a decision that they may regret in the future, especially because she is not certain that baby John will die in the near future. Because she cannot say that his death is imminent, she is hesitant to withdraw him from treatment.

Dr. Reid did tell Mr. and Mrs. Fitzer that she would bring the case before the hospital's ethics committee for review and consultation.

## Committee Discussion of the Case

Dr. Mary Collins:
(Chair)

Once again I want to thank all of you for taking time out of your busy schedules in order to attend an unscheduled meeting. The case that we have distributed to you was prepared by Dr. Paula Reid, a neonatologist who has recently joined our pediatric staff. She has been managing the care of this child since his birth. I have asked Dr. Reid to come to this meeting so that you can address your questions to her. I also have asked Mr. and Mrs. Fitzer to come to this meeting. These parties are in conflict and some tough choices need to be made. For a variety of reasons, I think that it would be inappropriate for the Fitzers to attend the entire meeting. They are waiting in my office. When we want them to join us, we will call them in.

| | |
|---|---|
| Prof. Carla Thomas: | Why have you chosen to exclude them from the first part of the meeting? I am not challenging your decision, but I would like to understand it. |
| Dr. Collins: | I want to encourage the free flow of information on this case, and I think that their presence would inhibit free and open discussion. In addition, this committee has only an advisory role, so our recommendations are not binding on any of the parties that are directly involved in the case. Therefore, there seems to be no requirement that the Fitzers have access to all of our deliberations. |
| Prof. Thomas: | My concern here is that there seems to be significant conflict between the parties involved in this case and I would not want to create the impression that we are biased in favor of Dr. Reid because we are hearing from her in the absence of the Fitzers. Dr. Reid may make statements in the first part of the meeting that the Fitzers may want to challenge. If they are not here, then they cannot do so. |
| Vivian Harris: | What is your problem, Carla? We have always proceeded by first securing information from the medical professionals and then deliberating on the ethical issues in the case. Are you suggesting that there is something wrong with our procedure? |
| Prof. Thomas: | Yes, I am concerned about a philosophical problem. Vivian, you say that we get our case information from the medical professionals and then proceed to make decisions about ethical matters. But doesn't it matter who gives us the information and whether the information is evaluated as objective? I am not saying that Dr. Reid will give us biased information, but the Fitzers may want to object to the way information is presented to the committee. Let me illus- |

trate what I mean. Reread paragraphs 4 and 5 in the case as it was presented to us. These paragraphs refer to the inner thoughts and feelings of Mr. and Mrs. Fitzer. These words were written by Dr. Reid. They seem to be Dr. Reid's impressions of the Fitzers. Furthermore, if we believe these words, then the Fitzers may be acting to relieve their own emotional stress rather than to secure the welfare of their baby.

The information that we take as accurate and objective will govern our advice, and it is, therefore, vitally important that we allow the Fitzers the opportunity to challenge this information. Perhaps the Fitzers would disagree with the claims made in these paragraphs or perhaps they would give a different interpretation of this information. I am trying to remind us that information is never neutral. It is always presented from someone's point of view. In this case the information is coming from Dr. Reid's point of view and not from the Fitzers.

Atty. John Quinn: I have practiced law for a long time, and what Carla is saying is the lawyer's religious creed. The first lesson of law school is "challenge the facts." But challenging the facts takes time. It takes people who will do the investigation. It takes a set of court rules as to what is admissible and what is not admissible. In short, challenging the facts requires an adversarial procedure. But our committee is not capable of following sophisticated procedures for the evaluation of information. We do not hear testimony under oath, nor do we allow cross-examination. We are not a court of law, and I do not think that we should pretend to follow a strict procedure.

Ms. Harris: Carla's claim has some merit, but I am totally uninterested in building a sophisticated, lawlike system for the evaluation of information. If that is the direction that the committee is going to take, then count me out. I am not convinced that the adversarial procedures of the courtroom yield anything like the truth. Courtroom procedures are effective for producing verdicts, but I am not sure they are effective for producing the truth. I believe that we can simply allow Dr. Reid and the Fitzers to present their sides of the case. I want to avoid any cross-questioning of either party. The family is in the middle of a tremendous personal crisis and I do not want to add to their misery by grilling them. Our job is not to probe them but to support them and assist them to manage this human crisis.

Rev. Richard Marcus:

I wish to echo Vivian's sentiments. The Fitzers are in a desperate emotional trauma and I think that we must assume that they are good-willed until it is proven otherwise. Hence, I will have no part in cross-examination of these people.

Prof. Thomas:

Vivian's point is well taken. But what is the role of this committee? Are we a support system for the family or a support system for the physician? I thought that our job was to yield advice on critical health care cases. Can we offer advice based on information that is not validated? If so, I think that our advice may be dubious. If the information that we get is in conflict, how do we determine whom to believe? If we do not have some means of determining who to believe, then it will be easy to produce hollow resolutions.

Dr. Collins:

I can see that my decision to allow the Fitzers to speak to the committee after our initial discussion of the case has opened up a can of worms. I think that we should postpone further discussion of this important topic until a later meeting. Perhaps we can develop a policy statement on this topic at that time. For now, however, the case at hand is our primary concern. I will bring the Fitzers into the meeting to make a presentation, and I will strongly discourage any questions that hint of cross-examination. However, I will not discourage challenging questions directed at Dr. Reid. So, let's begin with any questions that you might have for Dr. Reid.

Prof. Martin Fisk:   Dr. Reid, I am not sure about your reluctance to call this child terminal. The neonatal intensive care unit is an acute and temporary care facility. It was not designed to be a permanent home for ventilator-dependent patients. The child may not be terminal if we permanently care for him, but the question is, can he ever be expected to survive without intensive care?

Dr. Philip Davis:   Can you tell us what you know about bronchopulmonary dysplasia? Specifically, I am interested in quality-of-life considerations as well as survival rates. Also, how bad is the intercranial damage? Specifically, is there significant damage to the neocortex? I am concerned about whether we have reached the point where we can say that the child has lost the capacity for human interaction.

Marian Rhodes:   I am concerned about whether continued treatment is providing a net benefit to this child. Our application policy allows us to withdraw life-sustaining treatment, if such treatment does not provide a "net benefit." It seems to me that we are approaching this point.

Ms. Harris:   I am concerned with competence and the patient's best interest. Dr. Reid, I am uncertain about how we should understand paragraphs 4 and 5 of the case study that you have presented to us. Are you suggesting that because of the emotional stress associated with the birth of an impaired child, Mr. and Mrs. Fitzer are incompetent to make a decision about their child? Or are you suggesting that these parents may be making a decision based on the family's best interest rather than a decision based on the best interest of the child?

Mary Quigley:   The cost of this treatment must be very high. Who is paying for it?

Dr. Collins:   If there are no other questions, I will turn the floor over to Dr. Reid.

Dr. Reid:   You have asked some very difficult questions and I will do my best to answer them. The first question concerned the baby's prognosis for survival. I do not regard his chances as very high, but we have managed to pull him through the crises that he has so far faced and I *feel* that we can continue to pull him through future crises. I realize that our NICU is an acute treatment center and that it was not designed to function as a chronic care unit in which patients will be permanently cared for. I, too, would like to see John transferred to a technologically sophisticated nursing home that would care for him on a permanent basis. The two centers that I would recommend are currently full. Also, when I raised this possibility with the Fitzers, they told me that they did not want their baby put into a "high-tech medical warehouse" where a life would be "fabricated" for him.

Prof. Fisk:   So they will not approve a transfer, even if one were available. What then do you intend to do with the baby if the NICU becomes overcrowded? I know that our NICU is frequently full or near full. Are you going to continue to treat baby John, even if there is another baby that you might

|  | be able to save but cannot because baby John is a permanent resident of the facility? I guess what I am asking is "have you considered what to do if and when the resources of the NICU become scarce?" |
|---|---|
| Dr. Reid: | This is a real concern, and I think that our unit is considering the selection of a triage officer who would be charged with making these decisions. We have read the hospital's triage policy, and most of us are willing to abide by the rules laid down in that policy. At this point, however, the shortage problem has been avoided. |
| Dr. Collins: | Martin, I must remind you that Dr. Reid was trying to answer the questions placed before her. I hope that she can return to that task. |
| Dr. Reid: | The second question had to do with BPD and the survival rates and quality-of-life considerations. His pressures on the ventilator are typical for this condition and we seem to have stabilized him. But we cannot wean him from the ventilator. It is possible that he could survive this treatment for quite a long time. Regarding quality of life, he will be ventilator-dependent as far as I can tell for the remainder of his life. I have treated children in this condition who have lived quite a while. They have severe medical problems surrounding nutrition and hydration. They frequently have significant cognitive deficits. It would require substantial training to allow this child to live outside of a medical facility. Their lives are very limited. |

Regarding the capacity to interact as a human being, I am very uncomfortable with this criterion for withdrawal. I do not know what it means in that I do not know which patients would satisfy this criterion. Is a child born with Down syndrome capable of interacting as a human being? How do you tell if someone does or does not have this capacity? How much capacity is enough to satisfy this criterion? Because of this vagueness, I never get involved in debating these questions because they are purely philosophical and the medical facts do not yield an answer.

Dr. Davis:

I take it then that you do not think very much of our withdrawal policy because it grants to families and physicians the right to withdraw treatment from infants who have permanently lost the capacity to interact as persons. It seems to me that you do not have any real questions about the criterion; you simply reject it.

Dr. Reid:

Well, the idea of loss of capacity to interact as a person is just so vague. Has the Alzheimer's victim lost this capacity? If so, then at what point in the Alzheimer's disease process does he lose it? Has the child with severe Down syndrome lost this capacity? If so, then at what level of Down's does he lose it? Have patients with severe intercranial bleeds lost this capacity? If so, then how much neocortical tissue has to be destroyed before loss of capacity can be established? Without specific answers to these questions, I do not understand the meaning of the phrase "loss of capacity to interact as a person." I am very uncomfortable with this concept because it leaves unanswered the practical questions. With all this ambiguity the concept becomes practically useless. Regarding net benefit, I simply do not know if continued treatment will provide a net benefit to the child. I do not know whether anyone can answer this question. It is safer, I think, to continue to

|               | treat a patient if there is any chance that he will survive. |
|---------------|--------------|
| Prof. Thomas: | But Dr. Reid, do you seriously believe that medicine contains only precisely defined concepts and that any concept that has some vagueness in it must be eliminated from medicine? It sounds to me as if you would like to make medicine an exact science like mathematics. This couldn't be your view because so many diagnoses and treatment plans are based on less than exact information. |
| Dr. Reid:     | No! Medicine is by no means an exact science. And I do not mind making judgments on only partial evidence, but I raise my standards when it comes to withdrawing treatment that is life sustaining. In these cases, one needs to follow higher standards because death is so final. |
| Prof. Thomas: | It sounds to me, Doctor, as if you are not just raising your standards but dropping the entire net benefit approach to treatment in the context of death. It seems to me as if you do not think that net benefit applies to questions of withdrawal. |
| Dr. Davis:    | But it is certainly appropriate to require a physician to make a net benefit judgment as to whether continuing a life-saving treatment secures the net benefit of the patient. Dr. Reid, this is what clinical medicine is all about. Net benefit is the name of the medical game. You cannot say you never make end-stage clinical judgments based on net benefit to the patient. |
| Dr. Reid:     | What I am saying is that human life is so valuable that it ought to preserved, if there is the slightest chance that it can be preserved. It is possible that baby John will survive, and therefore I am reluctant to withdraw care from him. |

| | |
|---|---|
| Dr. Davis: | Do you mean that you disagree with any withdrawal order or with any "do not resuscitate" order? In most of these cases, there is a slight chance that the patient will survive. I think that you are confusing hope with justified belief. We hope that severely impaired children can recover, but parents need clinically justified advice, not just hope. |
| Dr. Reid: | Withdrawal is permissible when brain death is reached, and it may be permissible if a competent patient refuses this care, but I am very skeptical that we should ever get involved in the business of writing off certain babies with severe handicaps. |
| Ms. Quigley: | So you regard baby John as a handicapped person who needs to be protected from an uncaring and insensitive family and hospital. If so, then you must have a pretty low opinion of this committee's policy on withdrawal. |
| Dr. Reid: | I think that overstates my point, but I do think that the baby needs to be protected against those who understandably view him as a burden. |
| Dr. Collins: | Dr. Reid, you really think that our policy on withdrawal of treatment from infants is unethical, don't you? Why haven't you expressed these views to me or to other members of the committee before? |
| Dr. Reid: | This is the first time that I have come before this committee. I have only recently joined the staff, and these matters never came up when I interviewed for this position. |
| Dr. Collins: | Let's return to your answers to the questions at issue. |
| Dr. Reid: | Regarding the competency question, I think that it should be obvious that I do not consider Mr. and Mrs. Fitzer to be incompe- |

|  |  |
|---|---|
|  | tent. My concern is that they are acting in *their* best interest, not in the best interest of the baby. The stress of the situation has clouded their judgment as to what is best for the child. I do not blame them for this since I understand why they feel the way they do. But as a physician I need to protect the children in my care. |
| Dr. Davis: | So you think that they are acting in a way that violates the best interest of the child. |
| Dr. Reid: | In a sense, yes. |
| Dr. Davis: | But you just told us, Doctor, that you were uncertain about what is in the best interest of the child. Now you tell us that you know that the parents' decision is not in the child's best interest. How can you have it both ways, Doctor? How can you be ignorant of the child's best interest and also affirm that withdrawal from treatment is not in his best interest? |
| Dr. Reid: | Notice that I used the expression "in a sense." What I meant was that I think that the parents are acting for their best interest. Baby John is clearly becoming a profound burden for them. |
| Atty. Quinn: | But how do you know that they are not motivated by what they consider best for baby John? You claim to know something about their "true motives" and that is very relevant to this case. How do you know these real motives? Did they tell you or did one of the staff discover their "real motives"? |
| Dr. Reid: | My last three meetings with the Fitzers have been very emotional in that the two of them have expressed that they are growing very weary with the process of managing John. Both parents have cried in my office and expressed deep regret that they gave birth to such a profoundly handicapped |

child. Their focus seems to be on "what did they do wrong," rather than on what they need to do in order to manage their new life with a handicapped child. What they are going through seems to me very understandable. I would probably feel the same way if my own child were born with this handicap. However, I think it would be a big mistake if they were to act on these temporary feelings.

Dr. Davis:    Dr. Reid, are you trained in psychological evaluation? That is, do you have any special training in this field?

Dr. Reid:    No.

Dr. Davis:    My reason for asking is that you seem to be making your judgment on the basis of a psychological evaluation of these people, and I wonder whether your judgment is scientifically sound, given that you have no special training in this field. Have you called in one of the staff psychiatrists for a review of the case?

Dr. Reid:    I have spoken to the Fitzers about seeking psychological counseling, but they have refused. They claim that baby John is their baby and that they have the right to refuse continued treatment.

Atty. Quinn:    So it is your professional medical opinion that discontinuation of treatment is inconsistent with the medical best interest of the child?

Dr. Reid:    Absolutely! This child has a chance of surviving. The parents do not want to take that chance, and I do. I admit that the baby has a low probability of survival, but it is enough for me.

Ms. Quigley:    Now we have reached the real guts of the conflict between you and the Fitzers. The questions of competence and the question of whether they are acting for their own interests rather than the interest of the child were not the real issues at dispute, were they? You want to take the chance of saving this baby and they do not. They want to give up and you do not want to give up. Isn't it that simple, Dr. Reid?

Dr. Reid: No. We do disagree on this issue, but the motivation question is also a matter of conflict. I am very concerned that they are recommending a course of action based on their perceived best interest, not based on the actual best interest of this child.

Ms. Quigley: But, Dr. Reid, notice something about our policy on withdrawal of care for infants! It does give physicians the right to refuse to abide by the wishes of parents or guardians who are *obviously acting against the best interest of a child*. An example might help. We were thinking of the case of the Jehovah's Witness parents who wish to refuse a minor but life-sustaining surgical treatment for their child. They are being motivated by religious considerations, not by medical best interest. We were thinking of the clinical case in which the best interest of the child was clearly obvious. Is this such a clear case?

Dr. Reid: This case is not as obvious as the Jehovah's Witness case. But it is still clear to me that withdrawal of treatment is inconsistent with the best interests of the child.

Rev. Marcus: Notice, Doctor, that there is nothing in the policy that authorizes or obligates the physician to provide life-sustaining treatment if there is only the smallest chance of the treatment producing survival. The fact that a treatment can simply maintain the life is not viewed as sufficient in itself. The technology can prolong death as well as life.

The technology that we have developed, especially the NICU technology, is very effective at maintaining life. However, it frequently produces survivors whose quality of life is so awful that the treatment has produced a net loss to the patient rather than a net benefit to the patient. The policy grants the right to physicians, with the approval of the parents, to discontinue treatment in these cases. The first rule of medicine is to avoid harm, isn't it?

Dr. Reid: But my problem is how do you tell when you have reached the point when continued treatment is producing a net loss to the patient? There is no clear point.

Dr. Davis: That is where clinical science and clinical art unite to form the practice of medicine, Doctor. The hospital hired you to make the hard choices and advise parents or guardians regarding the probable course of a disease. The hospital does not require that your judgments be absolute and certain. We are not asking you to be a god. We only expect you to be a competent physician. May I finish by saying that you have a very different image of what a physician is than I do? You seem to want to play it very safe in medicine. I think that "playing it safe" produces vast amounts of harm to patients.

Dr. Reid: It sounds to me as if you are putting a lot of pressure on me to go along with the parents and order a withdrawal when, in my mind, this would involve a retreat from my commitment to my patient.

Dr. Collins: I need to say, Dr. Reid, that argument in this committee is often quite brisk and energetic. But our committee is advisory to the staff. The committee does not have the authority to require you to do anything that you consider inconsistent with your ethics.

| | |
|---|---|
| Rev. Marcus: | I think that I understand Dr. Reid's point of view on the case. I think that we need to speak to the Fitzers. I think that Dr. Reid should step outside so that we can have a good discussion with the parents. |
| Dr. Collins: | Dr. Reid, do you have any objections? |
| Dr. Reid: | I have no objections. |

Dr. Reid leaves, and the Fitzers are brought into the committee room and introduced to the members.

| | |
|---|---|
| Dr. Collins: | Mr. and Mrs. Fitzer, would you like to make a statement to the committee? |
| Mrs. Fitzer: | My husband and I are here because we have reached a very hard decision that we have agonized about for many weeks. We feel that our baby John should be allowed to die. This is a very hard thing for a mother to say. In some ways, I cannot even believe the words that are coming out of my own mouth. But yet my husband and I have thought about this very hard and we think that these machines are not helping our son. His brain damage is severe. He will never be able to enjoy life. There is nothing to compensate for the sufferings and humiliations that he will endure. Furthermore, we cannot care for him and so he will have to live his life in a hospital or a nursing home tied to a ventilator. This is a life that is unthinkable to us. We cannot allow this!

We know that Dr. Reid thinks that we are terrible people for wanting to let him die, but we think that we are right. |
| Dr. Collins: | I do not think that Dr. Reid thinks that you are terrible people. She disagrees with you about what is best for the baby. |
| Rev. Marcus: | You mentioned that John's life would be a life of suffering and humiliation. Why do |

|  |  |
|---|---|
|  | you feel that way? Does it have to be that way? |
| Mr. Fitzer: | Perhaps not. But we know that we cannot care for him and we know what nursing homes are really like. They are little more than warehouses for the "ought to be dead." John will never learn anything; he will never feel anything; he will never live in human society. Thirty or forty years ago he would have died. We would have mourned him and continued our lives. But thanks to this space age technology, he is on the borderline between life and death. He is little more than a hostage to this technology. We will not accept this. |
| Rev. Marcus: | But does his life have to be humiliating and degrading? Couldn't a more caring society find a place for John? Couldn't a more caring society treat him as an impaired brother? |
| Mr. Fitzer: | This society will probably not choose to spend its money taking care of the John Fitzers of the world. And I am not sure they should. Why should the country spend vast fortunes caring for John when he himself cannot benefit from this care? His brain has been damaged to the point where he cannot interact with others. He is not going to be just a little retarded. It looks like he's going to be a vegetable. Don't you understand that? |
| Mrs. Fitzer: | Perhaps, Reverend, you are suggesting that we are not a caring couple, or a generous family. We do not feel this way about ourselves. We just cannot see any sense in caring for a vegetable for the rest of our lives. Neither John nor our family would benefit from a life of devotion to him. We also have other children and they need us. They can receive something from us. We want the machines removed from him, not |

because we are selfish and won't give anything to him, but because *he cannot receive anything from us.*

Dr. Davis:    Dr. Reid is reluctant to remove John from continued treatment. Has she communicated to you her reasons for this reluctance and what are your reactions to her views?

Mr. Fitzer:    We feel that John's existence is a life in name only and that Dr. Reid disagrees with us about this. She has a different ethical view on this than we do. We hold no anger toward her, but she is not John's parent and we feel that we must decide and take the responsibility for this tragic choice. We will have to live with this choice, not her.

Dr. Davis:    But do you understand her reasons for refusing to withdraw him from further treatment?

Mrs. Fitzer:    Yes. She says that John has a chance of surviving. But that is precisely why we want him removed. You see, if he does survive this treatment, then he will survive in a way that is humiliating and degrading. You and your machines will save him for a life that is too awful for me to even think about. In our view, there are worse things than not surviving.

Dr. Collins:    What would you have this committee do for you, Mrs. Fitzer?

Mrs. Fitzer:    Speak to Dr. Reid and tell her to withdraw John from treatment. It is time to let him die.

Dr. Collins:    Are there any further questions that the members of the committee would like to ask the Fitzers?

Atty. Quinn:    Yes! Have you sought legal counsel on this conflict that you are having with Dr. Reid?

Mr. Fitzer:    No. It was only last week that we heard about this committee, and we wanted to see

| | |
|---|---|
| | whether you could resolve this conflict without going to the courts. However, we will contact an attorney if this committee cannot reach a satisfactory resolution. |
| Dr. Collins: | We would like to thank both of you for coming to our meeting. We will be in touch with you. |

The Fitzers leave the meeting.

| | |
|---|---|
| Dr. Davis: | This case is directly related to our policy. Let me read principles 3B and 3C. Principle 3B: If the treatment is of medically uncertain value and if the parents decide to forgo treatment, then the parents' wishes should be respected. If the parents choose to continue such treatment, then this decision should also be honored. Principle 3C: If the treatment is medically futile and if the parents wish to forgo treatment, then this wish should be honored. If the parents wish to continue with the medically futile therapy, then the pediatric ethics committee should be called upon to mediate this conflict between the parents and the health care providers. Community Hospital is not committed to providing medically futile treatment. The competent patient's right to refuse treatment does not imply that the patient or his guardian has a right to require the hospital to provide medically useless treatment. |
| Dr. Collins: | I take it, Dr. Davis, that you think that the Fitzers' request should be honored? |
| Dr. Davis: | I respect Dr. Reid's enthusiasm for protecting her patient, but our policy clearly is on the side of the family. |
| Prof. Fisk: | I am in agreement with you, Dr. Davis, but according to Dr. Reid, principle 3A is the operative rule and I think that our problem is to decide which is the rule most impor- |

tant in this case. Here is what 3A states: If parents make treatment decisions that are clearly inconsistent with what is medically berteficial to the infant, then the treatment should be continued and the institution should seek to have a guardian appointed by the court.

Ms. Rhodes:  Before we get into further discussion of this case, I think that we need to hear from nurse Martha Latour. She has been taking care of John since he was placed in the NICU. She is a first-rate professional with 15 years' experience in the field of neonatal medicine. Dr. Reid is relatively new to the practice of medicine. She is fresh out of her residency while Nurse Latour has had enormous experience caring for severely impaired children. She is anxious to speak to us and I think that she deserves to be heard.

Dr. Collins:  If there are no objections, I will request that Nurse Latour make a presentation.

Atty. Quinn:  I have no formal objections, but I want to remind the members of the committee that Nurse Latour does not have the primary responsibility for the medical management of this child. That belongs with the family and the physician.

Prof. Thomas:  Maybe legally she has no say in the matter, and I am not even sure of that, but nurses are on the front lines of patient manage-ment. If we don't listen to them we court disaster.

Nurse Latour joins the committee.

Dr. Collins:  Nurse Latour, thank you for coming to this meeting. You are aware of the purpose of this meeting, which is to assist the parties who are responsible for deciding the fate of John Fitzer. You are, I believe, also aware of the conflict between Dr. Reid and the parents. Can you offer us any further insight on these or related issues?

Nurse Latour:    I asked to come to this meeting for two reasons. First, as a nurse, I have a responsibility to my patient and, in this case, a responsibility to the parents of my patient. The responsibility is to be an advocate for quality care. This means forming a professional opinion regarding what constitutes "quality care" in a given context. Secondly, I am not the only nurse caring for this baby. There are at least five of us that have spent significant amounts of time with this baby, and we have discussed the case at length. This discussion has produced consensus among the staff and we believe this committee should be informed of our views.

The major fear that we have is that John Fitzer will be our next "Robbie." Most of you remember Robbie. He too was a BPD victim, and he lived his entire life at this hospital. Robbie lived for eight years up in pediatrics. He lived for eight months in the NICU, then for two years in the infant nursery, and then he lived the remainder of his life on the second floor pediatric wing. His entire life was spent tied to the ventilator. Robbie was the institution's child. His parents abandoned him, and he had no family except his hospital family. The professional and nonprofessional staff universally mourned when he died, and the experience has stayed with all of us. The nurses asked me to come and speak to you about the real possibility that John Fitzer may become our next Robbie. Many of us feel that we became Robbie's de facto parents and we think that we need to be consulted before we become the de facto parents of John Fitzer. We signed on to be

the acute care nurses of ill children, not to
be their permanent parents. It isn't fair to
the staff to require that they function as
permanent parents of BPD victims.

Dr. Collins:    But John's parents have not abandoned
him.

Nurse Latour:    The parents have spoken to three of the
nurses including me. To each of us they
have communicated their strong desire to
discontinue John's treatment. We fear that,
if the hospital refuses to grant their request,
then we, the nurses, will be left with the job
of not only being John's nurses but also his
parents. My point here is not to try to
coerce you to discontinue treatment but
rather to say that if you do decide to
continue treatment, then you must find a
solution other than keeping him as a
permanent resident of our hospital. When
Robbie died, it was as if all of us lost an
eight-year-old child. It was emotionally
devastating to the staff and it is not fair to
them.

The second reason for coming is the
consensus. We have cared for this baby for
12 weeks and we have seen the amount of
damage that he has suffered. We feel that
he has reached the clinical point where
discontinuation of treatment is a viable and
realistic option. We are not absolutely
certain that continued treatment is worthless to him, but we feel that the parents'
wishes are reasonable, given John's catastrophic clinical situation.

Dr. Collins:    Are there any questions for Nurse Latour?

Ms. Rhodes:    Yes. Are there any behavioral signs that the
baby is responding normally?

Nurse Latour:    John is nonresponsive to nearly all attempts
to interact with him. He is nothing like a

|              | typical 12-week-old baby in terms of his interaction with other people. |
|--------------|--------------------------------------------------------------------|
| Dr. Collins: | Thank you for coming to this meeting, Nurse Latour. We will give serious consideration to your views and the views of the staff. |

Nurse Latour leaves the meeting.

| Dr. Collins: | I think that it is time that we formulate a recommendation on this case. Does anyone want to make a first attempt at formulating a response? |
|--------------|--------------------------------------------------------------------|
| Dr. Davis: | I respect Dr. Reid's views, but I move that we recommend to the Fitzers that they ask Dr. Reid to transfer the case to another physician. I know that Dr. William Redman has had a lot of experience on cases of impaired newborns, and I think that perhaps he would be more willing to work with this family. |
| Atty. Quinn: | Does that mean that we are endorsing a withdrawal in this case? |
| Dr. Davis: | By all means. I think that this is a parental responsibility and that principle 3B applies. |
| Dr. Collins: | Hold on a minute! Do we have a motion? We need a second. |
| Prof. Thomas: | I second it. |
| Dr. Collins: | Now, discussion! |
| Atty. Quinn: | But you are disregarding Dr. Reid's belief that it is principle 3A that is operative in this case. She feels that it is not in the interest of this child to have life-sustaining treatment discontinued. I am reluctant to view her professional opinion as nonbinding. |
| Dr. Davis: | Let me be frank about my views. From my perspective, the BPD by itself is sufficient to |

allow the parents to withdraw treatment. If you add the intercranial bleeds and the resultant profound retardation, then I think that there is little doubt that the parents have the authority to withdraw. This is a parental call because it is an ethical issue, not a purely medical matter.

Prof. Thomas:    I agree with Dr. Davis. It seems to me that if principle 3B does not apply in this case, then it doesn't apply in any case and is therefore worthless and ought to be withdrawn from the policy. Furthermore, it seems to me that if it is worthless, then we ought to grant authority to physicians to call all the cases that are medically uncertain.

Dr. Collins:    What is your point, Carla?

Prof. Thomas:    It is a simple one. If we do not grant to parents the authority to refuse treatment in cases that are medically uncertain, then we should not have said that we are going to grant such authority to them. We should not contradict our words by our actions.

Prof. Fisk:    Carla, are you suggesting that we need not recommend that the Fitzers seek another physician and that we should recommend that Dr. Reid withdraw treatment from the child?

Prof. Thomas:    Dr. Reid seems to be violating principle 3B, so I wonder why we cannot hold her to the policy. Furthermore, she seems to hold treatment values that are at odds with the hospital's values contained in the pediatric withdrawal policy. What makes you think that this case is not going to repeat itself next week? I think that we have to address this problem.

## Committee Recommendations

| | |
|---|---|
| Prof. Thomas: | I move that the committee recommend to Dr. Reid that she remove herself from the case and recommend to the Fitzers that they seek Dr. Redman as their new physician. |
| Prof. Fisk: | Carla, what the hospital does regarding Dr. Reid is not relevant to this case at hand. I agree that her values and the committee's values seem to be at odds and this matter should be addressed at some later date. But our duty is to advise the parties in this case.<br><br>My concern is, will Dr. Redman take the case? |
| Dr. Davis: | I feel confident that he will, if he gets a formal request from the committee. I will inform him about the issues and tell him to expect a call from the Fitzers, if the committee approves. |
| Ms. Quigley: | How shall we proceed with Dr. Reid? |
| Dr. Collins: | If the committee agrees with the suggestion that is on the floor, that is, that we recommend that the Fitzers switch physicians, then I plan to merely advise the parties to end their doctor-patient relationship. Furthermore, I will advise the Fitzers to call Dr. Redman. Phil, I think that it is a good idea to call Dr. Redman.<br><br>Regarding Dr. Reid, I will speak with her. She and this committee are in significant ethical disagreement, and I think that this disagreement has to be managed with care and respect. I have no enthusiasm for coercing her to get in line with our values. |
| Ms. Quigley: | But what will you do in the future? |
| Dr. Collins: | That is an administrative problem, Mary. I will manage it. Perhaps I can engage in a longer ethical discussion with Dr. Reid.<br><br>But right now I want to reach some closure on this case. Are we in agreement that I should recommend to the Fitzers that |

they have the right to seek another physician and that we should mention Dr. Redman's name to them as someone who has a great deal of experience in these matters?

All the members of the committee except Atty. Quinn agree with this plan.

| | |
|---|---|
| Ms. Harris: | One final point. What do we do if Dr. Reid resists and seeks a court injunction to prevent either the transfer of care to Dr. Redman or the withdrawal, assuming that Dr. Redman approves of a withdrawal? |
| Atty. Quinn: | My sense is that if this happens we ought to be prepared to file an affidavit with the probate court attesting to the fact that we feel that withdrawal is ethically appropriate in this case. I, furthermore, recommend that Dr. Collins begin a dialogue with Dr. Reid immediately after this case is resolved. I am concerned about the ethical gulf that exists between the hospital's withdrawal policy and Dr. Reid's values on this matter. My experience tells me that it is the physician who most frequently raises the withdrawal issue with families. My concern is that given what Dr. Reid has indicated to this committee, she would hardly ever raise the nontreatment option with families, and this indicates a significant problem in her relationship with her patients. |
| Dr. Collins: | Once again this is a broader question that we are not asked to address in this case. I consider these questions as essentially administrative issues that I will deal with. If there are no further matters, I will direct Dr. Davis to speak to Dr. Redman and determine if he will take on the Fitzer case. If he agrees, then I will speak to the Fitzers and advise them of their right to change physicians. I will inform Dr. Reid of the actions of this committee.<br><br>If there is no further business, I think we are adjourned. |

436    Brendan Minogue

## Questions for Further Discussion

1. Should the committee have assigned an independent neonatologist to do a review of the case in order to assess the medical facts of the case? What would be the positive and negative implications of going this route? Think about all the possibilities this would open up!
2. Dr. Collins says that speaking to Dr. Reid about her ethical values and the disagreement that exists between her values and the committee's is an administrative matter. What should she say to Dr. Reid?
3. Nurse Latour is not the physician of record. Why should the committee listen to her report of the case? Evaluate this report.
4. Did the committee give serious attention to the possibility that principle 3A ought to be the operative principle in this case?
5. Should the committee have requested a psychiatric evaluation of the Fitzers in order to determine that they were acting in the best interest of their child?
6. Imagine that you are a handicapped-rights activist. How would you respond to this decision?
7. Imagine that you are a member of the National Right to Life Movement. How would you respond to this decision?
8. There is ambiguity in this case, and Dr. Reid wants to take what might be considered "the most cautious approach." Evaluate this approach.
9. What does the principle of autonomy have to do with this case? Or is it completely irrelevant to the case? If it is irrelevant, what is the main ethical principle of the case?
10. At the beginning of the case Mary Quigley asked about the cost of treatment and who was paying for it. This question did not receive much discussion. Is this matter relevant to the ethical issues in this case?

# More Cases Involving the Policy

## DNR and the Anencephalic Infant

Kevin Black has been in the neonatal intensive care unit for two hours. He is anencephalic and he is gasping for breath. Anencephalic children are born without parts of their upper brain, and all of them die within a very short period of time, usually less than two months. The parents had no warning of this condition and they are in a state of shock. The neonatologist approaches them with the aim of securing a "do not resuscitate" order. He notices that they are very upset and that they seem confused about the medical condition of the child. The physician asks them to approve the order and in the midst of their confusion they tell the physician that whatever she thinks is best is all right with them. The physician is concerned about the validity of the authorization but is anxious not to resuscitate the child, since she believes that resuscitation will only prolong his dying.

## Down Syndrome and Permission for Surgery

Michael is born with Down syndrome and his parents are devastated. They have three other children and they do not believe that they will be able to raise Michael. They also fear that if they give him up for adoption, he will not receive proper care. Such children are difficult to place into adoptive homes, and, with the decline in social services, they fear that he will not receive a decent minimum of care within the social services system. Because they fear that they will be unable to raise a mentally impaired child and they feel that a Down's child has a poor quality of life, they are both very concerned. Three days after the birth, the pediatrician calls them into his office and informs them that their child needs surgery. Michael has an esophageal fistula that prevents him from digesting food. Without surgery, he will surely die. The physician expects them to consent to the surgery. However, they refuse permission to operate. They claim that surgery will make possible a life that is not worth living and that it is really in Michael's best interest to be allowed to die. How should the pediatrician proceed?

## A Nurse Objects to Withdrawal

Two weeks ago infant Theresa was born premature at 30 weeks. She weighed 1,000 grams and is suffering from a grade III (moderately severe) intraventricular hemorrhage. There are risks that the child will be significantly retarded. In addition, she has a severely defective heart. Her left ventricle is so damaged that a transplantation may be her only chance of living. No transplants are available and, given Theresa's hemorrhage, it is not likely that she will be accepted for transplantation. Her parents request that all life-sustaining treatments be withheld or withdrawn and the pediatrician agrees. However, nurse Ruth Glenn, who is Theresa's nurse, disagrees. She has asked the ethics committee to convene a meeting, and she argues that they should wait and continue treatment in the hope that a heart will become available. How should the ethics committee respond to Ms. Glenn? She is also concerned that the baby is being discriminated against on the basis of the hemorrhage by transplantation committees that may exclude her from access to transplantation.

## Patients' Diverse Religious and Cultural Values

Muzafar is a 6-year-old boy with Lesch-Nyhan syndrome, a form of hyper-uricemia, an X-linked enzyme defect that results in urate overproduction. Lesch-Nyhan children exhibit self-mutilation, choreoathetosis, spasticity, mental and growth retardation, and high levels of serum and urine uric acid levels. They often develop uric acid stones and gouty nephropathy, which may lead to death from uremia. Most patients with Lesch-Nyhan syndrome die in childhood.

Muzafar was admitted to an intensive care unit at a tertiary care hospital for evaluation and treatment for pneumonia and bloody stools. His father works in a grocery store; his mother cares for his siblings. They are Muslims. Muzafar lives in an extended-care facility, where his family regularly visits.

At the time of admission, the ICU staff described Muzafar as "neurologically devastated" and "severely retarded." He has a feeding tube and a tracheostomy. The staff had difficulty placing IV lines and after several hours did a painful intraosseous (bone) line. The senior ICU physician who evaluated him at admission called Muzafar's father and explained his condition. He also asked whether, if the boy's condition suddenly worsened, the family would want to have CPR and other forms of resuscitation done. The senior physician reported that the father told him, regarding the possibility of DNR order, "Of course I don't want that. I will go to hell if I kill my son."

The ICU staff decided to invite the local Muslim clergyman, who serves as the Muslim chaplain at the hospital, to a meeting to discuss the case. The clergyman stated that some Muslims say we must do everything to save a patient. Others argue that God created us without machines, and that we must accept death. His own opinion based on his study of Islamic law is that if the doctors say there is no hope, we must "leave it to God" and let nature take its course. The clergyman added that to continue painful treatment that would not be effective would not be good for Muzafar. The clergyman concluded that he would talk with the father, whom he knows well.

The father continued to say that withdrawing treatment would lead him to hell and that he would never consent to it. Was the father acting in his own interest or in the interest of the child? Should the physician invoke the futility rule? How should patients from other cultures be assisted in managing ethical challenges?

## Further Reading

Frohock, Fred M., *Special Care: Medical Decisions at the Beginning of Life* (Chicago: University of Chicago Press, 1986).

Guillemin, Jeanne Harley, and Lynda Lytle Holmstrom, *Mixed Blessings: Intensive Care for Newborns* (New York: Oxford University Press, 1986).

Kuhse, Helga, and Peter Singer, *Should This Baby Live? The Problem of Handicapped Infants* (Oxford: Oxford University Press, 1985).

Lyon, Jeffrey, *Playing God in the Nursery* (New York: W. W. Norton, 1986).

McMillan, Richard C., H. Tristram Englehardt, Jr., and Stuart F. Spicker, eds., *Euthanasia and the Newborn: Conflicts Regarding Saving Lives* (Dordrecht: D. Reidel, 1987).

Murray, Thomas H., and Arthur L. Caplan, eds., *Which Babies Shall Live? Humanistic Dimensions of the Care of Imperiled Newborns* (Clifton, N.J.: Humana Press, 1985).

Shelp, Earl E., *Born to Die? Deciding the Fate of Critically Ill Newborns* (New York: Free Press, 1986).

Weir, Robert, *Selective Nontreatment of Handicapped Newborns: Moral Dilemmas in Neonatal Medicine* (New York: Oxford University Press, 1984).

## Notes

1. The President's Commission for the Study of Ethical Problems in Medicine and Biomedical and Behavioral Research: *Deciding to Forego Life Sustaining Treatment,* pp. 218–219.
2. Nurses also play a important role in the determination of best interests, but their legal status in making these determinations is still uncertain.
3. Allan Buchanan, "The Treatment of Incompetents," in *Health Care Ethics,* ed. Donald Van DeVeer and Tom Regan (Philadelphia: Temple University Press, 1987), p. 215.
4. H. Tristram Engelhardt, *The Foundations of Bioethics* (New York: Oxford University Press, 1986), p. 228.
5. Aristotle, *Politics,* in *The Basic Works of Aristotle,* ed. Richard McKeon (New York: Random House, 1941), p. 1302.
6. Engelhardt, op. cit., p. 107.
7. Robert Veatch, *A Theory of Medical Ethics,* (New York: Basic Books, 1981).
8. This concept that the authority of ethical judgments can be grounded in agreement or common consent has a number of sources. The major area of disagreement is over the nature of this agreement. For a variety of views about the nature of this agreement, see John Rawls, *A Theory of Justice* (Cambridge: Harvard University Press, 1971); Robert Nozick, *Anarchy, State and Utopia* (New York: Basic Books, 1974); and Kurt Beir, *The Moral Point of View: A Rational Basis of Ethics* (New York: Random House, 1965).

# Index